MEDICINE AND BIOLOGY RESEARCH DEVELOPMENTS

BENIGN DISEASE OF THE BREAST

DIAGNOSIS AND TREATMENT

MEDICINE AND BIOLOGY RESEARCH DEVELOPMENTS

Tsisana Shartava, M.D. (Series Editor)
(Tbilisi, Georgia)

Parasitology Research Trends
Olivier De Bruyn and Stephane Peeters (Editors)
2010. ISBN: 978-1-60741-436-0

General Anesthesia Research Developments
Milo Hertzog and Zelig Kuhn (Editors)
2010. ISBN: 978-1-60876-395-5

Venoms: Sources, Toxicity and Therapeutic Uses
Jonas Gjersoe and Simen Hundstad (Editors)
2010. ISBN: 978-1-60876-448-8

Biomaterials Developments and Applications
Henri Bourg and Amaury Lisle (Editors)
2011. ISBN: 978-1-60876-476-1

A Guide to Hemorrhoidal Disease
Pravin Jaiprakash Gupta (Author)
2010. ISBN: 978-1-60876-431-0

Type III Secretion Chaperones: A Molecular Toolkit for all Occasions
Matthew S. Francis (Author)
2010. ISBN: 978-1-60876-667-3

Recent Advances in BIS Guided TCI Anesthesia
David A. Ferreira, Luís Antunes, Pedro Amorim and Catarina Nunes (Authors)
2010. ISBN: 978-1-61668-627-7

TRP Channels in Health and Disease: Implications for Diagnosis and Therapy
Arpad Szallasi (Editor)
2011. ISBN: 978-1-61668-337-5

Biological Aspects of Human Health and Well-Being
Tsisana Shartava (Editor)
2011. ISBN: 978-1-61209-134-1

Tracing the Drainage Divide: The Future Challenge for Predictive Medicine
Enzo Grossi (Author)
2011. ISBN: 978-1-61209-232-4

Nanotechnology and Advances in Medicine
Maysaa El Sayed Zaki (Editor/Author)
2011. ISBN: 978-1-61209-640-7

Beneficial Effects of Propolis on Human Health and Chronic Diseases. Volume 1
Tahira Farooqui and Akhlaq A.Farooqui (Editors)
2012. ISBN: 978-1-62081-440-6

Beneficial Effects of Propolis on Human Health and Chronic Diseases. Volume 2
Tahira Farooqui, Akhlaq A.Farooqui (Editors)
2012. ISBN: 978-1-62081-483-3

Benign Disease of the Breast: Diagnosis and Treatment
Jaime de la Garza-Salazar, Claudia Arce-Salinas and Abelardo Meneses-Garcia (Editors)
2014. ISBN: 978-1-63321-624-2

MEDICINE AND BIOLOGY RESEARCH DEVELOPMENTS

BENIGN DISEASE OF THE BREAST

DIAGNOSIS AND TREATMENT

JAIME DE LA GARZA SALAZAR, M.D.
CLAUDIA ARCE SALINAS, M.D.
AND
ABELARDO MENESES-GARCIA, M.D., PH.D.
EDITORS

NOVA BIOMEDICAL

New York

For permission to use material from this book please contact us:
Telephone 631-231-7269; Fax 631-231-8175
Web Site: http://www.novapublishers.com

Library of Congress Cataloging-in-Publication Data

ISBN: 978-1-63321-624-2

Library of Congress Control Number: 2014945906

Published by Nova Science Publishers, Inc. † New York

We dedicate this book to all women who experience changes in their breasts at some moment in their lifetime.

Breast cancer is the most dreaded pathology. However, it is considered that around 90% of breast pathologies are benign diseases.

May this book be of service of physicians in general. Know these diseases in detail and help your patients to differentiate between cancer and these benign diseases.

An acknowledgment of our Mexican Institutes of Health, especially the Instituto Nacional de Cancerologia.

Jaime G. de la Garza-Salazar
Editor-in-Chief

Dedicamos este libro a todas las mujeres que experimentan cambios en algún momento de su vida en sus glándulas mamarias.

El cáncer de mama es la patología más temida, sin embargo se considera que alrededor del 90% de la patología mamaria son las enfermedades benignas, sirva este libro para los médicos en general, conozcan estas enfermedades con detalle y ayude a sus pacientes a diferenciarlas del cáncer con las enfermedades benignas.

Un reconocimiento a nuestras Instituciones de Salud de México en particular al Instituto Nacional de Cancerología.

Jaime G. de la Garza Salazar
Editor en Jefe

Contents

Editorial

We were invited to write a book on benign disease of the breast. The reason for this is that in the medical literature, all of the information that we have with respect to these tumors is found in fragmented publications in texts and in innumerable articles in the international literature. Of course, the information provided on the entity, in chapters as well as in reports, is very complete; however, some data of interest, such as, for example, the epidemiological ones, are not addressed extensively, nor are the conceptual problems of the diagnosis, which can come to be proposed by the histopathology of some lesions and, similarly, the overwhelming data of Imagenology for the diagnosis, and of course, the indicationsfor treatment.

As Editor-in-Chief, I have invited two experts in the theme, Dr. Claudia Arce-Salinas and Dr. Abelardo Meneses-García, to present to them a book that includes topics-of-interest on the theme.

Thus, we have collaborated to bring together a group of medical specialists with experience in the theme; institutional specialists who naturally have encountered the problems of the differential diagnosis of Benign Breast Lesions, with the accumulated epidemiological data, Infectologists, Gynecologists, General Surgeons, Oncological Surgeons, Pathologists, Radiologists, and Medical Oncologists.in order to prepare the chapters that we present in this text, including the embryology, anatomy, and physiology of the mammary glands, with special attention paid to the anomalies of breast development, chronic secretions of the nipple, inflammatory lesions, fibrocystic disease of the breast, proliferative lesions, gynecomastia, benign tumors, and mastalgia. In all of these we will address the differential diagnosis in terms of the clinic, the imaging, and the histopathology.

The most frequent pathologies of the breast, as observed by those of us devoted to Oncology, are of the benign type. However, this is not so for non-specialist physicians and the women who suffer from these and for whom they are a true cause for alarm. Therefore, it is very important for physicians who are not specialists in cancer to know the signs and symptoms of each of these in order for them to be able to emit a diagnostic impression and to suggest treatment.

Dr. Jaime G. de la Garza-Salazar
Editor-in-Chief

Acknowledgments

We would like to acknowledge the following persons: Maggie Brunner and Carlos Escobar (English translation and style correction), (style correction), Sandra Garnica (secretarial work), Edmundo Alvarez (computer systems advisor), and Carra Feagaiga (project manager).

In: Benign Disease of the Breast
Editors: J. de la Garza Salazar, C. Arce Salinas et al.
ISBN: 978-1-63321-624-2

Chapter 1

General Overview of the Benign Diseases of the Breast

Jaime G. de la Garza-Salazar[1] ***and Paula Juárez-Sánchez***[2]
[1]Clinical Research Department, Instituto Nacional Cancerologia-Mexico, Mexico City, DF, Mexico
[2]Pathology Department, Instituto Nacional Cancerologia-Mexico, Mexico City, DF, Mexico

Abstract

Breast complaints may be cause for alarm for both the patients as well as their primary care physicians. Thorough clinical history and physical examination can undoubtedly improve treatment results.

Breast developments begin in the utero as an epidermically derived structure from the skin arising from modified sweat glands in the dermis and the inductive interaction between ectoderm and mesenchyme. These are studied together as mammary glands are initially a skin specialization and are intimately related to the development of cutaneous tissue.

There are also other aspects related to breast embryology and its development that are also studied, but these may rarely be the cause of congenital diseases and subsequent medical consultation.

These conditions will include anatomical differences in numerous situations of mammary glands (polythelia, polymastia, amastia, or the presence of rudimentary breasts) and developmental alterations (juvenile hypertrophia, gynecomastia, hypoplasia of the breast, or umbilication of the nipple).

Accordingly, when the patient is seen by a medical specialist with the presence of a breast lump, which may or may not be associated with other symptoms, a detailed clinical history should then be obtained.

This ought to include: 1) The presence of accompanying pain and its characteristics. Is pain (mastodyinia) uni- or bilateral? Is the pain cyclical and related to or not with the menstrual period? With trauma? Is the pain incapacitating? Is it associated with the use of certain drugs? 2) Is there secretion from the nipple? Is this uni- or bilateral? Serous or bloody? Or is it milk? Can it be related to pregnancy or is it associated with breast feeding? 3) Are there cutaneous signs including nipple retraction, loss of breast profile, ulcerations or eczematiform lesions of the skin? 4) Are there other associated signs (fever, for example)? 5) Does the patient take drugs such as hormones (estrogen) or antidepressants? 6) Are there associated risk factors including any of the following: A) *Personal*: early age at menarche, number of pregnancies, age at first gestation, age at menopause, use of hormonal therapy, prior breast surgeries and the histopathologic diagnosis; and B) *Familial:* Family members with history of malignant conditions, including breast cancer and ovarian cancer and their age at diagnosis.

Introduction

Benign breast lesions, excluding the congenital diseases, represent the most common clinical entity present in young women. These benign lesions are often identified a few days prior to menstruation. When the woman then seeks medical help for this reason [benign lesions], she may describe the findings of increased breast consistency and pain.

As a result the patient on occasion may only refer to the unexpected and alarming findings as easily moveable nodules under the skin of the breast, which are almost always well defined, painless, and elastic in consistency. It is these benign lesions, with their large variety, that require to be classified due to their histological characteristics.

The precise classification of benign breast conditions presents certain difficulties due to the fact that different authors work with different classifications. For example, it has been proposed that one of the most frequent benign breast lesions, fibroadenoma, should be considered as a mastopathy based on diagnostic criteria.

Nonetheless, and with the purpose of adhering to a descriptive system, a proposal to classify what we consider acceptable for benign breast diseases based on histopathology and clinical findings is:

1 Fibrocystic mastopathy
2 Fibroadenoma
3 Adenoma of the breast or nipple
4 Benign phyllodes tumor or intracanalicular cellular fibroadenoma
5 Hamartoma or fibroadenolipoma
6 Lipoma
7 Fibrous histiocytoma
8 Granular cell tumor
9 Fibromatosis
10 Cutaneous marginal zone tumors
11 Ductal ectasia
12 Intraductal papilloma
13 Mammary cyst
14 Galactocele
15 Other benign lesions

1. Fibrocystic Mastopathy

Fibrocystic mastopathy includes Schimmelbusch adenoma, chronic cystic mastitis, dense cyst disease, benign mastopathy, also known as mammary dysplasia, and what the World Health Organization (WHO) denominates mammary dysplasia to differentiate the condition from another one that may be potentially malignant.

This is a frequent disorder in women over 30 years of age and is consistent with an increase in breast tissue in the upper and external zones of the breasts and augmented density in the affected areas.

It tends to be bilateral, although not of equal density and customarily present after menarche.

The woman usually refer to moveable nodular zones with an increased consistency and tissue irregularity, that at times can be accompanied by pain on days prior to the initiation of their menstruation.

Clinically, in addition to confirming the presence of increased density and irregularity, it is possible to confirm the presence of fluctuating and painful cystic lesions.

The recommendations for a diagnostic workup in these cases are as follows: if the woman is less than 40 years of age, a mammary ultrasound (US) should be performed, and if she is over 40 years of age a bilateral mastography with complimentary US is indicated. It is very important to identify potential risk factors and to keep in mind the possibility that there may be a malignant lesion, even though clinical workup suggests a benign disease.

2. Fibroadenoma

Fibroadenoma is the most frequent benign breast disease in young women (between 15 and 30 years of age). Its formation and often rapid growth is directly related to circulating hormone levels, whose variations are linked with the menstrual cycle, pregnancy and the ingestion of contraceptives with high hormone levels, especially estrogen.

On the other hand, when menopause sets in and circulating hormone levels decrease, existing fibroadenomas may shrink or even disappear.

Fibroadenomas are usually non-painful solid diseases with a round, ovoid or multilobulated contour. They [fibroadenomas] have shown to duplicate in size every 2 to 6 months until they reach between 3 to 4 cm in diameter. Tumor consistency is firm, moveable (not fixed to adjacent tissues) and they are easily detected by US.

A juvenile fibroadenoma is a variant of the common fibroadenoma. It is denominated "juvenile" because it is present in females less than 18 years of age. Histopathologically it exhibits great richness and cellular activity. They can reach a diameter of 10–20 cm in a very short time. In 10–15% of the cases lesions can be multiple. Imaging studies such as US and mammography are very useful and fibroadenomas typically present themselves with radio opaque borders, low density and are very well circumscribed [2].

The orthodox treatment modalities for fibroadenomas are to be addressed later in this book.

Nonetheless, it is to be noted that in 2001 the US Federal Drug Administration (FDA) approved cryoablation as a minimally invasive alternative in patients with a sonographically visible lesion of no more than 4 cm in size and with a histologically confirmed diagnosis of fibroadenoma.

This procedure is performed under local anesthesia and uses US imaging as a guide.

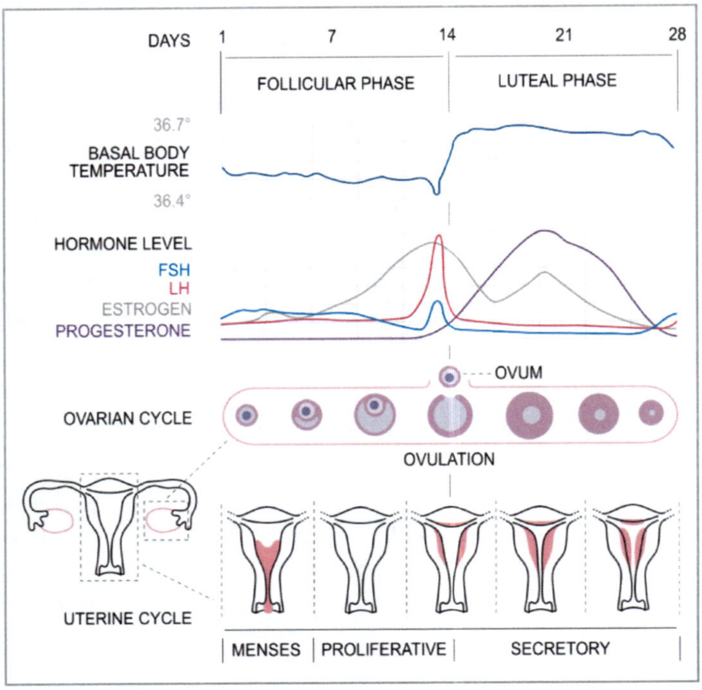

Figure 1. Feminine menstrual cycle (wikimedia commons). The diagnosis, as we have previously cited, is commonly that of a "benign disease." The exact cause of these lesions is unknown, but it is thought that the hormones produced during the sexual cycle from the hypothalamus-hypophysis-target organ axis (commonly between days 7 and 10 prior to the 28-day-cycle menstruation) can cause a woman's breasts to feel swollen, bulky, or painful prior to or during menstruation. It is known that around 50% of women experience this problem at some time during their gestational life, but are infrequent in postmenopausal women, at least for those taking estrogens. These symptoms, however, can last throughout the month and the breast can be thick or with protuberances [1].

3. Adenoma of the Breast or Nipple

Clinically there is no difference between adenoma and fibroadenoma. However, its epithelial characteristic, without the fibrous component, imprints upon it a different histology resulting in the diagnosis of anatomopathological.

Depending on the histology, there are various subtypes: ductal adenoma; tubular adenoma (frequently common in women aged more than 50 years); lactating adenoma, which occurs during the peripartum period; and the apocrine adenoma.

Other forms include adenoma of the nipple (papillary or erosive adenomatosis of the nipple), pleomorphic adenoma and mixed adenoma.

An adenoma of the nipple is an epithelial proliferation within the terminal collecting duct with a pseudo infiltrating pattern and is rarely capable of becoming malignant. A medical expert should carefully evaluate these lesions given that a different diagnosis may be made with solitary papilloma of the nipple, a lesion which may often be accompanied by in situ breast cancer.

In further stages of evolution, an adenoma should not be confused with Paget's disease. These lesions require surgical resection due to the existence of thickening, nipple retraction or ulceration.

4. Benign Phyllodes Tumor or Intracanalicular Cellular Fibroadenoma

Phyllodes tumor (from the Greek *phullon*, leaf), or cystosarcoma phyllodes, as it may also be called, is very rare (0.3–0.9% of the cases). It is reported with greatest frequency in women of over 40 years of age and is characterized by a painless, multinodular, firm growth with a smooth surface. It often measures 5 cm in diameter or more, even doubling the initial breast volume.

For a long time phyllodes tumors were considered malignant. However, from the histopathological point of view, they do not meet the microscopic criteria necessary for malignant classification.

When the tumor is not totally extirpated, it has a high degree of recidivism, but it does not have the potential to metastasize. Imaging studies show a well-defined solid mass. Simple mastectomy is recommended for large lesions [3].

5. Hamartoma or Fibroadenolipoma

This is a rare tumor (1% of cases). Clinically it is represented by an increase in breast volume or asymmetry between both breasts.

On palpation, its soft consistency may be confused with fibroadenoma as the Hamartoma is characteristically well circumscribed and encapsulated.

It usually is present in women between the ages of 40 and 55 years and, as its name indicates; its distinctive component is the presence of mature adipose tissue, muscle and fibrous tissue (common components of the breast).

These tumors range in size from 2 to 4 cm and may be associated with intermittent mastalgia in relation to the menstrual cycle. The most frequent clinical manifestation of these tumors is progressive and renders clinical diagnosis difficulties, making it necessary to employ imaging techniques. The role of fine or thick needle aspiration biopsy in its diagnosis is limited and requires clinical or radiological correlation.

These lesions tend to have pseudoangiomatous changes in the stroma. Correct histological identification of the Hamartoma is important because there can be apocrine metaplasia, cysts and adenosis [4]. Nonetheless, once the diagnosis is established, complete surgical extirpation is not recommended unless the tumor is very voluminous.

6. Lipomas

This is an example of a pure mesenchymatous tumor that can occur in the breast. It tends to be present in women between the ages of 40 and 50 years old. It is clinically characterized by a well-defined, mobile, soft nodule as it is composed exclusively of adipose tissue delimited by a fine fibrous covering. Lipomas can measure anywhere from 2 to 10 cm mammographically, its image is characteristic and its treatment is surgical. These adipose tissue-derived benign breast tumors are more frequent and can pose a problem for the radiologist during diagnosis with the malignant form (liposarcoma).

The lipoma tumors were classified in 2005 by the WHO as follows: lipoma; lipomatosis; nerve lipomatosis; lipoblastoma/lipoblastomatosis; angiolipoma; soft tissue myolipoma; chondroid lipoma; spindle cell lipoma/ pleomorphic lipoma; and hibernoma [5].

7. Fibrous Histiocytoma

Today it is considered that this group of lesions, with a poorly defined morphological aspect of histiocytic differentiation, should be diligently differentiated from malignant fibrous histiocytoma (MFH), a term that is currently substituted for sarcoma-like MFH.

The so-called benign fibrous histiocytomas poses a problem for histopathological interpretation and has given rise to controversy in recent years. Leiomyomas, histiocytomas and hemangiomas are examples of benign soft tissue tumors that can occur in the breast and, although they have low frequency, these pose a problem of diagnosis for pathologists and treatment for oncologists in terms of avoiding and compromising their optimal treatment.

Benign smooth muscle tumors (leiomyomas), that are extracutaneously localized, or those with extra uterine localization, have been the reason for the conceptual changes approved by the WHO and persisting at present.

The WHO recognizes the following types of leiomyomas: 1) angioleiomyoma; and 2) deep soft tissue leiomyoma. Clearly other benign tumors deriving from soft tissues may be found, such as striated muscle lesions (rabdomyoma), or vascular structures derived tumors, hemangiomas, epithelioid hemangiomas, lymphoangioma and angiomatosis. These afore mentioned benign vascular lesions are frequent and are generally localized on the skin. It is often difficult to differentiate between malformation, tumor, or reactive process.

8. Granular Cell Tumor

These tumors are rarely found in the breast and are nearly always benign. Most frequently the lesion is small, scarcely more than 2 cm in size, and is palpable and mobile, although sometimes it can be adhered to the skin or to the thoracic wall. These tumors can be confused in the clinical setting with a malignant lesion due to their consistency, especially if they seem fixed to the chest wall. Mammographically they may also represent a diagnostic challenge and therefore fine needle aspiration or thick needle biopsy is necessary for definitive diagnosis. Treatment is always surgical.

9. Fibromatosis

Desmoid tumor or fibromatosis of the breast was described at the beginning of the past century and is an infrequent benign tumor of mesenchymatous lineage (comprising scarcely 0.3% of solid tumors, according to some authors). It is characterized by locally aggressive clinical behavior.

This tumor tends to be present in females within a wide age range (between 14 and 80 years), although fibromatosis has also been reported in males. Clinically and radiologically, this tumor can simulate a carcinoma and therefore the diagnosis must be histopathological [6].

10. Cutaneous Marginal Zone Tumors

Cutaneous lymphoid hyperplasia (CLH) is a benign reactive lymphoid proliferation. These tumors share many histological and clinical features with cutaneous marginal zone lymphoma (MZL). Both lesions are similar in feminine preponderance and median age. The most common localizations are arm, head and neck, and trunk.

The histological appearance in both CLH and MZL is a dense lymphocytic infiltrate, bottom-heavy or top-heavy growth pattern, eosinophilia, and a grenz zone, equally observed in both disorders. Dutcher bodies were observed only in cutaneous MZL [7].

11. Ductal Ectasia

This type of lesion in which there is a dilation of terminal lactiferous ducts present in adult women, fundamentally during climacterium, manifest themselves by means of a thick and dark secretion that emerges from the nipple. Sometimes a retroareolar nodular zone can be palpated and the secretion's cytological evaluation, together with the culture, provide guidance towards medical or surgical treatment by excision of the nodule.

12. Intraductal Papilloma

The term papilloma includes lesions, a "tree-like" growth with a fibrovascular stem, exclude juvenile papillomatosis which are characterized by epithelial proliferation without a fibrovascular stem.

Strictly speaking intraductal papillomas have two microscopic cellular components, epithelial and myoepithelial, without atypia. Histologically, however, on occasion the intraductal papilloma can find some areas of cellular dysplasia which classify the lesion as an "atypical papilloma".

It is important to note that Carcinoma must always be ruled out in the presence of atypical papilloma.

The typical intraductal papilloma is unilateral and present in older women during menopause at ages between 40 and 60 years. Papillomas may either be asymptomatic or cause nipple discharge.

Nipple secretion may be serous, bloody and/or of a dark-brown or frankly black material and of pasty consistency.

Thelorrhagia (blood secretion) may also be present in association with other lesions, such as the existence of hyperplasia of the canicular epithelium itself, trauma, adenosis and angiomas.

Many authors lend importance to the presence of thelorrhagia because they indicate that the latter is an alarm signal for malignant affliction. (For example, in one report the authors cited 12 of 414 cases (3.4%) and Leschickter reported 4% in 2,393 cases analyzed). However, one must bear in mind that some cancers, such as papillary adenocarcinoma, can have clinical thelorrhagia as a manifestation.

Other secretions that can be emitted from the nipple are of a serous, purulent or milky character. All of these discharges are generally benign, except when a carcinoma or a sarcoma is involved. The cytology of these will often afford the diagnosis.

In addition to nipple discharge, papillomas may present as a solitary or multiple mass that occupies the larger caliber mammary ducts with subareolar localization. US is the best study to perform the diagnosis as dilatation of the retroareolar ducts is exhibited. Surgical treatment must also be considered.

13. Mammary Cysts

These are thin-walled nodules that contain liquid and can appear at any age. They are well circumscribed tumors and diagnosis can be made by means of palpation as well as by US, while direct guided puncture is diagnostic and comprises the best treatment.

The simple cyst, as its name indicates, is a dilatation of the deep ducts. The liquid that it contains can be clear, serous, purulent (abscess), or hemorrhagic (hematoma). The simple cyst is characterized by being ovoid, mobile, soft, and renitent in consistency. These cysts are frequently more than 2 to 3 cm in size. On puncture, the nodule disappears but its treatment should be surgical if it is found to be a complex lesion, that is, if the formation of bags and bubbles are present in an initially homogeneous medium.

14. Galactocele

The galactocele (from the Greek *gala* and *kéle*, tumor) contains liquid or thick milk and is associated with lactation.

Clinically it is a round and fluctuating tumor not fixed to adjacent tissue, well circumscribed, and in addition compresses around the nipple and often causes milk to be discharged.

US imaging shows a spherical image with precise borders, very similar to the images of simple cysts. Puncture is the indicated treatment.

15. Other Benign Lesions

Mondor's disease. This is a phlebothrombosis of a superficial vein of the breast which may be traumatic or spontaneous.

On inspection, it is easily visualized and on palpation there can be pain and heat in the entire trajectory of the vein. Treatment consists of antibiotic therapy, anti-inflammatory and analgesic medication. Care should be taken to avoid trauma in the affected breast.

Fat necrosis appears as a non-painful, isolated nodule that is sometimes accompanied by retraction of the skin of the breast, thus it is confused with breast cancer.

The history of previous breast trauma may aid in diagnosis, which is confirmed by fine-needle aspiration (FNA) or core biopsy.

Treatment is surgical.

Conclusion on the Treatment of Benign Breast Diseases

The treatment of benign breast tumors is surgical and as to be expected some are treated sooner than others. In general, however, no benign breast tumor is urgent and its size will determine the subsequent intervention, which always will be more conservative in adolescents.

Hence the phrase "Nodule diagnosed, nodule operated on" will always be complied with, but not necessarily in an urgent fashion.

Evaluation, diagnosis and treatment of benign breast diseases should always be performed by an experienced medical specialist.

References

[1] Pearlman, M. D., Griffin, J. L. Benign breast disease. *Obstet. Gynecol.* 2010; 116:747-758.

[2] Pons, M. J., Domínguez, P., Piña, L., et al. Fibroadenomas of the breast with atypia or carcinoma in its interior. *Radiología* 2005; 47(6):351-353.

[3] Aranda Flores, C., Olaya, G. E. J., et al. Tumor phyllodes: experiencia institucional. *Ginecol. Obstet. Mex.* 2009; 77(12):567-572.

[4] González Blanco, I., Rodríguez-Bújez, A. B., Román, A., et al. Los hamartomas de la mama. *Ginecol. Obstet.* 2004; 31(6).

[5] Torrecabota, J., Tejedor, A. Cambios fibroquísticos de la mama. Hiperplasia epitelial/Breast fibrocystic changes. Epithelial hyperplasia. *Cienc. Ginecol.* 2004; 8(1):21-26.

[6] Qureshi, N. A., Tahir, M., Carmichelo, A. Tumor de células granulares de los tejidos blandos. Reporte de un caso y revisión de la literatura. *Int. Semin. Surg. Oncol.* 2006; 3:21.

[7] Baldassano, M. J., Bailey, E. M., Ferry, J. A., et al. Cutaneous lymphoid hyperplasia and cutaneous marginal zone lymphoma. Comparison of morphologic and immunophenotypic features. *Am. J. Surg. Pathol.* 1999 Jan.; 23(1):88-96.

In: Benign Disease of the Breast
Editors: J. de la Garza Salazar, C. Arce Salinas et al.
ISBN: 978-1-63321-624-2

Chapter 2

Epidemiology

Nancy Reynoso-Noveron * ***and Alejandro Mohar-Betancourt***
Epidemiology Unit; Instituto Nacional Cancerologia-Mexico,
Mexico City, DF, Mexico

Abstract

Benign breast alterations are lesions with high prevalence and potentially cancerogenous. There are relatively few studies with respect to their epidemiology and etiology. The most prevalent benign lesions comprise fibrocystic diseases and dominant masses, which include fibroadenomas, cysts, and galactoceles. According to the American Cancer Society (ACS), 9 of every 10 women exhibit benign changes in microscopically examined breast tissues. The incidence of the disease has not been widely studied, but in general these lesions arise during the second decade of life, with peaks in the fourth and fifth life decades, in contrast with malignant diseases. The purpose of this chapter is to describe the epidemiological information available, including frequencies and risk factors, with the aim of providing the reader with useful information for the management and control of this group of diseases.

Introduction

Benign breast alterations represent a group of heterogeneous lesions that merit special attention due to their high prevalence, their impact on women's Quality of life (QOL), and because some histological types are potentially cancerogenous. The great majority of breast lesions are benign. It has been estimated that one of every two women can develop some form of fibrocystic breast disease during their lifetime, and that one of five can develop fibroadenoma [1].

Although the benign disease is frequent, there are relatively few studies with respect to the epidemiology and etiology of the former; in addition, only isolated and nonrelated studies

* Corresponding author.

exist. The literature of breast lesions has focused on the most frequent neoplasm in Western women: breast cancer. Likewise, there are only some descriptions of factors related with benign disease in which endocrine factors have been broadly studied, and these have demonstrated a weak and inconsistent relationship, similar to that of smoking, consumption of exogenous hormones, alcoholism, and the consumption of caffeine, while obesity has been identified as a consistent risk factor [2, 3].

One cause of the difficulty regarding epidemiological knowledge of the disease is its diversity with respect to its presentation, symptomatology, and histopathologic characteristics. Many efforts have been made with the purpose of standardizing the classification and of reducing the proportion of underregistration through the capture of nonconfirmed lesions, notwithstanding that the information possessed continues to be deficient, with differences between that reported by clinics with that registered by Pathologists. To mention only a few numbers, by means of autopsy studies, estimated prevalence is nearly 50%, while prevalence obtained by biopsies, that is confirmed biopsies, is only 10–20% [4–12]. Thus, a greater effort should be made to confirm the existence of this group of diseases, which tends to be poorly feasible at the population level.

Fortunately, at present the use of mammography, Ultrasound (US), and magnetic resonance as breast imaging methods, in addition to the extensive use of the biopsy, has facilitated the diagnosis of benign disease without the need for surgery in the majority of patients, allowing Pathologists, Radiologists, and Oncologists to recognize benign disease, disease *in situ*, or advanced disease, and to establish the management in each of the modalities.

Within this concept, the purpose of this chapter is to describe the epidemiological information that is available, including frequencies and risk factors, with the aim of providing the reader windows of opportunity through which the appearance of this group of diseases can be controlled.

Epidemiology

At a center specialized in mammary gland diseases, appointments involving benign pathology are around 90%. This is due to the great anxiety and worry in women in the face of the signs and symptoms related with the mammary gland, because its differential diagnosis will always be breast cancer.

The term benign breast lesions includes a great number of physiopathological lesions of the different components of breast tissue (epithelial, stroma, adipocytes, or blood vessels). Classification of these lesions has been at issue for some time, due to the separation between pathological and physiological changes of the breast. However, there have been two important moments for the understanding and classification of these lesions. The first, in 1985, represents the adoption by general agreement of the College of American Pathologists (CAP) of the histological classification based on the work of Dupont and Page [13], in which these authors define benign proliferative disease as the clinical characteristics with cancerogenous potential and in which they specify nonproliferative lesions without atypia and hyperplastic lesions with atypia. The second, in 1987, corresponds to the consideration of the

Aberrations of Normal Development and Involution (ANDI), providing a total framework for benign breast conditions, including the pathogenesis as well as the degree of abnormality.

In this manner, benign breast diseases encompass a heterogeneous group of lesions that can present a broad gamma of symptoms or that can be detected by means of a microscopic finding. The incidence of benign lesions begins to rise during the second decade of life, with peaks in the fourth and fifth decades, in contrast with malignant diseases, whose incidence continues to increase after menopause, although more slowly [14].

Benign breast lesions are sufficiently common among women; according to the American Cancer Society (ACS), 9 of every 10 women exhibit benign changes in microscopically examined breast tissues [15–17]. The most prevalent benign lesions comprise fibrocystic diseases and dominant masses, the latter defined as persistent lesions without change, which include fibroadenomas, cysts, and galactoceles.

As previously mentioned, despite the extensive presence of benign breast lesions, the incidence of the disease has not been widely studied. In some reviews, the authors mention that the subjective nature of the disease renders it nearly impossible to measure the incidences, or in those in which data do exist, these are highly distinct [17,18]. One of the epidemiological studies that has permitted obtaining the greatest amount of evidence in this respect is the Nurses' Health Study II (NHS II), which describes a self-reported incidence of fibrocystic disease or some other benign lesion of 30.9 per 1,000 person-years (3.9%). This study also reported an increase with age of 22.6 per 1,000 person-years in women aged 25–29 years and of 35.6 per 1,000 person-years in women aged 40–44 years [19,20]. Other sources estimate that the accumulated incidence of fibrocystic disease is 60% of the feminine population, and yet others state that the incidence is unknown, but these estimate that fibrocystic changes can be identified in 54% of clinically normal breast autopsies, in 34% of breast biopsies, and in 40% of breasts with cancer [19]. These generally tend to present in older population –during the third and fourth decades of life-, reporting a dominant mass in 15% of postmenopausal women [19]; this is the most frequent condition that has suggested that perhaps this is not properly a disease, but rather an alteration of normal breast development (ANDI) [21]. Some references indicate that this process is observed clinically and histologically in >50–90% of women, respectively [22].

For many years, the presence of cysts in breast tissue has been considered a risk factor for the development of breast cancer. The precancerous nature of fibrocystic mastopathy is the matter of very much debate, accepting that its malignant transformation is low. Simple, nonproliferative fibrocystic mastopathy does not imply having a greater risk for having breast cancer. On the other hand, proliferative mastoplasy without atypia (which includes hyperplasia, fibroadenoma sclerosing adenosis, and intraductal papilloma) entertains a Relative risk (RR) for cancer of 1.5–2, and proliferative mastopathy with atypia has an RR for breast cancer of 4–5, both compared with nonproliferative lesions (Table 1) [5]. According to Hartmann et al., the risk for breast cancer in young women with a diagnosis of atypical epithelial cancer is twice that of women >55 years of age. In the same study, familial history of breast cancer is an independent factor for increase of the risk, even in patients with nonproliferative lesions [23, 24]. Habor et al. analyzed 677 surgical breast interventions, and in 115 of these (17%), the authors found the coexistence of cancer with fibrocystic breast disease. These findings suggest that breast cancer can begin initially as an epithelial hyperplasia, which corroborates that these hyperplastic changes are a risk factor for cancer [25]. Compared with general population, women with nonproliferative lesions experienced no increase in risk, while those with proliferative disease without atypia and with ductal or lobular atypia did have a risk, increasing to 1.3–1.9 and to 3.9–13.0, respectively [24, 26, 27]. In addition to histological characteristics, age at biopsy and familial history of breast cancer have been reported as the greatest determinants of risk for breast cancer after diagnosis of a benign disease [26]. According to Hartmann et al., the risk for breast cancer in young women with a diagnosis of atypical epithelial proliferation is twice that observed in women aged over 55 years with a diagnosis of atypical epithelial proliferation. In this same study, it was cited that familiar history of breast cancer comprises an independent risk factor and that this can increase the risk for breast cancer in patients with nonproliferative lesions. The absolute risk for both atypical and not atypical is relatively low. More than 80% of patients with a diagnosis of atypical hyperplasia do not develop invasive cancer during their lifetime.

Table 1. Fibrocystic changes, proliferative lesions, and the risk of breast cancer

Nonproliferative lesions (70% of cases): Relative risk (RR) of cancer = 1
Adenosis
Cystic or apocrine changes
Mammary duct ectasia
Usual slight epithelial hyperplasia
Proliferative lesions without atypia (26% of cases): RR of cancer = 1.5–2
Usual moderate or florid hyperplasia
Papillomas
Sclerosing adenosis
Proliferative disease with atypia (4% of cases): RR of cancer = 4–5
Atypical ductal hyperplasia
Atypical lobular hyperplasia

Modified from Dupont WD, Page DL.

On the other hand, in reports on the incidence of dominant masses, fibroadenomas present in women aged <35 years are rarer; these occur in 25% of asymptomatic women, it is usually a disease that appears during early reproductive life, and it has been considered an aberration and involution of normal breast development. Various studies have considered fibroadenoma a risk factor for breast cancer; a systematic review in this respect showed that the RR for fibroadenomas without hyperplasia was 1.48–1.7, with hyperplasia, of 3.47–3.7, and with hyperplasia and with atypia, of 6.9–7.29, persisting during >20 years [28].

In addition to this type of lesion, there is the phyllodes tumor, a rare fibroepithelial lesion that presents in <1% of all mammary neoplasms. Papillomas, which are exophytic proliferations adhered to the walls of the galactophorous ducts, formed of epithelial cells without atypia, are another type of benign disease, among which the solitary intraductal papilloma of the breast is a strange benign tumor of the large ducts that tend to appear 1 or 2 cm from the nipple. Their principal clinical manifestation is the secretion from the nipple of serous, hematic, or another liquid. Mean age at presentation is 48 years, and 40 years for multiple papillomatosis. It grows slowly and is rarely palpable. And finally –to mention the most frequent lesions- intraductal papillomas measure around 0.5 cm in diameter and can reach up to 4 or 5 cm. Multiple intraductal papillomas are most frequent in young patients and are associated with less frequency in secretion by the nipple in contrast with solitary intraductal papillomas of the breast [29, 30]. More information in this respect will be found described in subsequent chapters.

As has been noted, assessment of the incidence of benign disease is difficult in general population, due to the heterogeneousness of the clinical and pathological definitions and the non-necessity of receiving medical attention and treatment throughout the lifetime. Women who receive medical treatment in reality tend to represent a low proportion of all of the cases; thus, the detection rate is not known in full. A real approach can be to obtain this through autopsy studies. In this regard, there are reports carried out between 1919 and 1957 in which the prevalence of fibrocystic disease (defined as macrocysts, microcysts, or epithelial hyperplasia) among asymptomatic women was 58.5% (424 cases/725) of the total number of autopsies. Some more recent studies have been consistent with this result; another 12 studies conducted since 1937, and two even more recent publications, report a prevalence of fibrocystic disease of between 54 and 61%, this in Caucasian women. Prevalence of fibroadenoma was reported by another four studies conducted after 1980 as between 15 and 23%. These reports also show a greater prevalence in Black than in Caucasian women. Therefore, it has been estimated that one of every two women can develop some form of fibrocystic breast disease throughout their lifetime, and that one of every five can develop fibroadenoma.

With respect to incidence rates calculated in cohort studies, seven studies were found that had been published between 1976 and 1986, five of which only included cases confirmed by biopsy and an additional two that compared the nonbiopsied and biopsied asymptomatic disease rate. Incidence by specific groups obtained by biopsy for fibrocystic disease and for fibroadenoma was consistent among the studies, but this was when the designs were heterogeneous, because one of these reported the hospitalization rate in a cohort of 67,500 women, another was a population-based case-control study with 485 women, yet another was performed in a series of cases of Australian women, and the fourth study showed the hospitalization rates of fibrocystic disease in a cohort of menopausal women of a health cooperative. These studies report an incidence rate of 100,000 person-years of fibrocystic disease of 137 with women aged between 25 and 29 years, of 411 of those aged between 20 and 44 years, and of 387 in women aged between 45 and 49 years, with fair diminution from this latter age. On the other hand, the incidence peak of 115 per 100,000 person-years presented in women between the ages of 20 and 24 years, with a fair decrease up to 45–49 years, observing nearly a 5 in older women. The accumulated incidence obtained through biopsy for fibrocystic disease prior to the age of 65 years was 8.8%, and for fibroadenoma, 2.2%. One must recall that, according to autopsy studies, only between 10 and 20% of cases of benign disease are diagnosed histologically; thus, the statistics reported could entertain strong problems of validity [31].

In Mexico, there are unfortunately no national registries of benign breast diseases. In this regard, we only retain the experience of the Nacional Institute of Cancerology that, despite its being a concentration hospital of patients with cancer, during the year 1983 at the Breast Tumor Service, 50% of patients receiving a histopathological diagnosis had benign disease. Distribution by specific type shows that 41% were fibroadenomas, 37% were identified as dysplasias, 8% as papillomas, 6% as cysts, 3% as phyllodes tumors, 0.3% as lipomas, and 0.1% as hemangiomas. In another analysis conducted with data collected between 1980 and 1985 in adolescent patients, the most frequent benign lesion was fibroadenomas (63.7%), followed by fibrocystic mastopathy (14.9%), with the remainder being gynecomastia, mastitis, other dysplasias (papillomatosis, cysts, fibrosis), phyllodes tumors, and lipomas. For 2001, of the total biopsies, fibrocystic disease and fibroadenomas were the most frequent, with a total of 63 and 16.5% of the total biopsies performed, respectively. The tendency was similar to that of 2002–2003, when 58% of biopsies performed were fibrocystic changes and 16%, fibroadenomas. Although these data are not at all representative of Mexican population, they do coincide with that reported in the literature concerning the identification of the most frequent benign breast lesions.

Risk Factors

Despite the well-established association between benign proliferative lesions and the risk for breast cancer, which has been confirmed by a risk model based on the NHS II, showing that women who had benign breast disease present a greater incidence of breast cancer while young, and even after considering the known risk factors, little is known about the etiology of benign breast disease. The result of epidemiological studies has been inconsistent, due in part to publications with different methodologies, the lack of systematic reviews, and the discrepant classification of benign pathology. Additionally, the greater part of these studies has focused only on risk factors at adult age, precisely prior to the biopsy, which cannot be the most relevant etiological period.

Some authors, such as Baer et al., suggest that given the evidence that some early lifestyles are implicated in the development of breast cancer, it is plausible to think that these also play a role in the etiology of benign breast disease. Two previous analyses of the information gathered by the NHS II support this hypothesis. One of these was in the prospective analysis of alcohol consumption at different life moments, in which this same group of investigators observed that recent alcohol consumption was not related with the incidence of benign breast disease, but that alcohol consumption between the ages of 18 and 22 years was associated with a significant increase of risk for proliferative as well as for nonproliferative lesions. On the other hand, it also has been reported that in the population providing retrospective information on diet in school, it was shown that diets based on vegetable fats, vitamin E, and fiber during adolescence had an inverse association with the incidence of benign proliferative breast lesions; in contrast, this association was not found in adult population, suggesting that exposure at early life stages can exert an influence on benign breast disease, basing this on the analysis that Baer et al. conducted with the purpose of determining the association among early factors and the risk for breast cancer, childhood and adolescent obesity, physical activity during adolescence, birth weight, and the history of having been breastfed, in relation to the incidence of histologically confirmed benign proliferative breast cancer among NHS II participants [32].

These possible associations were analyzed among 71,896 postmenopausal women, who were questioned about body fat when they were young women, physical activity in adolescence, birth weight, and the history of being breastfed. Between 1991 and 1997, 901 of these women were identified as having benign breast disease; the RR with its 95% Confidence interval (95% CI) was estimated by means of Cox proportional hazard models. Body fat during infancy (5–10 years of age) was associated with a decrease in the risk of presenting benign proliferative breast disease; the RR (95% CI) of those who had overweight compared with those who were the most slender was 0.61 (range, 0.44–0.86; p <0.001), these factors continuing to be significant after adjusting for present Body mass index (BMI). BMI at age 18 years was inversely associated with the incidence of benign proliferative disease, with an RR (95% CI) of 0.67 (range, 0.52–0.88) for those with a BMI of ≥25 compared with those with a BMI of <19 (p = 0.001). A clear association was not found among physical activity on adolescence, birth weight, or having been breastfed. These results indicate that the premenopausal woman with greater weight in her youth had a lesser incidence of benign proliferative breast disease, compatible with previous conclusions for breast cancer [31].

Similarly, in the literature there are some reports found of other factors associated with benign disease: clinical observations of women who received estrogens and antiestrogens give rise to the thinking that hormonal events play an important role in the development of these diseases. In a subanalysis carried out in >6,000 women aged 40–59 years who were participants in the Canadian National Breast Screening Study (CNBSS), who by means of self-report were questioned about lifestyles and diet, the association was evaluated in postmenopausal women between hormone replacement therapy and benign breast disease. During the follow-up period, a total of 691 women were diagnosed by biopsy with benign breast disease, and on comparing these with a control group, a positive association was reported between duration of hormone replacement use and benign disease. During this study, the incidence rate adjusted for postmenopausal women who utilized hormones for >8 years was 1.70 (95% CI, 1.06–2.72) [33]. Additionally, it has been reported that the use of Tamoxifen, an antiestrogen, when employed for the prevention of cancer, is associated with a 28% reduction of benign disease (RR (95% CI) = 0.72 (range, 0.65–0.79), including those classified as adenosis, cysts, mammary duct ectasia, and hyperplasia [34].

Likewise, some genetic factors have been associated with the presence of benign lesions; loss of heterozygosity, as the result of the loss of small segments of DNA, is a common finding in benign lesions. In addition, women with *BRCA1* or *BRCA2* gene mutations also have a greater frequency of multiple benign lesions or malignant breast lesions [35].

Within this context, the hypothesis is interesting of the role that the risk factors play in breast cancer as possible factors also associated with benign lesions. However, greater scientific evidence continues to be lacking in this respect.

Prevention

Therefore, given the enormous frequency of this type of lesion and its relation with breast cancer, benign breast pathology should be studied with care.

Unfortunately, the level of evidence existing on the risk factors for benign disease is very poor. Thus, it is difficult for primary prevention strategies focused on this group of diseases to be implemented.

For its part, early identification of these diseases by means of clinical exploration, together with imaging techniques, is often not conclusive, requiring histopathological evaluation of the lesions to discard a malignancy process with certainty. This does not appear to be a simple process, because cancer will always be thought of as a differential diagnosis and clinical management and follow-up of the woman will require correct definition.

At present, there is a great increase in the incidence of breast biopsies practiced in all breast pathology units; the majority of these, fortunately, are histologically benign, but this incidence causes enormous anxiety and the sensation of disease in the women.

Thus, it is necessary to establish an adequate detection process of the lesions, which of course depends in its totality on the first-contact physician; this person is indispensable for being capable of optimizing the management of benign lesions, hand in hand with that of breast cancer. Thus, with the evidence available, the strategies that we can propose as preventive alternatives of malignant lesions, include improvement in the prevention of benign lesions, their form of presentation, symptomatology, and in the associated risk, with the purpose of correctly identifying and treating those who present a risk of having breast cancer.

References

[1] Goehring C, Morabia A. Epidemiology of benign breast disease, with special attention to histologic types. *Epidemiol Rev* 1997;19:310-327.

[2] England P, Skinner S. Sex hormones in breast disease. *Br J Surg* 1975;62:806.

[3] Hartmann L, Sellers T, Frost M. Benign breast disease and the risk of breast cancer. *NEJM* 2005 July 21;353:229-237.

[4] Page DL, Vander Zwaag R, Rogers LW, Williams LT, Walker WE, Hartman WH. Relation between component parts of fibrocystic disease complex and breast cancer. *J Natl Cancer Inst* 1978:61:1055-1063.

[5] Dupont WD, Page DL. Risk factors for breast cancer in women with proliferative breast disease. *NEJM* 1985;312:146-151.

[6] Page DL, Dupont WD, Rogers LW, Rados MS. Atypical hyperplastic lesions of the female breast: a long-term follow-up study. *Cancer* 1985;55:2698-2708.

[7] Fitzgibbons PL, Henson DE, Hutter RVP. Benign breast changes and the risk for subsequent breast cancer. An update of the 1985 Consensus Statement. *Arch Pathol Lab Med* 1998;122:1053-1055.

[8] Bartow SA, Pathak DR, Black WC, Key CR, Teaf SR. Prevalence of benign, atypical, and malignant breast lesions in populations at different risk for breast cancer: a forensic autopsy study. *Cancer* 1987;60:2751-2760.

[9] Ory H, Cole P, MacMahon B, Hoover R. Oral contraceptives and reduced risk of benign breast diseases. *NEJM* 1976;294:419-422.

[10] Cole P, Elwood JM, Kaplan SD. Incidence rates and risk factors of benign breast neoplasms. *Am J Epidemiol* 1978;16:112-120.

[11] Fleming NT, Armstrong BK, Sheiner HJ. The comparative epidemiology of benign breast lumps and breast cancer in Western Australia. *Int J Cancer* 1982;30:147-152.

[12] Jick SS, Walker AM, Jick H. Conjugated estrogens and fibrocystic breast disease. *Am J Epidemiol* 1986;124:746-751.

[13] Page DI, Dupont WD. Anatomic indicators (histologic and cytologic) of increased breast cancer risk. *Breast Cancer Res Treat* 1993;28:157-166.

[14] Donegan WL. Common benign conditions of the breast. In: Donegan WL, Spratt JS, Editors. *Cancer of the Breast.* Fifth ed. St. Louis, MO, USA: Saunders; 2002. pp. 67-110.

[15] Shaaban AM, Sloane JP, West CS, et al. Histopathologic types of benign breast lesions and risk of breast cancer. *Am J Surg Pathol* 2002;26:421-430.
[16] American Cancer Society, 2002. Benign Breast Conditions. http://www.canceer.org /docroot/CRI/content/CRI_2_6X_Benign_Breast_Conditions_59.asp (accessed December 2013).
[17] Johnson C. Benign breast disease. *Nurse Pract Forum* 1999;10(3):137-144.
[18] Marchant DJ. Benign breast disease. *Obstet Gynecol Clin North Am* 2002;29(1):1-20.
[19] U.S. Cancer Statistics Working Group. United States Cancer Statistics: 1999 Incidence. Atlanta, GA, USA: Department of Health and Human Services, Centers for Disease Control and Prevention and National Cancer Institute, 2002.
[20] Webb PM, Byrne C, Schnitt SJ, Connolly JL, Jacobs T, Peiro G, Willet W, Colditz GA. Family history of breast cancer, age and benign breast disease. *Int J Cancer* 2002;100(3):375-378.
[21] Hughes L, Mansel R, Webster D. Aberrations of Normal Development and Involution (ANDI): a new perspective on pathologenesis and nomenclature of benign breast disorders. *Lancet* 1987;6:5-36.
[22] Santen RJ, Mansel R. Benign breast disorders. *NEJM* 2005;353:275-285.
[23] Dupont WD, Parl FF, Hartmann WH, et al. Breast cancer risk associated with proliferative breast disease and atypical hyperplasia. *Cancer* 1993;71:1258-1265.
[24] Hartmann LC, Sellers TA, Frost MH, Lingle WL, Degnim AC, Ghosh K, et al. Benign breast disease and the risk of breast cancer. *NEJM* 2005;353:229-237.
[25] Habor V, Habor A, Copotolu C, Pantiru A. Fibrocystic breast disease- breast cancer sequence. *Chirurgia* (Bucur) 2010;105:191-194.
[26] Palli D, Rosselli Del Turco M, Simoncini R, et al. Benign breast disease and breast cancer: a case-control study in a cohort in Italy. *Int J Cancer* 1991;47:703-706.
[27] Marshall LM, Hunter DJ, Connolly JL, et al. Risk of breast cancer associated with atypical hyperplasia of lobular and ductal types. *Cancer Epidemiol Biomarkers Prev* 1997;6:297-301.
[28] El-Wakeel H, Umpleby HC. Systematic review of fibroadenoma as a risk factor for breast cancer. *Breast* 2003;12:302-307.
[29] Page DL, Anderson TJ. Diagnostic histopathology of the breast and related lesions. New York: Churchill Livingstone; 1987.
[30] Carter D. Intraductal papillary tumors of the breast. A study of 78 cases. *Cancer* 1977;39:1689.
[31] Baer HJ, Willett WC, Schnitt SJ, Rosner B, Connolly JL, Byrne C, Colditz GA. Early life factors and incidence of proliferative benign disease *Cancer Epidemiol Biomarkers Prev* 2005;14:2889-2897.
[32] Baer HJ, Schnitt SJ, Connolly JL, et al. Adolescent diet and incidence of proliferative benign breast disease. *Cancer Epidemiol Biomarkers Prev* 2003;12:1159-1167.
[33] Rohan TE, Miller AB. Hormone replacement therapy and risk of benign proliferative epithelial disorders of the breast. *Eur J Cancer Prev* 1999;8:123-130.
[34] Tan-Chiu E, Wang J, Costantino JP, et al. Effects of tamoxifen on benign breast disease in women at high risk for breast cancer. *J Natl Cancer Inst* 2003;95:302-307.
[35] Hoogerbrugge N, Bult P, de Widt-Levert LM, et al. High prevalence of premalignant lesions in prophylactically removed breasts from women at hereditary risk for breast cancer. *J Clin Oncol* 2003;21:41-45

In: Benign Disease of the Breast
Editors: J. de la Garza Salazar, C. Arce Salinas et al.
ISBN: 978-1-63321-624-2

Chapter 3

Development, Anatomy, Physiology, and Developmental Abnormalities

***David Isla-Ortiz*[*1] and *Eduardo Charco-Lopez*[2]**
[1]Surgical Oncology Department
Instituto Nacional Cancerologia-Mexico,
Mexico City, DF, Mexico
[2]Medical Oncology Department
Instituto Nacional Cancerologia-Mexico,
Mexico City, DF, Mexico

Abstract

The breast is a tubuloalveolar gland that undergoes several modifications during the person's lifetime. It has the specific function of synthesizing and secreting. During a woman's life, the female mammary gland goes through drastic changes in composition, architecture, size, and function, mediated by changes in gene expression and subsequently, physiological stages of development. The breasts of a newborn consist of rudimentary ducts that regress soon after birth. The breasts of nulliparous women contain more type 1 lobules than the parous breast, which contains more differentiated type 3 lobules. During the pregnancy and lactancy cycle, the breast becomes a fully mature functional organ and its maximal branching capability is expressed: the secretory acinus that is formed during pregnancy represents a terminal outgrowth that marks the full extent of glandular differentiation. Postmenopausal involution is triggered by declining ovarian function, thus of declining circulatory levels of sex-steroid hormones (estrogen, progesterone).

Prior to puberty, there are no functional or structural differences between the male and female breast. With the onset of puberty, a striking sexual dimorphism becomes manifest as dramatic changes ensue in the morphology and function of the female breast.

Throughout the menstrual cycle, healthy women are exposed to frequent changes in the hormonal milieu through monthly cycling levels of estradiol and progesterone. After the initial conditioning of the mammary secretory tissue by estrogen and progesterone,

[*] Corresponding author.

there is a specific need for lactogenic hormone alongside the permissive actions of glucocorticoids, insulin, and thyroxin for successful milk production.

The breast is composed of glandular (secretory) and adipose tissue supported by a loose framework of fibrous connective tissue. The secretory tissue is drained by a ductal system that stores and transports milk to the nipple during lactation.

The multiple, but rare, congenital anomalies of the breast may be associated with various other syndromes, including polythelia, polymastia, hypoplasia, amastia, amazia, Poland syndrome, and anomalies of breast size such as megalomastia and gynecomastia, which will be described in this chapter.

Development of the Breast

During life, the female mammary gland undergoes drastic changes in composition, architecture, size, and function, which are mediated by changes in gene expression and subsequently, physiological stages of development. The mammary gland developmental stages (Figure 1) are the following: fetal growth; infant (prepubertal) growth; pubertal expansion; pregnancy and lactation-associated remodeling a postlactational and postmenopausal involution [1].

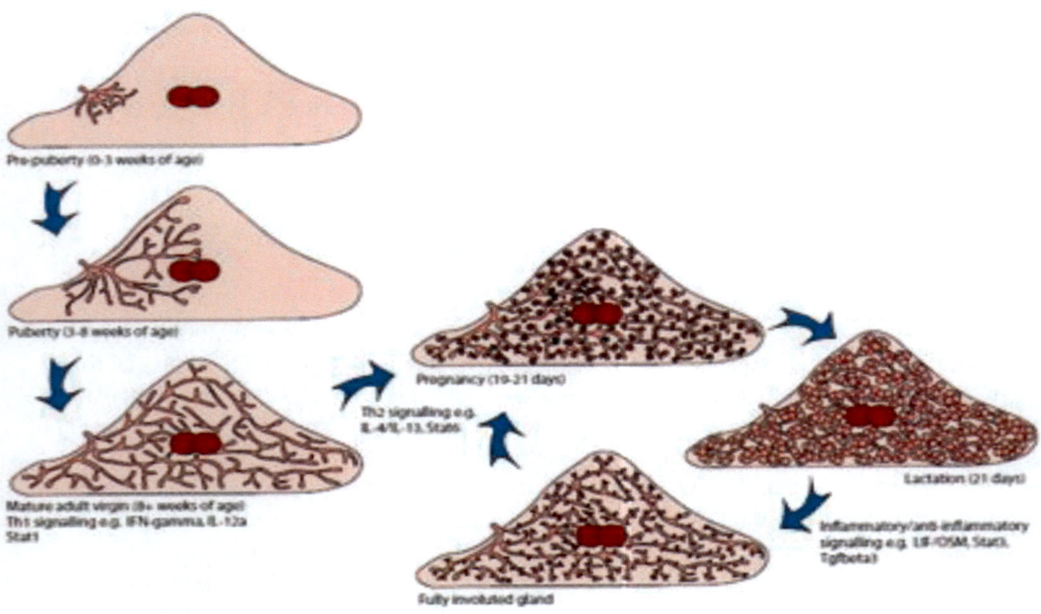

Figure 1. Schematic diagram of mammary gland development in the adult. Reproduced with permission [2].

Fetal Development

The breasts arise from the skin, perhaps in response to signaling by Fibroblast growing factor (FGF) [3]. Embryonic development of the breast is initiated during the sixth week from a thickened, ectodermal ridge extending along the milk line (from the groin to the axilla on the anterior surface) (Figure 2).

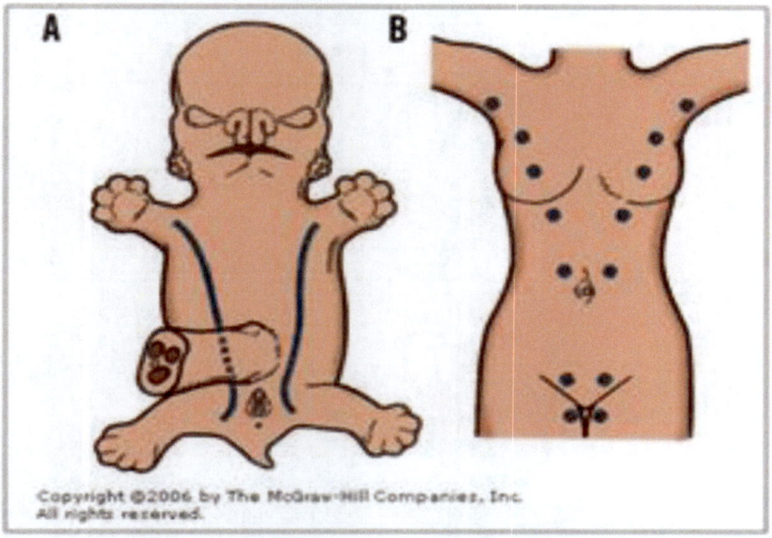

Figure 2. The milk lines in an embryo. Mammary glands form along these lines. B. Common sites of formation of supernumerary nipples or mammary glands in the human. Reproduced with permission [4].

During week 7, the mammary parenchyma invades the stroma, forming the mammary crest, and the mammary vascular system initiates as mesenchymal cells. During weeks 10–12, differentiation between males and females begins: the female ovoid vs. the male's spherical budding shape. The smooth musculature of the areola and nipple are formed between weeks 12 and 16. During weeks 13–19, a depression is formed on the surface of the buds and proliferation of epithelial progenitor populations results in secondary bud formation and initial branching (arborization). After week 32, branching and canalization of the arms result in the formation of the lactiferous ducts that open in the area of the nipple [5].

Neonatal and Prepubertal Development

The breasts of a newborn consist of rudimentary ducts that regress soon after birth. Maternal lactogenic hormones can produce colostrum in the product. Regression of the infant's gland occurs within 4 weeks postpartum [1]. The mammary gland remains at an immature resting state with virtually no differences in structure between those of males and females.

Puberty

This begins at around the 10th–12th years of life under the influence of hypothalamic hormones as follows: the anterior pituitary gland releases follicle-stimulating hormone and luteinizing hormone, which promote maturation of the ovarian follicles and their secretion of estrogens, primarily 17beta-Estradiol (17β-E2). Changes in the trajectory from puberty to adulthood can be defined by the appearance, the number of structures, and the degree of branching or differentiation of structures [6]. External appearance from childhood to maturity has been divided into five phases by Tanner (Figure 3).

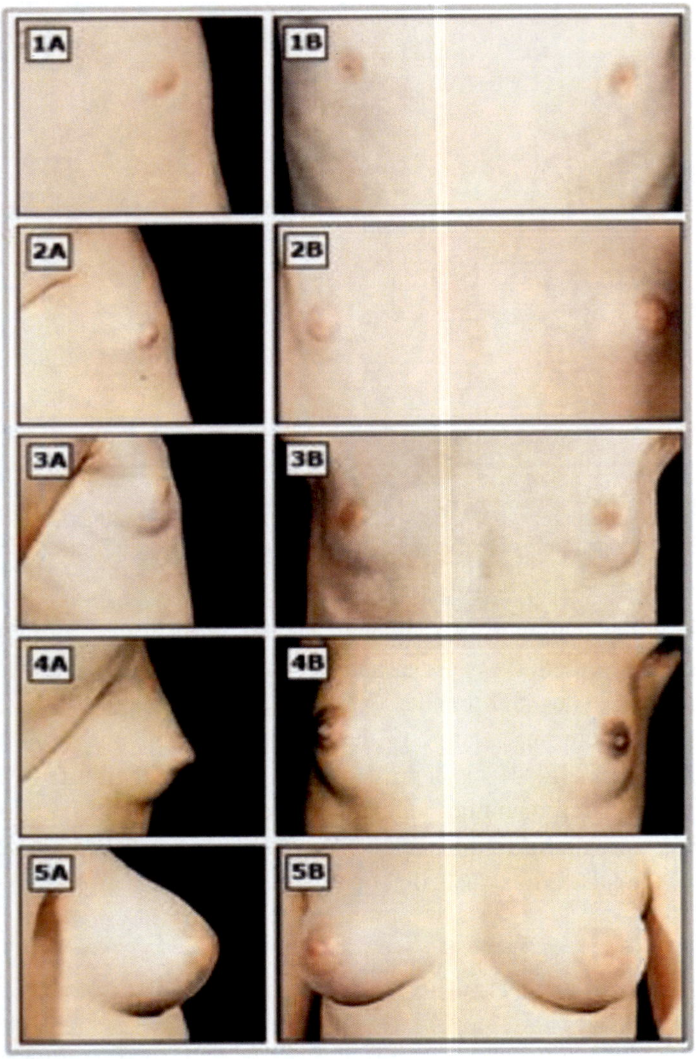

Figure 3. Tanner staging of female breast. 1A, 1B: Stage 1, Prepubertal with no palpable breast tissue. 2A, 2B: Stage 2, Development of breast bud: elevation of the papilla and enlargement of areolar diameter. 3A, 3B: Stage 3, Enlargement of the breast, without separation of areolar contour from breast. 4A, 4B: Stage 4, areola and papilla project above the breast (secondary mound). 5A, 5B: Stage 5, recession of the areola to match the contour of the breast; the papilla projects beyond the contour of the areola and breast. Reproduced with permission [7].

Adipose tissue increases breast size [6]; there is elongation of the initial ducts and branching into secondary ducts (Figure 4) in which bilayered epithelial buds appear and form clusters called lobules [1, 8].

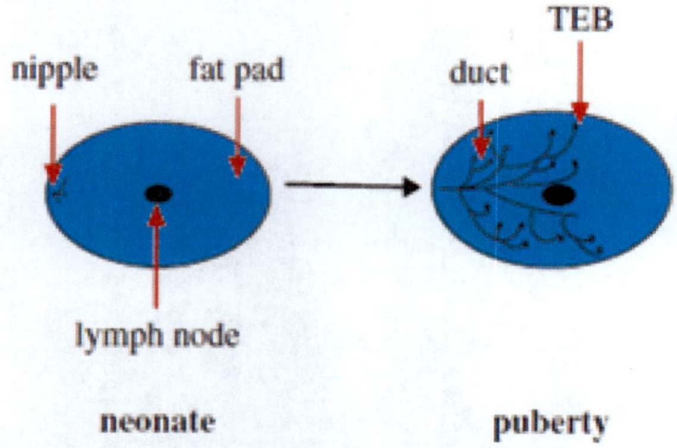

Figure 4. After birth, the mammary gland is a fat pad with a primitive epithelial network extending from the nipple. Terminal end buds (TEB) appear at puberty and drive expansion and invasion of the fat pad by the ductal network. Reproduced with permission [9].

The branched alveolar duct system presents histological differences from puberty to pregnancy, giving rise to the classification of breast lobules into the following four types:

- Lobule 1: This type is dominant in the nulliparous (beginning 1–2 years after menarche), characterized by high proliferation and poor differentiation (Figure 5A). It is made up of 11 alveolar buds that cluster around a terminal duct.
- Lobules 2 and 3 (Figures 5B and 5C). Estrogen and progesterone stimulate the type 1 lobule to sprout new alveolar buds. From 11 buds, this increases to 47 in the type 2 lobule and to 80 in the type 3 lobule.
- Lobule 4 (Figure 5D). These lobules appear during pregnancy (maximal breast development) through the combined action of Prelatic (PRL) and placental lactogen. There are poorly differentiated and highly proliferative epithelia, with large amounts of Terminal duct lobular units (TDLU).

The breast of a nulliparous woman contains more type 1 lobules (65–80%) than the parous breast, which contains more differentiated type 3 lobules (70–90%).

Pregnancy

During the pregnancy and lactancy cycle, the breast becomes a fully mature, functional organ and maximal branching capability is expressed. The secretory acinus formed during pregnancy represents a terminal outgrowth that marks the full extent of glandular differentiation [10-12].

The breasts reach their maximal development in two phases: in the early stage (first trimester of pregnancy), proliferation of mammary stem cells in the terminal end bud leads to branching, formation, and expansion of terminal buds (lobule type 4) [13], and in late pregnancy (second half), PRL levels increase and stimulate cellular differentiation (secretory differentiation), which occurs at around week 24 and which is often accompanied by colostrum.

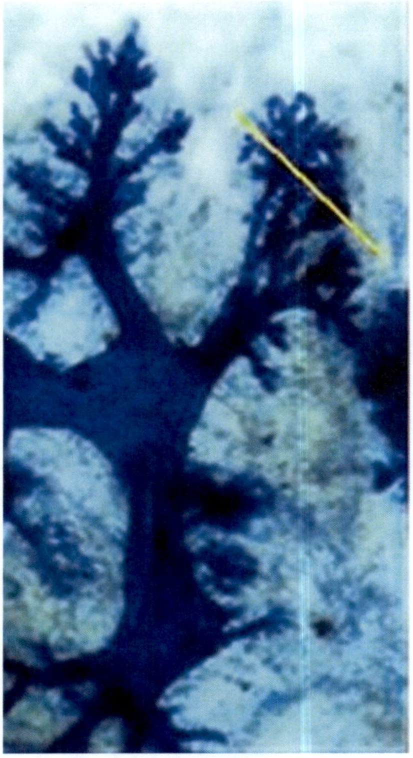

A. Lobule, type 1

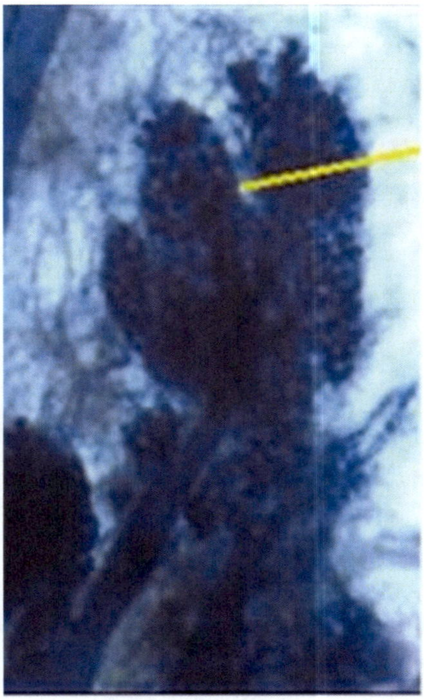

B. Lobule, type 2

Figure 5. (Continued).

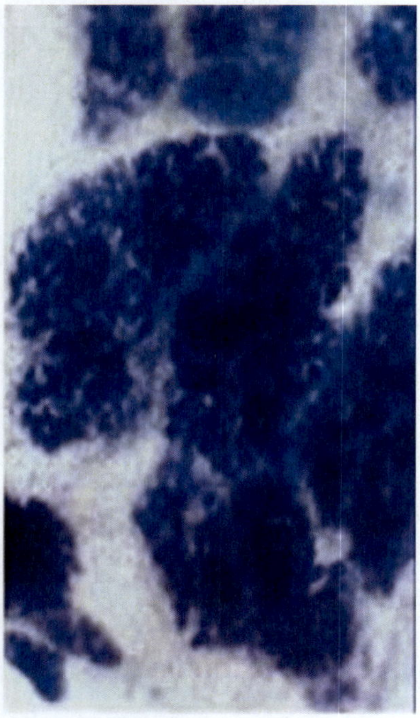

C. Lobule, type 3

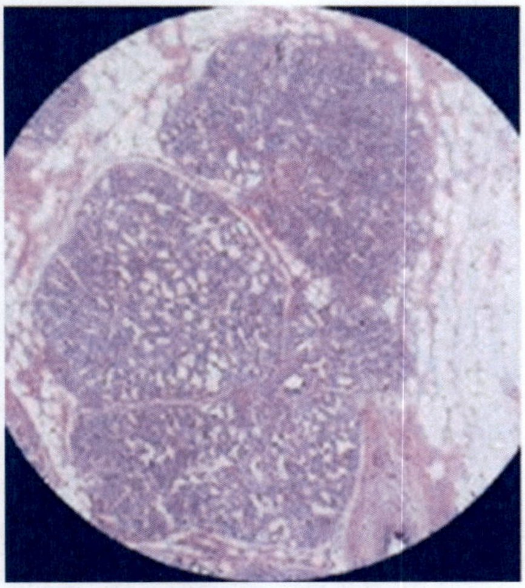

D. Lobule, type 4

Figure 5. Breast lobules. Reproduced with permission from: Russo J. Development of the human breast [1].

Postlactational Involution

Involution comprises two distinct phases. Phase I lasts up to 2 weeks, is characterized by programmed cell death and regression of both epithelial and stromal tissues, and is reversible (removal of milk can re-establish the milk supply). Phase II is irreversible and is characterized by luminal cell loss and extensive stromal remodeling [14]. Even at the conclusion of involution, the structure and morphology of the gland is not identical to that of the prepregnancy state [1] and considerably more Lobule (Lob) 2 and Lob 3 structures are present in the parous gland.

Postmenopausal Involution

Postmenopausal involution is triggered by declining ovarian function, thus declining circulatory levels of sex steroid hormones (estrogen, progesterone). This results in further regression and atrophy of the glandular tissue of the breast and in a concurrent increase in adipose tissue [15]. Reduction of glandular tissue can be up to approximately one third of its original volume and starts at the breast periphery [15]. Table 1 depicts the stages of the breast.

Table 1. Stages of mammary development

Stage	Hormonal regulation	Description
Fetal embryogenesis	Fibroblastic growth factor (FGF)?	Epithelial bud develops from week 6; blind ducts appear
Prepubertal	Estrogen growth hormone	Ductal extension into mammary fat pad; branching morphogenesis
Puberty	Estrogen, progesterone?, Prolactin (PRL)	Lobular development with formation of Terminal duct lobular unit (TDLU)
Pregnancy	Progesterone, PRL, human Placental lactogen (hPL)	Alveolus formation, partial cellular differentiation. Stage I, midpregnancy Stage II, parturition
Lactation	PRL, oxytocin	Ongoing milk secretion
Involution	PRL withdrawal	Alveolar epithelium undergoes apoptosis and remodeling; gland reverts to prepregnant state

Physiology of the Breast

Prior to puberty, there are no functional or structural differences between the male and female breast. With the onset of puberty, a striking sexual dimorphism becomes manifest as dramatic changes ensue in the morphology and function of the female breast. These changes are the result of hormonal influences [16], including estrogen, progesterone, PRL, placental lactogen, epidermal Growth factor (GF), and stromal paracrine factors, whereas insulin, growth hormone, glucocorticoids, and FGF are involved indirectly [10-12].

Throughout the menstrual cycle, healthy women are exposed to frequent changes in the hormonal milieu by monthly cycling levels of estradiol and progesterone. The follicular phase of the cycle is associated with a peak of circulating estradiol and is followed by the luteal phase, during which a prominent peak of serum progesterone and a second peak of serum estradiol occur. This luteal phase of the cycle is characterized by the increasing complexity and size of the breast lobules, which reflects proliferative activity within the epithelial compartment when mitosis is highest [17]. Typically, mammary miniremodeling at each menstrual cycle does not fully regress at the end of the cycle. Thus, compounding epithelial development continues gradually during adolescence through to adult life until approximately the age of 35 years [1, 8]. The effects of these hormones on the breast are discussed briefly.

Estrogen

In premenopause, serum estrogens are produced in the ovaries (mainly) and peripheral organs, such as aromatization of androgens (fat and muscle tissue), and it is noteworthy that there is a third source: the mammary gland. In fact, 17β-E2 concentrations present in breast cancer tissues did not differ between pre- and postmenopausal women, while 17β-E2 circulating levels are 90% lower in postmenopausal women [18].

The normal breast contains receptors for estrogen and progesterone. An Estrogen receptor (ER) belongs to the steroid receptor superfamily-thyroid, and there are two types: ERβ, and ERα. They are encoded by different genes; however, they have similar chains with certain structural polypeptide differences that confer individual characteristics on each. ERα is localized mainly in terminal duct lobular epithelial breast cells, while ERβ is localized in the fat and stromal myoepithelial cells. ERα govern mammary development, together with progesterone [19]. The two ER have distinct functions and act antagonistically in multiple pathways: ERα plays an important role in growth and proliferation [20], while ERβ exerts antiproliferative, differentiative, and apoptotic actions in the breast [21].

Progesterone

Mitotic activity in the breast occurs during the luteal phase, which is dominated by progesterone. Progesterone is the major hormonal stimulus for breast growth and differentiation. At menopause, when estrogen concentration is very low and progesterone is absent, mitotic activity is very low [22]. The effect of the administration of progestins on the breast is different and depends on whether it is given cyclically or continuously. Studies in mammalian cells *in vitro* showed that cyclic progestins increase DNA synthesis and cell cycle progression, while the cells are inhibited during continuous administration [23].

Lactation

Endocrine regulation of milk synthesis is complex. After initial conditioning of the mammary secretory tissue by estrogen and progesterone, a specific need arises for the lactogenic hormone, in addition to the permissive actions of glucocorticoids, insulin, and thyroxin for successful milk production [24].

There are two lactogenic hormones: I) Prolactin (PRL), which is secreted by the lactotrophs in the anterior pituitary gland, and II) human Placental lactogen (hPL), which is produced by the maternal placenta. Secretion of the latter reaches a peak during the final weeks of gestation and this prepares the breast for milk production. At this stage, there is no significant milk secretion because the high levels of estrogen and progesterone in maternal blood exert an inhibitory effect on milk production [25].

Another hormone that plays an important role in lactation is oxytocin, a polypeptide that is synthesized in the hypothalamus and stored in the posterior pituitary (neurohypophysis). Milk ejection occurs only during nursing. The sucking stimulation of the breast sends neural impulses to the hypothalamus. The hypothalamus stimulates oxytocin secretion by paraventricular nuclei cells and suppresses the release of the PRL-inhibiting hormone.

Oxytocin stimulates the myoepithelial cells of the breast's secretory alveoli, effecting milk passage through the lactiferous ducts. The act of sucking stimulates the release of oxytocin, which in turn mediates the secretion of PRL.

Anatomy of the Breast

Mature Nonlactating Breast

The breast is composed of glandular (secretory) and adipose tissue supported by a loose framework of fibrous connective tissue denominated Cooper's ligaments. The secretory tissue is drained by a ductal system that stores and transports milk to the nipple during lactation [26] (Figure 6).

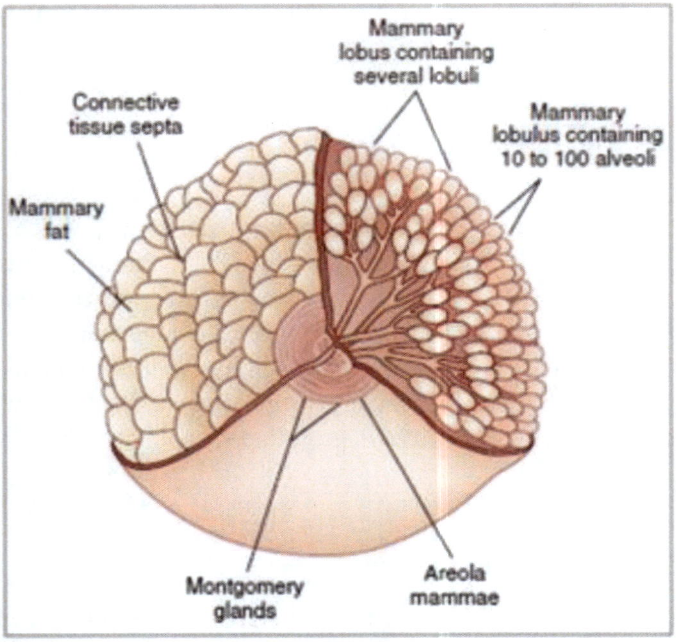

Figure 6. A diagram of a dissection reveals mammary fat and duct system. Modified and reproduced with permission [27].

Nipple and Areola

The nipple is a conical elevation in the areola at the fourth intercostal space. The nipple contains smooth muscle fibers and is richly innervated with sensory and pain fibers. It has a verrucous surface and has sebaceous and apocrine sweat glands, but not hair. The areola is slightly pigmented. The average diameter is 15–16 mm, but this may even exceed 5 cm during pregnancy.

The Corpus Mammae

This is an orderly conglomeration of a number of independent glands known as lobes (lobes are made up of lobules containing 10–100 alveoli that are approximately 0.12 mm in diameter [24]. Each lobe is considered a single entity [28]. The corpus mammae also includes the stroma, which is composed of connective tissue, fat tissue, blood vessels, nerves, and the lymphatic system. The mammary fat pad is essential for the proliferation and differentiation of ductal arborizations (branching) (Figure 6).

Breast Ductal System

This is composed of numerous, small ductules that drain the alveoli to culminate in one main duct that dilates slightly to form a lactiferous sinus (2–4.5 mm) [29]. Generally, dilated ducts in the nonlactating breast identified by Ultrasound (US) imaging are associated with pathologies such as ductal ectasia, fibrocystic disease, intraductal adenoma, or malignancy [30].

Lactating Breast

There are some differences. Nipple size typically increases during pregnancy and is related with plasma PRL levels. [31] Documented nipple diameters range from 9–23 mm. The breast ductal system has 15–20 ducts. Enlargement of the ducts does not necessarily occur. Variation in duct diameter among women is likely due to the amount of milk contained or synthesized at any time within the breast [32]. The volume of glandular tissue in the breast has not been quantified. Semiquantitative measurement of both glandular and adipose tissue in US images reported that the ratio of glandular to adipose tissue is approximately 2:1 [33].

Blood Supply

The breast's main blood supply is derived from the internal mammary artery (anterior and posterior medial branches) in 60% (Figure 7). Approximately one third of the blood supply (mainly to the upper outer quadrant) is provided by the lateral thoracic arteries (lateral mammary branch) [34]. Minor sources of arterial blood also include the posterior intercostal arteries and the pectoral branch of the thoracoacromial artery.

The rapid growth phase in pregnancy is reflected by a doubling in Mammary blood flow (MBF) at 24 weeks of gestation, after which it remains constant during lactation [35]. The ratio of blood flow-to-milk yield is approximately 500:1.

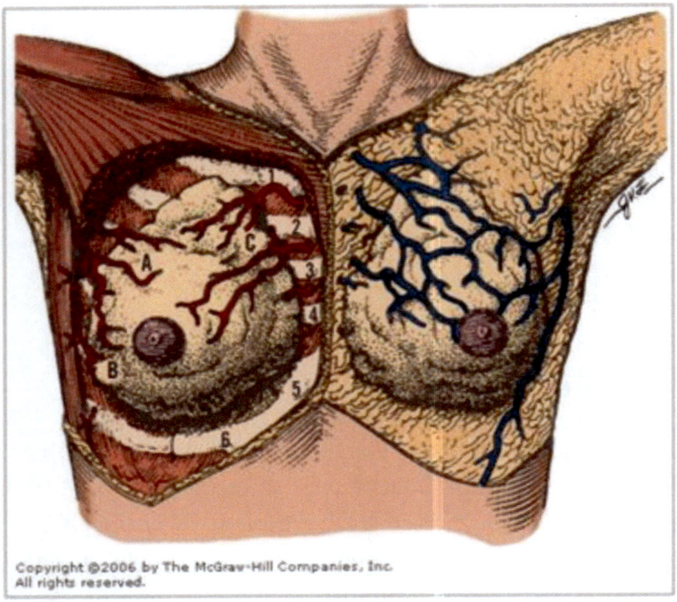

Figure 7. The arterial supply is derived from (A) mammary branches of the axillary artery; (B) branches of the lateral thoracic artery, and (C) perforating branches of the internal thoracic artery. Venous drainage is illustrated on the right side of the drawing. Modified and reproduced with permission [36].

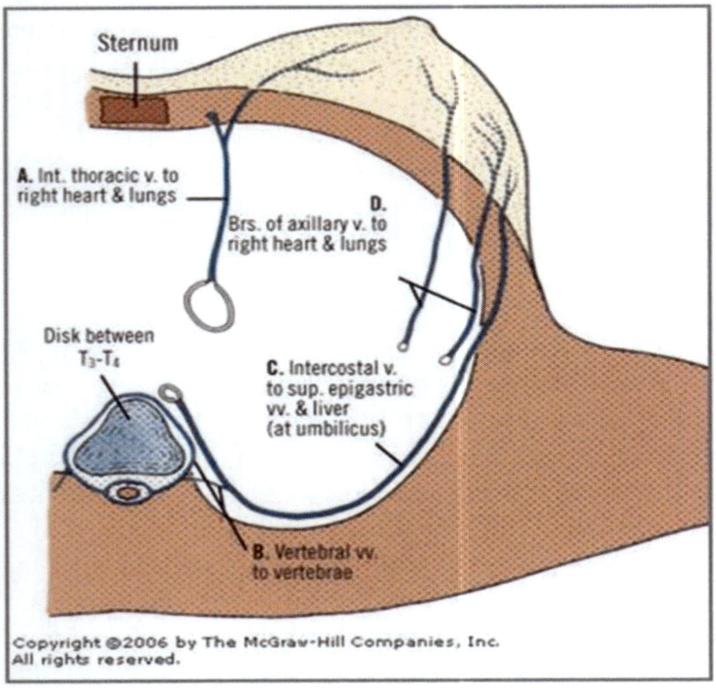

Figure 8. Pathways of venous drainage. A. Medial drainage through internal thoracic vein to the right heart. B. Posterior drainage to vertebral veins. C. Lateral drainage to intercostal, superior epigastric veins, and liver, and D. Lateral superior drainage through axillary vein to the right heart. Modified and reproduced with permission [36].

Venous Drainage

There are different drainage pathways, including the following: 1) perforating tributaries from the medial half of the breast enter the internal thoracic vein, which joins the brachiocephalic vein; 2) the axillary vein receives one or two pectoral branches from the breast; 3) intercostal veins communicate posteriorly with the vertebral venous system and anteriorly, with the brachiocephalic vein. Metastases of the breast readily reach the lungs by means of the first two pathways. Metastases can travel to the skeleton and the Central nervous system (CNS) by means of the third pathway (Figure 8).

Lymphatic Drainage

Lymphatic drainage of the breast is through both superficial (subepithelial and subdermal) and deep lymphatic vessels, and the lymph flows unidirectionally from the superficial to the deep plexus. The axillary nodes receive >75% of the lymph from both the medial and lateral portions of the breast [37]. The internal mammary nodes receive lymph mainly from the deep portion of the breast [38].

Breast lymphatics drain through three major routes: axillary; transpectoral, and internal mammary. The regional lymph nodes are presented here as follows (Figure 9):

1. Axillary (ipsilateral): nodes are divided into the following levels:

Level I (low axilla): lymph nodes lateral to the lateral border of the pectoralis minor muscle.

Level II (midaxilla): lymph nodes between the medial and lateral borders of the pectoralis minor muscle and the interpectoral (Rotter's) lymph nodes

Level III (apical axillary): lymph nodes medial to the medial margin of the pectoralis minor muscle.

2. Internal mammary (ipsilateral): lymph nodes in the intercostal spaces along the edge of the sternum in the endothoracic fascia.

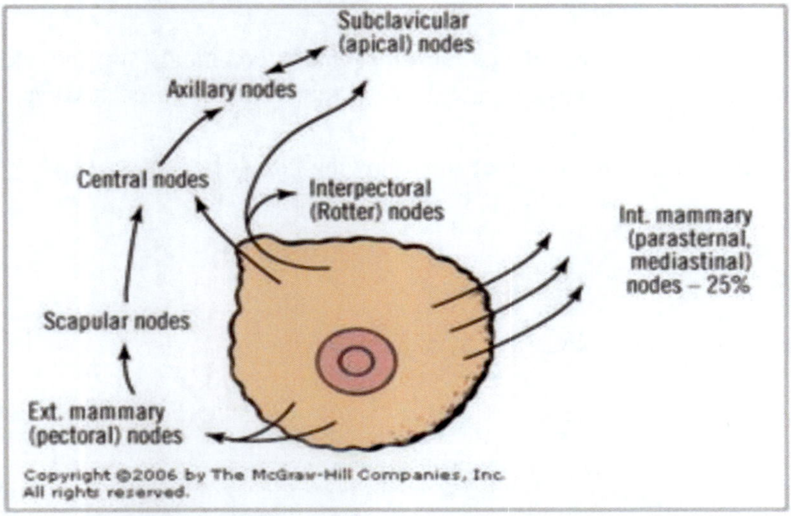

Figure 9. Diagram of lymphatic drainage of the breast. Modified and reproduced with permission [36].

Innervation

The second to sixth intercostal nerves innervate the breast and are localized superficially in the gland [26]. The nipple and glandular tissue are supplied by the deep branches, and the nipple and areola, by superficial branches, with complex and variable distribution. Detailed descriptions of the course of the branches are conflicting. These nerves are sensory in nature and, together with the lack of motor innervation of both the lactocytes or myoepithelial cells, suggest that both the synthesis and secretion of milk is independent of neural stimulation. In fact, the ejection reflex was demonstrated clinically to be caused by the release of oxytocin by the pituitary [39].

Abnormalities in Breast Development

Congenital

The multiple but rare congenital anomalies of the breast may be associated with various other syndromes.

Polythelia

This is an accessory or supernumerary nipple, ectopic nipple tissue may occur at any point along the milk streak from the axilla to the groin.

Supernumerary nipples have been associated with an increased risk of genitourinary abnormalities, malignancies, segmentation defect of the vertebrae, Becker's nevus, and other developmental abnormalities [40-44].

Polymastia

True accessory mammary glands develop, most commonly in the axilla. During pregnancy and lactation, an accessory breast may swell, and if an associated nipple is present, it may secrete milk.

Rare anomalies of the breast include the following [45, 46].

Hypoplasia

Underdevelopment of the breast.

Amastia

Congenital absence of the breast.

Amazia

Absence of breast tissue but a normal nipple-areola complex is present.

Unilateral hypoplasia may be accompanied by a normal, hypoplastic, or hyperplastic contralateral breast. Amazia usually presents as a component of a developmental syndrome and can be diagnosed during infancy or at the beginning of puberty [45].

The most severe of these deformities, amastia or severe unilateral hypoplasia, is associated with hypoplasia of the pectoral muscle in 90% of cases. However, the reverse does not apply; in women with pectoral muscle abnormalities, 92% have a normal breast [47].

Poland Syndrome

This syndrome includes abnormalities ranging from unilateral hypoplasia to the absence of the breast and pectoral muscle, and these frequently occur in combination with distal hypoplasia of the upper limb and anomalies of the hand (syndactyly, brachydactyly, oligodactyly) [48-50]. These anomalies may result from diminished blood flow in the subclavian artery during early fetal development.

Anomalies of Breast Size

In megalomastia, the breast is extremely enlarged. According to Anastassiades and colleagues [51], unilateral megalomastia is extremely rare. However, Netscher reported massive asymmetric virginal breast hypertrophy in a 13-year-old girl. In micromastia, the breast is very small, failing to develop beyond its prepubertal state [52].

Gynecomastia

Gynecomastia refers to enlargement of the male breast. Guvenc reported on the incidence of pubertal gynecomastia in 646 Turkish boys in Ankara [53]. Highest incidence was at age 14 years (61.1%). The incidence of gynecomastia at various pubertal stages and ages was 34.6%. The incidence of unilateral gynecomastia was 19.6%. A study of healthy young men aged 18–26 years found an incidence of 40.5% [54]. In a study of 115 men attending a dermatologic clinic, Seibel found an incidence of 27.8% with a skinfold exceeding 2–3 cm and an areolar diameter of >3 cm. [55].

References

[1] Russo J and Russo IH. Development of the human breast. *Maturitas,* 2004;49(1):2-15.

[2] Watson CJ, Oliver CH, Khaled WT. Cytokine signalling inmammary gland development. *J Reprod Immunol.* 2011;88(2):124-9.

[3] Veltmaat JM, Mailleux AA, Thiery JP, et al. Mouse embryonic mammogenesis as a model for the molecular regulation of pattern formation. *Differentiation*. 2003;71(1):1-17.

[4] Carlson B. Editor. Human Embryology and Developmental Biology. 2nd ed. St. Louis, MO, USA: *Mosby;* 1999.

[5] Tobon H and Salazar H. Ultrastructure of the human mammary gland. I. Development of the fetal gland throughout gestation. *J Clin Endocrinol Metab.* 1974;39(3):443-56.

[6] Russo J and Roi L. Influence of age and gland topography on cell kinetics of normal human breast tissue. *J Natl Cancer Inst* 1987,78(3):413-8.

[7] Roede MJ and van Wiering JC, Editors. Growth Diagrams 1980: Netherlands Third Nation-wide Survey. Vol. 63:1. 1995, *Tijdschr Soc Gezondheids.* 1995;63(1).

[8] Russo J, Tay LK, Russo IH. Differentiation of the mammary gland and susceptibility to carcinogenesis. *Breast Cancer Res Treatment.* 1982;2(1):5-73.

[9] McNally S and Martin F. Molecular regulators of pubertal mammary gland development. *Ann Med.* 2011;43(3):212-34.

[10] Pang WW and Hartmann PE. Initiation of human lactation: secretory differentiation and secretory activation. *J Mammary Gland Biol.* 2007;12(4):211-21.

[11] Medina D. The mammary gland: a unique organ for the study of development and tumorigenesis. *J Mammary Gland Biol.* 1996;1(1):5-19.

[12] Czank C and Kent J. Hormonal control of the lactation cycle. Textbook of Human Lactation. Amarillo, TX, USA; *Hale Publishing;* 2007.

[13] Sternlicht MD. Key stages in mammary gland development: the cues that regulate ductal branching morphogenesis. *BCR Breast Cancer Res,* 2006;8(1):201.

[14] Monks J and Henson PM. Differentiation of the mammary epithelial cell during involution: implications for breast cancer. *J Mammary Gland Biol.* 2009.;14(2):159-70.

[15] Williams P, Editor. Gray's Anatomy. 38 ed. New York: *Churchill-Livingstone*, Inc.: 1996.

[16] Ellis H, Mahadevan V. Anatomy and physiology of the breast. *Surgery* (Oxford). 2013;31(1):11-14.

[17] Hilton HN, Santucci N, Silvestri A. Progesterone stimulates progenitor cells in normal human breast and breast cancer cells. *Breast Cancer Res Treat.* 2014;143(3):423-33.

[18] van Landeghem AA, Poortman J, Nabuurs M, et al. Endogenous concentration and subcellular distribution of estrogens in normal and malignant human breast tissue. *Cancer Res.* 1985;45(6):2900-6.

[19] Mueller SO, Clark JA, Myers PH, et al. Mammary gland development in adult mice requires epithelial and stromal estrogen receptor alpha. *Endocrinology.* 2002;143(6):2357-65.

[20] Ewan KB, Oketch-Rabah HA, Ravani SA, et al. Proliferation of estrogen receptor-alpha-positive mammary epithelial cells is restrained by transforming growth factor-beta1 in adult mice. *Am J Pathol.* 2005;167(2):409-17.

[21] Lazennec G, Bresson D, Lucas A, et al. ER beta inhibits proliferation and invasion of breast cancer cells. *Endocrinology.* 2001;142(9):4120-30.

[22] Potten CS, Watson RJ, Williams GT. The effect of age and menstrual cycle upon proliferative activity of the normal human breast. *BJC Br J Cancer.* 1988;58(2):163-70.

[23] Vering A, Vockel A, Stegmuller M. Immuno-biochemical assay for determination of nuclear steroid receptors during tamoxifen therapy. *J Cancer Res Clinical Oncol.* 1993;119(7): 415-20.

[24] Hartmann PE. The breast and breast-feeding. Scientific Foundations of Obstetrics and Gynaecology. 4th ed. Philipp EE, Setchell M, Ginsburg J, Editors. Oxford, U.K. 1991; pp. 378-90.

[25] Delgado BH. Hormones en la mama; de la fisiología a la enfermedad. *Rev Venez Endocrinol Metab* 2008;6(2):9-14.

[26] Hassiotou F and Geddes D. Anatomy of the human mammary gland: current status of knowledge. *Clin Anat.* 2013;26(1):29-48.

[27] Lawrence RA, Editor. Breastfeeding: A Guide for the Medical Profession. 7th ed. St. Louis, MO, USA: *Saunders;*2010. Vol. 28.

[28] Going JJ and Moffat DF. Escaping from Flatland: clinical and biological aspects of human mammary duct anatomy in three dimensions. *J Pathol.* 2004;203(1): p. 538-44.

[29] Venta LA, Dudiak CM, Salomon CG, et al. Sonographic evaluation of the breast. *RadioGraphics.* 1994;14(1):29-50.

[30] Stavros AT and Parker SH, Editors. Breast Ultrasound. Philadelphia, PA, USA: *Lippincott Williams & Wilkins;* 2004.

[31] Cox DB, Kent JC, Casey TM, et al. Breast growth and the urinary excretion of lactose during human pregnancy and early lactation: endocrine relationships. *Exp Physiol.* 1999,84(2):421-34.

[32] Ramsay DT, Mitoulas LR, Kent JC, et al. Milk flow rates can be used to identify and investigate milk ejection in women expressing breast milk using an electric breast pump. *Breastfeed Med.* 2006;1(1):14-23.

[33] Ramsay DT, Kent JC, Hartmann RA, et al. Anatomy of the lactating human breast redefined with ultrasound imaging. *J Anat.* 2005;206(6):525-34.

[34] Doughty JC, McCarter DH, Kane E, et al. Anatomical basis of intra-arterial chemotherapy for patients with locally advanced breast cancer. *Br J Surg.* 1996;83(8):1128-30.

[35] Geddes DT, Aljazaf KM, Kent JC, et al. Blood flow characteristics of the human lactating breast. *J Hum Lactation.* 2012;28(2):145-52.

[36] Skandalakis JE, Editor. Skandalakis' Surgical Anatomy. 2006. *McGraw-Hill.*

[37] Borgstein PJ, Meijer S, Pijpers RJ, et al. Functional lymphatic anatomy for sentinel node biopsy in breast cancer: echoes from the past and the periareolar blue method. *Ann Surg*. 2000;232(1):81-9.

[38] Aukland K and Reed RK. Interstitial-lymphatic mechanisms in the control of extracellular fluid volume. *Physiolog Rev*. 1993;73(1):1-78.

[39] Newton N and Newton M. Psychologic aspects of lactation. *NEJM.* 1967;277(22):1179-88.

[40] Lewis EJ, Crutchfield CE, Ebertz MJ, et al. Report of a nipple nevus and an overview of accessory mammary tissue. *Cutis.* 1998;62(5):243-6.

[41] Grimshaw EC and Cohen PR. Supernumerary nipple and seminoma: case report and review of polythelia and genitourinary cancers. *Dermatol Online j.* 2013;19(1):4.

[42] Ferrara P, Giorgio V, Vitelli, O, et al. Polythelia: still a marker of urinary tract anomalies in children? *Scand J Urol Nephrol.* 2009;43(1):47-50.

[43] Sadove AM and van Aalst JA. Congenital and acquired pediatric breast anomalies: a review of 20 years' experience. *Plast Reconstr Surg.* 2005;115(4):1039-50.
[44] Bygum A, Petkov Y, Graakjaer J, et al. Phylloid hypermelanosis in a child with psychomotor delay, cicatricial alopecia, hearing loss and polythelia. *Acta Derm-Venereol.* 2012;92(2): 191-2.
[45] Nso-Roca AP, Aguirre-Balsalobre FJ, Juste Ruiz M Isolated unilateral amazia: an exceptional breast anomaly. *J Pediatr Adoles Gynecol.* 2012;25(6): e147-e148.
[46] Chan W, Mathur B, Slade-Sharman D, et al. Developmental breast asymmetry. *Breast J.* 2011;17(4): 391-8.
[47] Trier WC. Complete breast absence. Case report and review of the literature. *Plast Reconstr Surg*. 1965;36(4):431-9.
[48] Ravitch MM. Poland's syndrome- a study of an eponym. *Plast Reconstr Surg.* 1977;59(4):508-12.
[49] Beals RK and Crawford S. Congenital absence of the pectoral muscles. A review of twenty-five patients. *Clin Orthop Rel Res.* 1976;119:166-71.
[50] Jones KL del Campo M, Editors. Smith's Recognizable Patterns of Human Malformation. 7th ed. Philadelphia, PA, USA: *Saunders;* 2013.
[51] Anastassiades OT, Choreftaki T, Ioannovich J, et al. Megalomastia: histological, histochemical and immunohistochemical study. *Virchows Arch A Pathol Anat Histopathol.* 1992;420(4):337-44.
[52] Netscher DT, Mosharrafa AM, Laucirica R. Massive asymmetric virginal breast hypertrophy. *South Med J.* 1996;89(4): 434-7.
[53] Guvenc H, Yurdakok M, Kinik E, et al. The incidence of pubertal gynecomastia in boys living in the Ankara region. *Turk J Pediatr.* 1989;31(2):123-6.
[54] Georgiadis E, Papandreou L, Evangelopoulou C, et al. Incidence of gynaecomastia in 954 young males and its relationship to somatometric parameters. *Ann Hum Biol.* 1994;21(6):579-87.
[55] Seibel V, Muller HH, and Krause W. [Incidence of gynecomastia in dermatology patients]. *Der Hautarzt.* 1998;49(5):382-7.

In: Benign Disease of the Breast
Editors: J. de la Garza Salazar, C. Arce Salinas et al.
ISBN: 978-1-63321-624-2

Chapter 4

Physical Exploration of the Breast

Carlos Robles-Vidal**, *Miguel Lazaro-Leon, Robin Shaw-Dulin and Osvaldo Armando Quiroz-Sandoval

Surgical Oncology Department,
Instituto Nacional Cancerologia-Mexico,
Mexico City, DF, Mexico

Abstract

Breast examination is an important component of both primary and specialized care. Early diagnosis is essential in the management of breast cancer. Clinical breast examination is an integral component of breast screening when performed by trained health professionals and is particularly important in countries where resources for mammograms are insufficient and where breast cancer usually presents at an advanced stage at the time of diagnosis.

Introduction

Breast complaints are one of the most frequent causes for medical consultation, with breast pain and identification of breast lumps accounting for up to 80% of appointments. One in four women will present for a medical appointment for this reason at some time in their life[1].

In addition, poor or incomplete evaluation of breast conditions is the most frequent cause for lawsuits in the U.S.

A first-contact physician should be able to determine if they are capable of resolving the situation or if the problem requires additional specialized management.

* Corresponding author.

Clinical breast exploration (CBE) is used with greater frequency for detection of breast cancer than for diagnosis. Of a total of 14,859 CBE performed in a cohort of 2,400 women during a 10-year period, 73% were for detection and 26% were for diagnosis [2].

There are medical, ethical, and legal reasons why CBE should be performed and integral part of patient care [3]. Physicians who do not carry out a careful exploration can become the object of lawsuits.

Anatomy of the Mammary Gland

The feminine mammary gland is made up of glandular, fibrous, and fatty tissue. The normal human breast is composed of 12-20 sections called lobes, which in turn are made up of smaller functional milk-producing units called lobules. Both lobes and lobules are connected by ducts and irradiate from the nipple. The mammary tissue is surrounded by superficial fascia, which is joined to the skin and to the pectoral fascia by means of support ligaments. The fat surrounding the breast lobes is found predominantly in superficial and peripheral portions [4]. Breast tissue extends medially from the sternum toward the mid-axillary line and above the clavicle toward the inter-mammary cleft. The normal breast does not have a homogeneous texture, but is usually nodular on palpation. In Figure 1, a basic anatomical model is presented, designed by the National Cancer Institute (NCI) of the U.S. National Health Institutes of Health (NIH) [4, 5].

Duration of the CBE correlated significantly with accuracy of the detection of nodules in experiments with silicon models. In five studies, the average duration of the exploration was always greater for examiners with greater sensitivity [6–11]. The highest sensitivity described in studies with humans (69%) was obtained in the National Breast Screening Study (NBSS), in which the examiner took between 5 and 10 minutes to carry out a complete exploration in both breasts [12, 13].

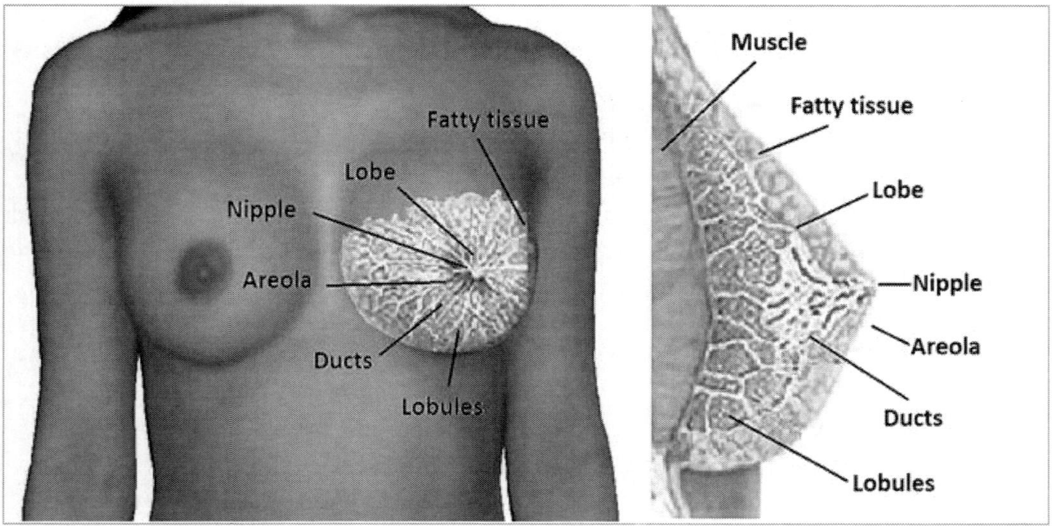

Figure 1. Basic anatomical model of a normal breast.

Experience of the Explorer

Experience in abnormal breast nodules can be important. Even when controlling for differences in technique, medical residents found more nodules in silicone models than women who had received special training [14, 15].

Among medical residents, previous experience predicted greater sensitivity. After practicing on silicon models, the skill of the women improved and surpassed that of the physicians. Two studies found no difference between the two categories [16, 17]. It is evident that devoting adequate time to the CBE and using the appropriate techniques improve the detection of breast nodules [18–21].

Technique

Correct use of the CBE technique (a systematic search for patterns, attention to detail, variation of palpation pressure, use of three fingers, fingertips, and circular motion) also correlated with greatest sensitivity in exploration of silicon models [22–25].

Patient Factors

On average, younger women have denser breast tissue, which renders the detection of masses more difficult, while in older women, breast tissue has a larger amount of fat, making detection of tumors easier [20]. In one study, the sensibility of the examiner was 86% among women aged 20–49 years and 96% among women aged 50 years and over.

Two studies with a large amount of participants arrived at a different conclusion, even among women in narrowly defined age ranges. The Breast Cancer Detection and Demonstration Project (BCDDP) found that complete CBE has a sensitivity of 53% among women aged between 40 and 49 years and one of 48% among those aged between 50 and 59 years [26].

NBSS79 reported that the CBE has greater sensitivity in women aged 40–49 years (68%) in comparison with those aged 50–59 years (63%), among women who had mammography and complete CBE. More assays are required with respect to this theme.

Characteristics of the Breast

CBE sensitivity is slightly inferior in women with large breasts [20]. Breast tissue also varies with respect to the amount of glandular nodularity, which is a normal characteristic of the mammary gland. Many women experience poorly defined areas of fibrocystic changes (FCC) which make their breasts feel irregular in consistency; physicians and women themselves find it difficult to detect breast cancer in markedly nodular breast tissue.

Characteristics of Cancer

Breast cancer varies in size, consistency, mobility, and location in the breast. CBE sensitivity probably varies according to these characteristics.

Prognosis generally depends on the size of the cancer at diagnosis; thus, it is important to determine the accuracy of the CBE for small tumors, that is, those of 2 cm or less.

In the BCDDP, sensitivity for non infiltrating cancer was 35%, for infiltrating cancers <1 cm, 36%, and for infiltrating cancers ≥1 cm, 52% [22, 27].

To date, the majority of information on CBE accuracy regarding breast characteristics derives from experiments conducted in silicone breast models with imbedded nodules that vary in size, consistency, and location. In these studies, sensitivity was calculated for detection with respect to tumor characteristics such as size and the consistency. An increase was reported in the sensitivity of in regards to average size (14% for 3-mm nodules and 79% for 1-cm nodules) and hardness (42% for tumors of 20-durometer tumors and 72% for 60-durometer tumors [20].

Durometers are a unit of measurement for the resistance of a material to localized deformation under pressure, and therefore usefull in determinging the hardness of nodules: 20 durometers correspond to soft-to-medium, and 60 durometers is nearly as hard as calcified bone. Medium or deep location of the mass in the model does not, apparently, alter the sensitivity [12, 27–29].

In sum, the woman's age and breast size can affect the examiners' capacity for detecting cancer. Similarly, the size and hardness of the malignant nodule affect sensitivity during the performance of CBE.

From the propedeutic, methodological viewpoint, the physical exploration should begin with the inspection; however, given the greater relevance of the palpation phase, the approach of the technique will begin with that exploratory section. Many books on diagnosis provide instructions for the performance of the breast examination. All of these implicate inspection and palpation, but investigation has placed an emphasis on palpation. The focus described next derives from a review of the research literature and is greatly indebted to Baines et al., due to their objective of standardizing the breast examination [12, 13, 24, 25, 27–29].

This recommendation incorporates the practices of the MammaCare [29] method because its components have proven valid in independent investigations of the CBE technique.

Palpation

Important variables in correct breast palpation include the patient's position, the limits of the breast, the pattern of the examination, the movement and pressure of the fingers, and the duration of the examination.

Position of the Patient

CBE requires flattening of the breast against the thoracic wall of the patient; in addition, the patient should be in supine position during the examination. The importance of the maneuvers for flattening the breast depends on breast size, and these are particularly useful in women with large breasts. To flatten the lateral part of the breast, the examiner should rotate the patient onto her contralateral hip, turn her shoulders in the decubitus supine position, and place her ipsilateral hand on her forehead or resting on top of her head (Figure 2). To flatten the middle part of the breast, the woman should lie down on her back and move her elbow upward until it remains at shoulder level [12, 13, 20].

Limits of the Breast

Breast tissue extends laterally toward the axilla and above toward the clavicle. To ensure that all of the breast tissue is examined, it is better to cover rectangular areas bordered above by the clavicle, medially by the sternum, laterally by the mean axillary line, and below, by the support line.

Inspection

The importance of the inspection has been demonstrated. More commonly, guidelines for the inspection suggest that the women should be in front of a mirror with her arms by her sides. The breasts are inspected to detect nipple abnormalities, collapses, retractions, or immobilization of the skin.

There is a lack of sufficient evidence to support examination of women in other positions, such as with their hands over their head, or placing their hands on their hips while leaning downward (to contract the pectoral muscles), or leaning forward to allow the breasts to hang over the thoracic wall [12, 13, 20].

In a series of 296 patients, breast cancer was found by CBE; 96% of these breast cancers were discovered by palpation, 1% with retraction, and 3% by visible abnormalities in the nipple.

It is suggested that physicians treating asymptomatic women should concentrate on breast palpation, carrying out visual inspection simultaneously. If the patient is found to be symptomatic or if an anomaly is discovered during the palpation of asymptomatic patients, the performance of a careful inspection should be added [30, 31].

Pattern of Exploration

Palpation initiates at the axilla and extends toward the axilla in a straight line of the mid axillary line to the inframammary fold (Figure 2). Next, the fingers are moved toward the inside and palpation continues in a straight line up to the clavicle. The entire breast is covered in this manner, from up to down between the clavicle and the inframammary fold. To examine all of the breast tissue, vertical palpation should be superimposed. It was found that vertical palpation is more complete than the circular or radial examination pattern [20, 26, 28, 29].

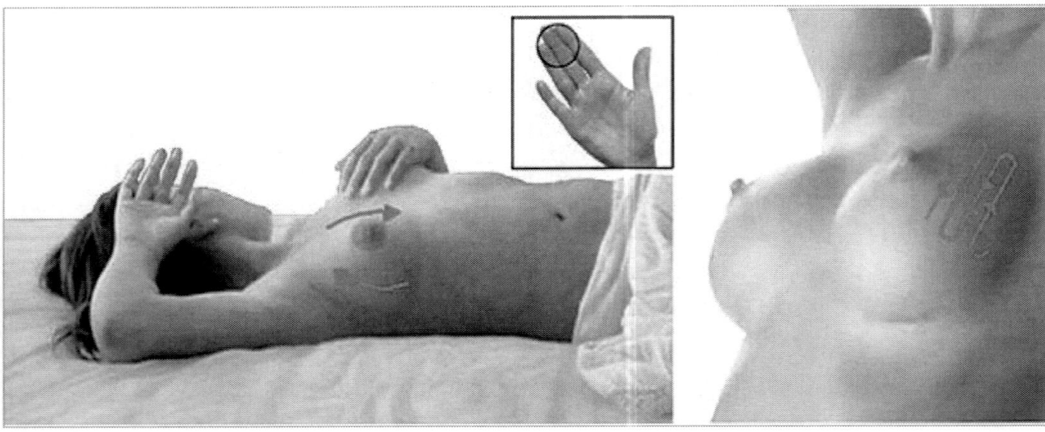

Figure 2. Position of the patient and direction of the exploration.

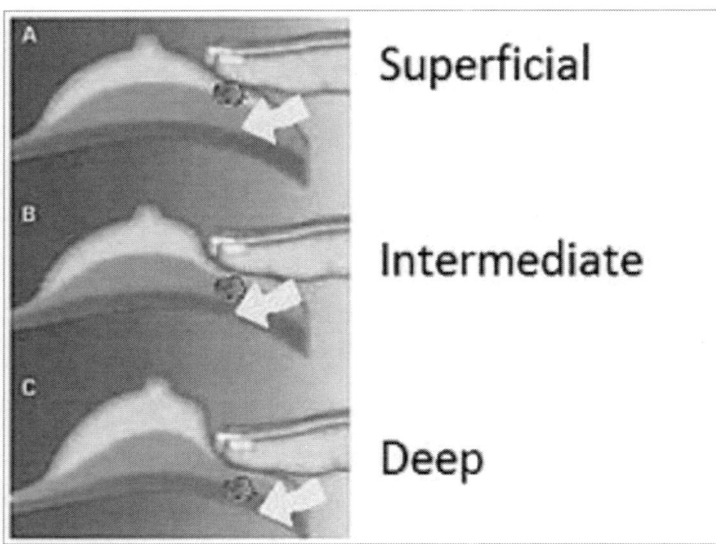

Figure 3. Palpatory technique, degrees of digital pressure (*adapted from Barton* [30].

The majority of texts scarcely describe what the fingers should do during palpation, an ironic situation because the fingers should detect and differentiate abnormal tumors in the breasts. Behavioral psychologists have demonstrated that the finger can detect a soft nodule (of 20 dm) in the breast tissue when the specific techniques are used. Investigators have developed a palpation technique (the MammaCare method) that combines the vertical band-like pattern and specific techniques for the fingers, for improving detection. Their method is explained next [20, 24, 25, 27–29].

The middle three fingers are kept together, with the metacarpo-phalangeal joint slightly flexed. The fleshy parts of the fingers comprise the examining surface (confusion about the definition of the fingertip arises, even among experienced examiners). Each area is palpated, making small circles as if following the edge of a coin. At each site, three circles are traced with different pressures (slight, medium, and deep) to ensure palpation at all levels of the tissue [20, 29] (Figure 3).

Duration

Careful examination of a medium-sized breast (size B) takes at least 3 minutes (6 minutes for both breasts). This is much more than the average 1.8 minutes that physicians utilize, reported in a study based on both breasts and giving instructions for self-examination. Physicians should inform patients of the time necessary for performing a complete self-examination and communicate the procedure to the patient during an examination [20, 30–33].

Regional Lymph Nodes

Palpation of the axillary and infraclaviculra and supraclavicular regions to detect adenopathies is a standard part of the CBE (Figure 4).

Breast cancer was found in a minority of women with axillary adenopathies and a normal breast exploration in two series (12 and 29%, respectively) [20].

Palpation of the zone of the nipple is carried out in the same way as in the remainder of the breast, although some texts suggested squeezing the nipple to assess whether there is a discharge (Figure 5).

Among 448 women who referred nipple secretion, the emergence of fluid was not employed as a prognostic sign of breast cancer. In women with a normal clinical examination result, only three (2%) of the 151 women with spontaneous nipple secretion were later diagnosed with cancer, while none of the women with only secretion were diagnosed with cancer [20].

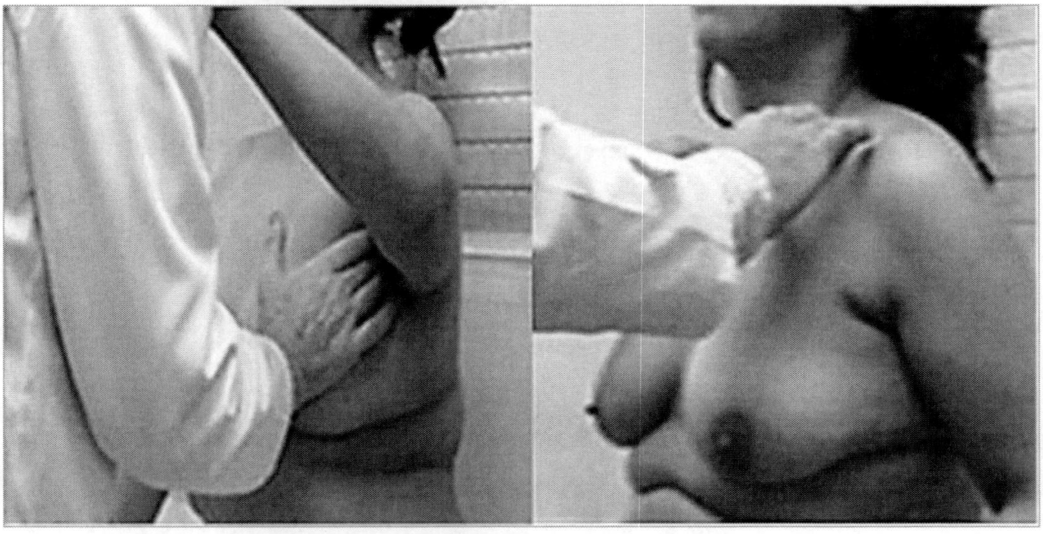

Figure 4. Palpation of the axillary and supraclavicular regions.

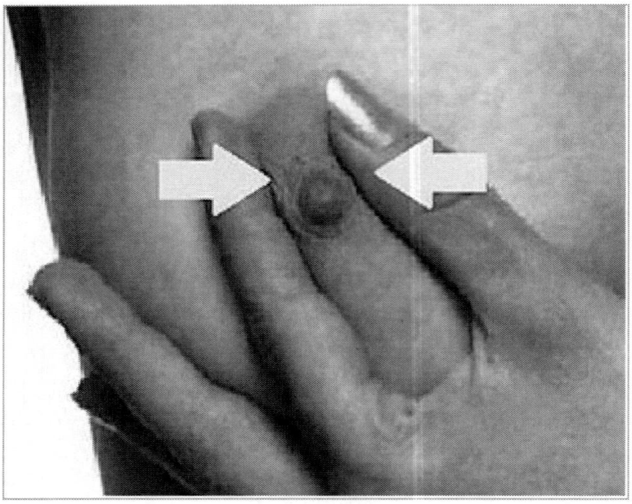

Figure 5. Palpation of the areola-nipple complex.

Final Recommendation (Mammacare Clinical Breast Examination Method) [28]

Fingers

- Use the three middle fingers
- Use the distal fleshy parts (not the whole finger)

Pattern of examination

- Vertical grid (rather than circular)
- Rotate the three fingers in circular fashion, such as when fingering a coin

Pressure

- Use three levels of pressure: superficial, moderate, and deep

Position

- Seated

Observe for asymmetries and depressions in four positions

- Hands by sides
- Hands on hips
- Hands above the head
- Leaning forward

Palpate the axillary lymph nodes

- Hold the patient's arm
- Patient lying down face up
- Palpate the breast in its totality, with the patient's arm above her head
- Oblique
- Palpate the outer upper quadrant (OUQ) of the breast with the patient's arm on her forehead
  - Examination time: 5 minutes
  - Expected sensitivity: 3–5 mm
  - Remember: 15% of breast cancers that can be palpated cannot be visualized with mastography [30, 31].

Teaching the Technique

What is the evidence that use of the MammaCare [28] method improves global detection capacities and that the technique can be taught?

Three randomized assays used silicon models for evaluation by Internal Medicine residents, nurses, medical students, and patients [17–20, 25, 26, 29–31]. All three showed that practice improved the sensitivity of CBE when it was measured in silicon models.

In the sum of the results of clinical studies, training improved the sensitivity by 13 percentage points (95% Confidence interval [95% CI], 10–16%), from 46 to 59%, while specificity diminished nonsignificantly by an average of four points (95% CI: –8.9 to 0.7%), from 61 to 57% [30]. In the majority of cases, sensitivity improved to a greater degree than specificity.

Can Breast Nodules Be Normal?

Normal breast are frequently unequal or nodular. Thus, the task of the physician is to distinguish the normal from the abnormal, above all in breast nodules. Cancer is typically characterized as hard, fixed, and irregular, while benign breast tumors are the contrary: soft; cystic, moveable, and regular. However, many cancers do not present with the classical image, and likewise, benign lesions can mimic cancers [20, 31].

As certain physical findings can be associated with both being and malignant growths, physicians rarely diagnose breast pathology using physical breast examination as an exlcusive clinical tool. Although careful exploration of the breasts can localize abnormalities, additional evaluation with other examinations is required [32, 33].

References

[1] Elmore JG, Barton MB, Moceri VM, Polk S, Arena PJ, Fletcher SW. Ten-year risk of false-positive screening mammograms and clinical breast examinations. *NEJM*. 1998;338:1089-1096.

[2] Physician Insurers Association of America. Breast Cancer Study- June 1995. Washington, D.C., USA: Physician Insurers Association of America; 1995.

[3] Baines CJ. Physical examination of the breasts in screening for breast cancer. *J. Gerontol.* 1992;47:63-67.

[4] Manual de Exploración Clínica de las Mamas. Programa de prevención y control del cáncer de mama. 1a ed. Secretaría de Salud; 2007. ISBN 979-970-721-456-9.

[5] Consenso Nacional sobre diagnóstico y tratamiento del cáncer mamario. 5a rev. Colima; México; 2013.

[6] Ries LAG, Kosary CL, Hankey BF, Miller BA, Edwards BK, Editors. SEER Cancer Statistics Review. National Cancer Institute Bethesda, MD 1999; 1973-1996. http://www.seer.cancer.gov/csr/1975_2010/

[7] Baines CJ, Miller AB, Bassett AA. Physical examination: its role as a single screening modality in the Canadian National Breast Screening Study. *Cancer*. 1989;63:1816-1822.

[8] Shapiro S, Venet W, Strax P, Venet L. Periodic Screening for Breast Cancer: The Health Insurance Plan Project and Its Sequelae, 1963–1986. Baltimore, MD, USA: The Johns Hopkins University Press; 1988.

[9] Collette HJA, Rombach JJ, Day NE, de Waard F. Evaluation of screening for breast cancer in a nonrandomized study (the DOM project) by means of a case-control study. *Lancet*. 1984;1:1224-1226.

[10] Alexander FE, Anderson TJ, Brown HK, et al. The Edinburgh Randomised Trial of Breast Cancer Screening. *Br. J. Cancer*. 1994;70:542-548.

[11] Tabar L, Fagerberg CJ, Gad A, et al. Reduction in mortality from breast cancer after mass screening with mammography. *Lancet*. 1985;1:829-832.

[12] Miller AB, Baines CJ, To T, Wall C. Canadian National Breast Screening Study, 1. *CMAJ*. 1992;147:1459-1476.

[13] Miller AB, Baines CJ, To T, Wall C. Canadian National Breast Screening Study, 2. *CMAJ*. 1992;147:1477-1488.

[14] Andersson I, Aspegren K, Janzon L, et al. Mammographic screening and mortality from breast cancer. *BMJ*. 1988;297:943-948.

[15] Palli D, Del Turco MR, Buiatti E, et al. A case-control study of the efficiency of a non-randomized breast cancer screening program in Florence (Italy). *Int. J. Cancer*. 1986;38:501-504.

[16] Verbeek ALM, Holland R, Sturmans F, Hendriks JHCL, Mravunac M, Day NE. Reduction of breast cancer mortality through mass screening with modern mammography. *Lancet*. 1984;1:1222-1224.

[17] UK Trial of Early Detection of Breast Cancer Group. First results on mortality reduction in the UK trial of early detection of breast cancer. *Lancet*. 1988;2:411-416.

[18] Thomas LB, Ackerman LV, McDivitt R. Report of NCI Ad Hoc Pathology Working Group to Review the Gross and Microscopic Findings of Breast Cancer Cases in the

HIP Study. Bethesda, MD, USA: National Cancer Institute; 1977. Publication NIH 77-1400.

[19] Seidman H, Gelb SK, Silverberg E, LaVerda N, Lubera JA. Survival experience in the Breast Cancer Detection Demonstration Project. *CA Cancer J. Clin.*1987;37:258-290.

[20] Baines CJ, Miller AB. Mammography versus clinical examination of the breasts. *J. Natl. Cancer Inst.* 1997;22:125-129.

[21] Mahoney L, Csima A. Efficiency of palpation in clinical detection of breast cancer. *CMAJ.* 1982;127:729-730.

[22] Fletcher SW, O'Malley MS, Earp JL, Morgan TM, Lin S, Degnan D. How best to teach women breast self-examination. *Ann. Intern. Med.* 1990;112:772-779.

[23] Campbell HS, Fletcher SW, Lin S, Pilgrim CA, Morgan TM. Improving physicians' and nurses' clinical breast examination. *Am. J. Prev. Med.* 1991;7:1-8.

[24] Saunders KJ, Pilgrim CA, Pennypacker HS. Increased proficiency of search in breast self-examination. *Cancer.* 1986;58:2531-2537.

[25] Bates B. A Guide to Physical Examination and History Taking. Philadelphia, PA, USA JB Lippincott Co.; 1998.

[26] Welch HG, Fisher ES. Diagnostic testing following screening mammography in the elderly. *J. Natl. Cancer Inst.* 1998;90:1389-1392.

[27] Pilgrim C, Lannon C, Harris RP, Cogburn W, Fletcher SW. Improving clinical breast examination training in a medical school. *J. Gen. Intern. Med.* 1993;8:685-688.

[28] MammaCare - Clinical Breast Exam Certification and Breast Self – Examination.

[29] Barton MB, Harris R, Fletcher SW. Does This Patient Have Breast Cancer? The Screening Clinical Breast Examination: Should It Be Done? How? *JAMA.* 1999;282(13):1270-1280.

[30] Thistlelwaite J, Stewart RA. Clinical breast examination for asymptomatic women. Exploring the Evidence. *Australian Family Physician.* (Mar) 2007;36:145-150.

[31] McDonald S, Saslow D, Alciati MH. Performance and reporting of clinical breast examination: a review of the literature. *CA Cancer J. Clin.* 2004;54:345-361.

[32] UK Trial of Early Detection of Breast Cancer Group. Specificity of screening in UK Trial of Early Detection of Breast Cancer. *BMJ.* 1992;304:346-349.

[33] Chamberlain J, Clifford RE, Nathan BE, Price JL, Burn I. Error-rates in screening for breast cancer by clinical examination and mammography. *Clin. Oncol.* 1979;5:135-146.

In: Benign Disease of the Breast
Editors: J. de la Garza Salazar, C. Arce Salinas et al.
ISBN: 978-1-63321-624-2

Chapter 5

Nipple Discharge and Secretions

Robin Shaw-Dulin*[*1] and Juan Enrique Bargallo-Rocha[2]
[1]Surgical Oncology Department
Instituto Nacional Cancerologia-Mexico,
Mexico City, DF, Mexico
[2]Breast Surgery Department
Instituto Nacional Cancerologia-Mexico,
Mexico City, DF, Mexico

Abstract

Nipple discharge is a common complaint, accounting for approximately 5% of breast related symptoms. Manipulation of the breast may elicit fluid secretion from the nipple in the majority of healthy women; however, discharge may also be a cause for alarm as it is often associated with underlying breast pathology.

Nipple discharge is classified as benign or pathologic on the basis of clinical characteristics. Benign discharge may be physiologic, related to endocrine disorders, pharmacologically induced, or idiopathic. Pathologic discharge is most commonly associated with intraductal papillomas, ductal ectasia or, in some cases, *in situ* or invasive breast carcinoma.

A thorough clinical evaluation should be performed in the patient presenting with nipple discharge, including complete medical history, physical examination, laboratory testing, and imaging studies, in order to determine the underlying cause and proper treatment strategies.

Introduction

Nipple discharge is the one of the most commonly encountered breast complaints [1], occurring in up to 80% of women in their reproductive years. Discharge can be bothersome

[*] Corresponding author.

for some patients, especially if it is abundant or persistent, and it can also elicit fear, particularly when it is bloody. The majority of nipple discharges are caused by benign conditions, although up to 15% may have an underlying malignancy, rendering appropriate evaluation and management imperative [2–4].

Nipple Discharge Classification

Based on the characteristics of clinical presentation, nipple discharge is classified as normal milk production (lactation), physiologic nipple discharge, or pathologic discharge.

Lactation

The normal secretory products of the breast are milk and colostrum. During pregnancy and the postpartum period, the mammary glands produce milk in response to hormonal and physical triggers [5,6]. Lactogenesis can continue for at least 6 months after delivery or after cessation of breastfeeding.

Bloody nipple discharge can be observed in 20 percent of women during the second or third trimester of pregnancy and lactation, and is usually benign.

Physiologic Nipple Discharge

Physiologic nipple discharge or galactorrhea is a nonpathologic nipple discharge unrelated to pregnancy or breastfeeding. Galactorrhea is usually a bilateral milky or clear nipple discharge involving multiple ducts. Less commonly, the discharge may be unilateral and a variety of colors, including yellow, green, brown, or gray.

Nonpuerperal galactorrhea is frequently caused by inappropriately elevated prolactin levels (hyperprolactinemia), which may be secondary to medications, endocrine tumors (pituitary adenoma), endocrine abnormalities (hypothyroidism), chronic breast stimulation, or a variety of medical conditions including renal failure [4]. The normal value for serum prolactin in the majority of laboratories is 20 ng/mL and, depending on the cause of hyperprolactinemia, may vary greatly.

Pharmacologic Causes of Galactorrhea

Pharmacologic agents that cause lactotroph stimulation or inhibit dopamine are a common cause of galactorrhea. Under normal circumstances, dopamine inhibits prolactin secretion [7]. Several drugs, such as antipsychotics and gastric motility promoters, are known dopamine D2 receptor antagonists and as such raise serum prolactin. Other drugs inhibit dopamine synthesis (Methyldopa) or storage (Reserpine). Yet other drugs, such as Verapamil, raise serum prolactin concentrations by unknown mechanisms.

Typical Antipsychotics Phenothaizines (Chlorpromazine, Clomipramine, Fluphenazine, Prochlorperazine, Thioridazine Holoperidol Pimozide
Atypical Antipsychotics Risperidone Molindone Olanzapine
Antidepressants Clomipramine Desipramine Selective serotonin reuptake inhibitors – Fluoxetine, Fluvoxamine, Dialproex
Gastrointestinal Drugs Cimetidine Metoclopramide
Antihypertensive Agents Methyldopa Reserpine Verapamil
Opiates Codeine Morphine

Neurogenic Stimulation

Neurogenic stimulation represses the secretion of the hypothalamic prolactin inhibitory factor, presumably via a neural pathway, resulting in hyperprolactinemia and galactorrhea [8]. Examples of neurogenic stimulation include chronic breast stimulation from manipulation or clothing (for example, a poorly fitting brassiere).

Often, women will see a drop or two of discharge associated with a warm bath or shower. Patients should be reassured that approximately two thirds of nonlactating women have a small amount of fluid secreted from the nipple, especially upon manual compression. These women should be advised to avoid frequent checking for nipple discharge, because repeated stimulation of the nipple will promote the production of more discharge. Discharge due to neurogenic stimulation generally resolves with resolution of the inciting factor [8–10].

Post-thoracotomy syndrome is a rare disorder in which the healing chest wound simulates the effect of a suckling infant. It can be associated with elevated prolactin concentration, breast pain, and milk production. A similar effect can be observed with other forms of chest wall injury, including burns [11], cervical spine lesions, and herpes Zoster.

Other Causes of Physiologic Nipple Discharge

Any disease in or near the hypothalamus or pituitary that interferes with secretion of dopamine or its delivery to the hypothalamus can cause hyperprolactinemia. Stresses such as trauma, surgical procedures, and anesthesia may also inhibit dopamine release, thereby causing hyperprolactinemia and inducing galactorrhea. Purulent nipple discharge can be observed in association with periductal mastitis.

Pathological or Suspicious Nipple Discharge

Secretion of fluids other than milk may be due to a pathological process in the breast. The discharge is usually unilateral and localized to a single duct, persistent, and spontaneous. It can be serous, bloody, or serosanguineous.

The most common cause of pathologic nipple discharge is a papilloma, present in 52–57% of cases presenting with this symptom [12–14]. A papilloma is a papillary tumor growing from the lining of the breast duct. The discharge associated with a papilloma can be clear or grossly bloody. Solitary papillomas can harbor areas of atypia or Ductal carcinoma *in situ* (DCIS). The standard recommendation for management of papillomas is that they be excised whenever they are diagnosed by CNB [15–19].

The remaining cases of secretion of products other than milk are caused by ductal ectasia or by other benign changes (14–32%).

Malignancy is found in 5–15% of cases of pathological nipple discharge. The most common malignancy associated with nipple discharge in the absence of other findings is DCIS [20–22].

Clinical Evaluation of Nipple Discharge

A thorough history and physical examination should be performed in all women with nonlactational nipple discharge.

Age

Age is predictive of the risk of cancer in women with nipple discharge. Malignancy may be present in up to 3% of those <40 years of age, 10% of those 40–60 years of age, and 32% of those aged >60 years [23].

Medical History

A complete medical history, including medication use, should be obtained. Specific areas to address are the appearance of the discharge, whether the discharge is spontaneous or provoked by manipulation of the breast, and whether it is unilateral or bilateral. Cancers generally present with spontaneous, unilateral, uniductal, frankly bloody, or hemoccult-positive discharge. Bilateral nipple discharge is usually due to an endocrinologic or physiologic process, although bilateral synchronous cancers can occur. A history of recent trauma should also be documented.

A complete gynecologic history should be elicited, including pregnancy and recent childbirth. A personal history of breast cancer or benign breast conditions should be excluded. Recent onset of amenorrhea or other symptoms of hypogonadism or menopause (hot flashes, vaginal dryness) should prompt endocrinologic work up. A family history of malignancy, especially breast and ovary, should also be obtained.

Physical Examination

The physical examination should include not only a complete examination of the breast, but also an evaluation of the eyes for visual field deficits (bitemporal field loss in chiasmal syndrome associated with pituitary adenomas) and a search for signs of hypothyroidism or hypogonadism. The thyroid should be palpated to evaluate for enlargement or a palpable mass.

The breast examination should include the four breast quadrants, subareolar areas, axillae, supraclavicular, and infraclavicular areas. Focus should be placed on inspection for detection of asymmetry, irregular breast contour, nipple position, presence of vascular patterns, skin changes including hyperpigmentation or depigmentation, retraction, dimpling, and edema or erythema should be noted.

In particular, the skin covering the breast and nipple areolar complex should be examined for lesions that may be staining the woman's clothes and mimicking nipple discharge. In such cases, crusty lesions with serosanguineous scabs are sometimes found on the nipple or areola. Some examples are Paget disease, insect bites, local infections, and eczema.

Upon palpation, an attempt should be made to elicit discharge from the nipple and to identify the involved duct or ducts. Pressure in a clockwise direction around the areola can help identify a specific site or duct that is producing the discharge [24]. A warm compress placed on the breasts will enhance the chances of detecting mammary secretion. Gentle, firm pressure should be applied at the base of the areola (not on the nipple). Massage from the periphery towards the nipple areolar complex may also help. Any discharge elicited from the nipple should be tested for blood with a hemoccult or guaiac test.

Palpation should also focus on the detection of enlarged regional lymph nodes and breast masses.

Bilateral Discharge

Although commonly associated with benign conditions, bilateral discharge should be evaluated for gross blood or guaiac positivity. In the case of a guaiac-positive nipple discharge, an abnormal mammogram or breast US, or in the presence of a breast mass, evaluation by a breast surgeon will be required. Bilateral multiductal secretion that tests negative for blood is usually normal. Medical evaluation and endocrine workup may be required, but surgical intervention is usually not indicated.

Unilateral Discharge

Uniductal unilateral discharge is more likely to represent underlying pathology, such as papilloma or intraductal breast carcinoma. This is true even if the discharge is guaiac-negative, because the sensitivity of guaiac testing has been shown to be only about 50% [25].

In contrast, multiductal discharge, even if unilateral, is less likely to represent significant breast disease, and should be investigated similarly to bilateral discharge.

Color of Discharge

The color of nipple discharge can provide a tool for differential diagnosis, as it has shown to be an indicator of the risk of underlying malignancy. A meta-analysis of eight studies including 3,110 patients showed that patients with bloody nipple discharge had a 52% risk of breast cancer compared with the 19% risk of patients with nonbloody nipple discharge [26].

Clear Discharge

Yellow or clear serous nipple discharge is typically due to a papilloma, although malignancy must always be excluded. Papillomas nipple discharge occurs when the increased pressure on lymphatic and vascular structures in the narrow pedicle causes plasma transudate.

Bloody Discharge

Bloody or guaiac-positive nipple discharge simply means that a lesion in the duct is bleeding. The bleeding can be caused by an intraductal carcinoma (*in-situ* or invasive), a bleeding papilloma, or benign fibrocystic changes with an active intraductal component (e.g., plasma cell mastitis, ductal ectasia, intraductal hyperplasia, or papillomatosis).

Bloody or guaiac-positive nipple discharge can also be observed in approximately 20% of women during pregnancy and lactation. The cause is usually hypervascularity of developing breast tissue, which is benign and requires no treatment [27, 28]. However, evaluation of breast complaints in pregnancy and lactation can be complicated by the changing breast examination. Referral for surgical evaluation and biopsy is warranted for evaluation and management of bloody nipple discharge [29].

Nipple secretion that is not grossly bloody, but that is guaiac-positive, is usually also caused by intraductal pathologies (e.g., papilloma, papillomatosis, and hyperplasia) or plasma cell mastitis with duct ectasia, which is a chronic inflammatory condition and occasionally, breast carcinoma.

Staining of the Bra without Obvious Nipple Discharge

A woman may report finding a stain or spot of blood on her brassiere or underclothing [30]. Careful examination of the skin around the nipple and nipple areolar complex should be performed. Dermatosis such as contact dermatitis or eczema may be the cause; however, it is important to rule out Paget disease of the nipple with a skin biopsy and radiologic evaluation if the lesions persist after conservative treatment. Paget disease is an *in situ* adenocarcinoma of the nipple sometimes associated with *in situ* or invasive underlying breast cancer, which is clinically characterized by eczematoid changes, nipple crusting, or erosion.

Diagnostic Evaluation

After clinical evaluation and physical examination, all women with pathologic nipple discharge should undergo a breast US. A mammogram should be performed for women ≥30 years of age [31].

Histopathologic evaluation with percutaneous or excisional biopsy is indicated if there is a breast mass, any imaging abnormality, a positive occult blood test, or if the discharge is spontaneous, uniductal, and/or bloody. Surgical evaluation of pathologic nipple discharge is required for diagnosis and treatment even if imaging results are negative.

If physical examination and imaging is normal and the discharge is multiductal and negative for occult blood, then the patient will require laboratory tests, medical evaluation, and galactorrhea workup.

A guide to management for the general practitioner is exemplified in the following figure:

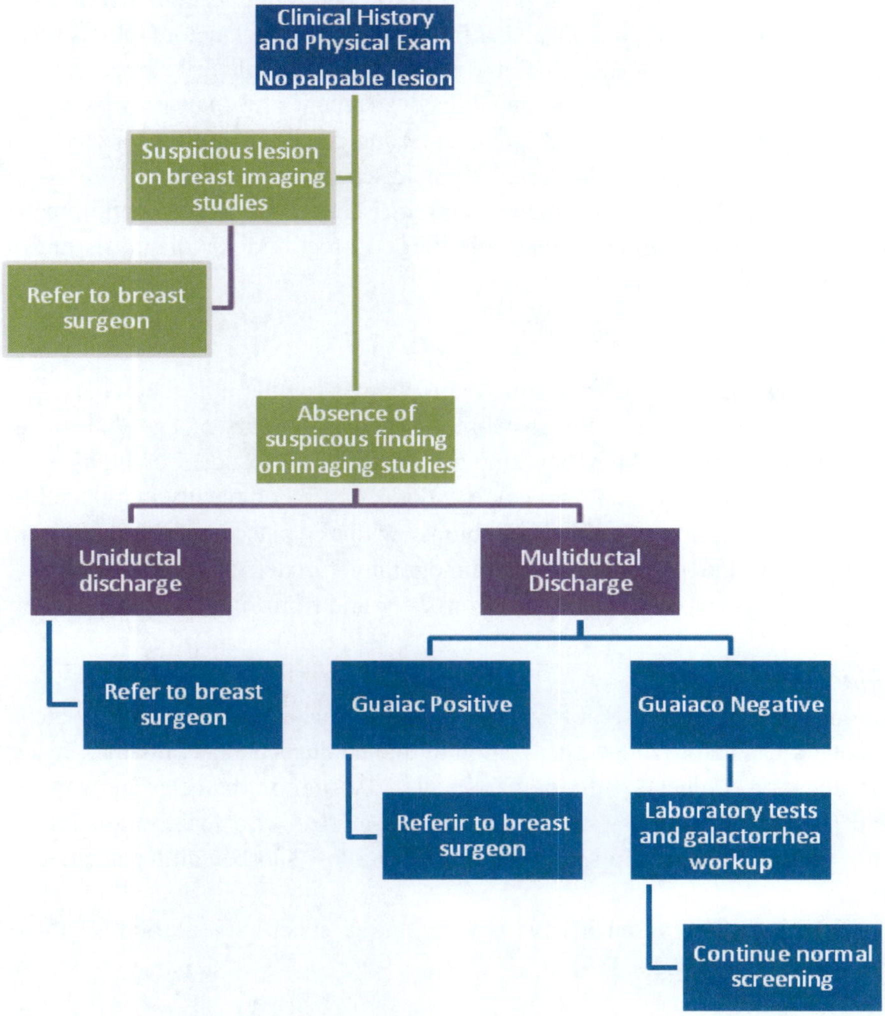

Figure 1. Guide to management of the patient with nipple discharge for the general practitioner.

Laboratory Examination

Multiductal discharge should be evaluated with a pregnancy test, prolactin levels, renal and thyroid function tests, and referral to an endocrinological specialist if there are abnormal findings. These tests are not indicated for evaluation of uniductal discharge. Endocrinological evaluation is also important in the presence of menstrual irregularity, infertility, headaches, visual disturbances, or symptoms of hypothyroidism.

Imaging

Imaging studies may reveal an underlying abnormality in the duct or breast tissue and help direct the surgical evaluation.

Mammography and US examination should be included upon initial imaging workup. The sensitivity of mammography is low; however, it is the best modality for identifying suspicious lesions in the breast. US is most useful for identifying lesions within the ducts that can be subjected to core biopsy or localized for surgical biopsy. Ductography is often used to identify an intraductal filling defect that may be causing the nipple discharge.

Other diagnostic testing, including breast magnetic resonance imaging, magnetic resonance ductography, ductal lavage, and ductoscopy can be helpful in selected women, but are not always necessary for the workup of nipple discharge.

Imaging does not identify all cancers or high-risk lesions, such as papilloma or atypia. Surgical evaluation of pathologic nipple discharge is required for diagnosis and treatment even if imaging results are negative.

Mammography

Mammograms should be performed in women with nonlactational spontaneous discharge. The study is most useful in women at least 30 years of age due to high breast density in younger patients. Mammograms may not identify cancers or high-risk lesions if they are small, are not associated with calcifications, or are completely intraductal [32]. If an abnormality is detected, image-guided core biopsy with clip placement should be performed.

The sensitivity and specificity of mammography for detection of cancer or high-risk lesions such as papilloma or atypia ranges from 7–10 and from 94–100%, respectively [33].

Ultrasound

Ultrasound (US) is very useful for the diagnosis of ductal disease as it may be directed to the periareolar area and provides visualization of dilated ducts and any nodules inside these. It allows visualization of ductal pathology as small as 0.5 mm in diameter and can be used for US-guided percutaneous biopsy of lesions and US-guided wire localization for surgery. If core biopsy is performed, a clip should be placed to allow subsequent localization if surgery is required.

Ultrasonography has a sensitivity of 97% and a specificity of 60% with a Positive predictive value (PPV) of 95% [34].

Ductography

Ductography is a study that requires installation of iodine containing contrast medium into the discharging duct [35]. The intraductal lesion will appear as an intraductal filling defect, a complete ductal obstruction, or a wall irregularity. Ductography can only be performed if the nipple discharge can be elicited on physical examination and if the duct can be cannulated.

Ductography has been associated with a sensitivity of 76% and a specificity of 11% [36], with PPV on ductography in this series of 19%.

The absence of a lesion on ductogram does not exclude a cancer. Ductography should not be performed in patients with mastitis or a breast abscess. Ductography can cause mastitis if too much contrast material is injected or if too much pressure is used during injection, resulting in perforation of the duct and extravasation of contrast material.

Magnetic Resonance Imaging

Magnetic resonance imaging (MRI) is a relatively sensitive imaging modality with low-to-moderate specificity [37]. The significant false-positive rate and somewhat limited availability of Magnetic resonance (MR)-guided biopsy limits the utility of this modality. If MR is going to be used, it should be performed at a facility that has MR biopsy capabilities.

MR Ductography

MR ductography uses heavy T2 weighting, which accentuates the visibility of fluid-containing structures, providing a three-dimensional image that can show the precise shape and location of the abnormal duct and lesion in the breast. This technique will not reveal ducts that are not dilated or those with low signal intensity on heavily T2-weighted images, due to hemorrhage or the presence of proteinaceous contents within the duct [38].

Cytologic Examination

No definite benefits have been identified for routine use of cytology in the evaluation of nipple discharge. Systematic cytologic examination of all nipple discharges is not cost-effective [39].

At one time, it was recommended that nipple discharge be sampled during examination and sent for cytologic evaluation. Recent studies have suggested that cytology of nipple discharge has poor sensitivity and specificity (16.7 and 66.1%, respectively) and does not add merit to clinical decision making [40]. It is, therefore, no longer routinely recommended.

Ductoscopy

Ductoscopy can be utilized as a minimally invasive method for evaluation and treatment of nipple discharge [41]. As with ductography, ductoscopy requires a reproducible discharge and the ability to cannulate and dilate the discharging duct [42].

Ductoscopy involves placing a small fiberoptic cannula into the discharging duct. The newest scopes have an outer diameter of 0.9 mm with a 0.2-mm working channel attachment that can be employed for insufflation and tissue sampling. Ductoscopic biopsy is also possible in some cases.

Supporters of this procedure point out that ductoscopy allows visualization of more peripheral lesions and may serve to decrease surgical duct excisions in the case of benign lesions. Further study and refinement of this technique is needed [43–45].

Ductal Lavage

Ductal lavage is used to increase the cellularity of specimens obtained by expression or aspiration of nipple discharge for cytology. The procedure requires cannulation of each fluid-yielding duct with a single lumen catheter and instillation of saline solution. The effluent is immediately fixed and centrifuged to recover a cell pellet. The effectiveness of this technique has been questioned, because the cancer-filled duct may not always yield fluid, and even if cells are obtained on lavage, this does not help localize the lesion. This technique has the same limitations as cytology and is, in general, not useful [46].

Treatment

Medical Treatment for Physiologic Nipple Discharge

If the patient is taking a medication that has been associated with galactorrhea, the patient should be educated that physiologic nipple discharge is a side effect of the medication. In some cases, continuing the medication is necessary. If the nipple discharge is bothersome to the patient, the medication can be changed if underlying conditions so permit.

Surgical Treatment for Pathologic Nipple Discharge

Once a full evaluation has ruled out malignancy, pathologic nipple discharge in nonlactating women may be managed by a terminal duct excision. If a Core needle biopsy (CNB) or an excisional biopsy has demonstrated ductal carcinoma *in situ* or invasive breast cancer, appropriate oncologic treatment will ensue.

If a core biopsy was not possible or was nondiagnostic, a terminal duct excision is necessary to treat the nipple discharge and to confirm the diagnosis [47]. A terminal duct excision is usually performed through a circumareolar incision and removes tissue at least 2–3 cm distal from the nipple. When a single duct can be implicated, the surgeon should direct the resection to the site of concern, possibly cannulating the affected duct. When preserving unaffected ducts, lactation may still be possible.

An intraductal papilloma may be resected by selective excision of the abnormal duct, assisted by preoperative ductography or needle-guided localization. This helps limit the dissection to the area of the intraductal lesion and to increase the likelihood of excising the lesion [48, 49].

Central (total) terminal duct excision is occasionally used for persistent discharge from multiple ducts that is causing significant distress to the patient. It is important to discuss with premenopausal women that this will preclude lactation in the future.

Intraductal Papillomas

Solitary intraductal papillomas may be identified as a mass on a mammogram, US, MRI, ductogram [50], or as an incidental finding on core biopsy [51]. Nipple discharge is a frequent clinical presentation.

Solitary papillomas consist of a monotonous array of papillary cells that grow from the wall of a cyst into its lumen. Solitary papillomas can harbor areas of atypia or Ductal carcinoma *in situ* (DCIS). Although there is some debate in the literature, the standard management of papillomas diagnosed by CNB is surgical excision [52–57], as up to 15% may be upgraded to malignancy following a surgical excision [58].

Diagnosis of malignancy is even higher when the papilloma contains atypical cells. However, if an intraductal papilloma is incidental and is ≤2 mm, an excision may not be necessary as associated malignancy is rarely encountered. If the patient remains radiographically stable, surveillance is safe in this setting. [59].

Once the diagnosis of solitary papilloma is confirmed by excisional biopsy, no additional treatment is needed. Unless there is associated atypia, there is no increased risk of subsequent breast cancer.

Multiple Papillomas

Diffuse papillomatosis (multiple papillomas) may present as breast masses, nodules on US, or may be the cause of nipple discharge and can be observed on ductography. Diffuse papillomatosis is defined as a minimum of five papillomas within a localized segment of breast tissue [60,61]. After excision, additional treatment is not required for diffuse papillomatosis.

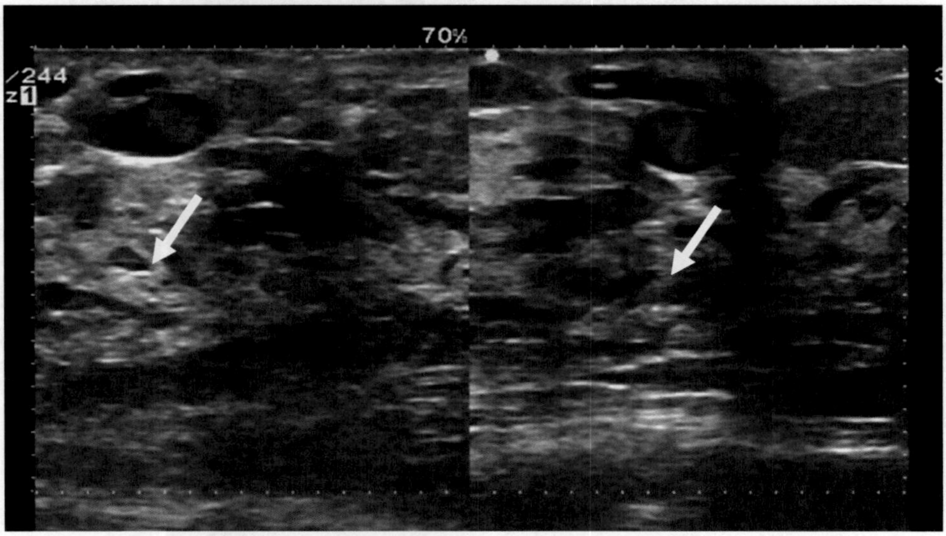

Figure 2. Case 1. A 47-year-old female presenting with unilateral blood-tinged nipple discharge. Ultrasound imaging of the retroareolar region showed nodular lesions associated with ductal ectasia. Histopathologic evaluation with percutaneous biopsy reported papillary neoplasia. The surgical specimen after needle-guided excision was positive for ductal carcinoma *in situ* associated with papilloma.

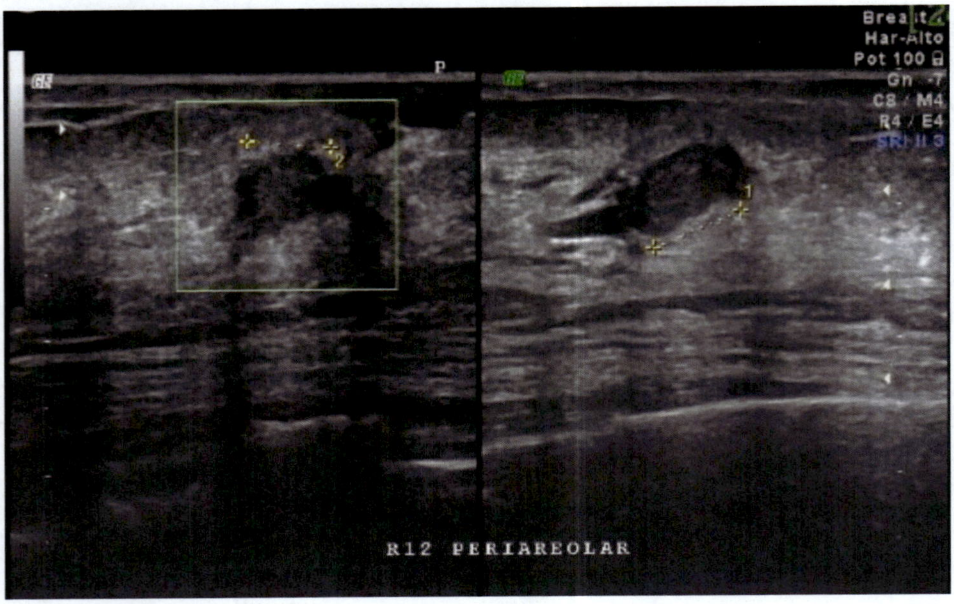

Figure 3. Case 2. A 47-year-old female with unilateral serous nipple discharge who, upon US imaging, was found to have a retroareolar, 11-mm, irregular intraductal lesion, with no vascularity or posterior acoustic shadowing. Histopathologic study by percutaneous biopsy and later excisional biopsy confirmed intraductal papilloma.

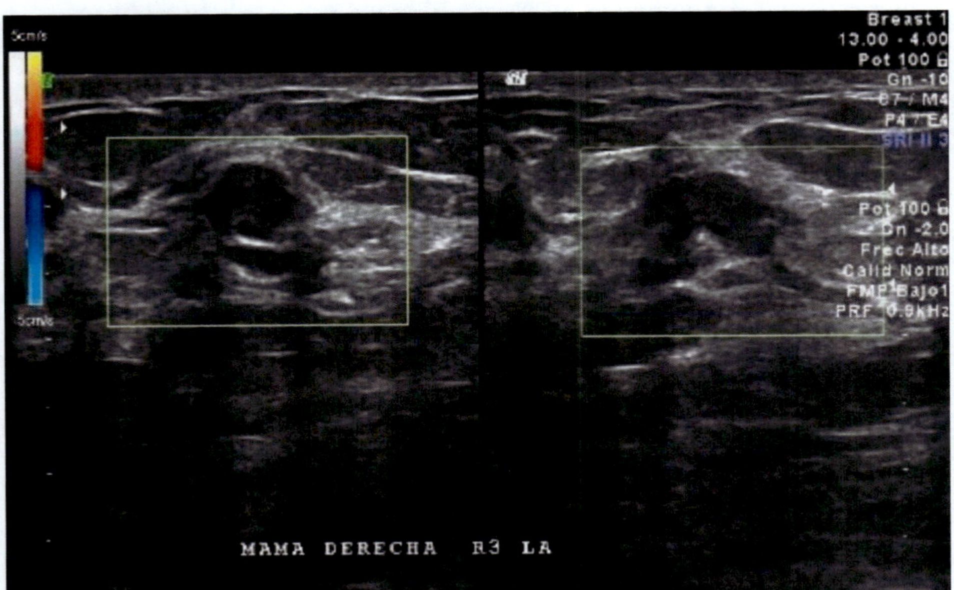

Figure 4. Case 3. A 33-year-old female with unilateral single duct serous nipple discharge who, upon US imaging, was found to have an 8-mm ectasic duct occupied by an irregular echogenic lesion with no apparent vascularity. Histopathologic analysis of an excisional biopsy reported papillomatosis.

References

[1] Hussain AN, Policarpio C, Vincent MT. Evaluating nipple discharge. *Obstet Gynecol Surv* 2006;61:278-283.

[2] Hughes, L, Mansel, R, Webster, D, Gravelle, I. Benign Disorders and Diseases of the Breast. London, UK: *WB Saunders*; 2000.

[3] Santen RJ, Mansel R. Benign breast disorders. *NEJM* 2005;353:275-285.

[4] Onstad M, Stuckey A. Benign breast disorders. *Obstet Gynecol Clin North Am* 2013;40:459-473.

[5] Neville MC, McFadden TB, Forsyth I. Hormonal regulation of mammary differentiation and milk secretion. *J Mammary Gland Biol Neoplasia* 2002;7:49-66.

[6] Buhimschi CS. Endocrinology of lactation. *Obstet Gynecol Clin North Am* 2004;31:963-979.

[7] Molitch ME. Drugs and prolactin. *Pituitary* 2008;11(2):209-218.

[8] Leung AK, Pacaud D. Diagnosis and management of galactorrhea. *Am Fam Physician* 2004;70:543-550.

[9] Kuerer HM. Kuerer's Breast Surgical Oncology. New York: *McGraw-Hill;* 2010.

[10] Falkenberry SS. Nipple discharge. *Obstet Gynecol Clin North Am* 2002;29:21-29.

[11] Morley JE, Dawson M, Hodgkinson H, Kalk WJ. Galactorrhea and hyperprolactinemia associated with chest wall injury. *J Clin Endocrinol Metab* 1977;45:931-935.

[12] Gioffrè Florio M, Manganaro T, Pollicino A, et al. Surgical approach to nipple discharge: a ten-year experience. *J Surg Oncol* 1999;71:235-238.

[13] Vargas HI, Vargas MP, Eldrageely K, et al. Outcomes of clinical and surgical assessment of women with pathological nipple discharge. *Am Surg* 2006;72:124-128.

[14] Nelson RS, Hoehn JL. Twenty-year outcome following central duct resection for bloody nipple discharge. *Ann Surg* 2006;243:522-524.

[15] Lewis JT, Hartmann LC, Vierkant RA, et al. An analysis of breast cancer risk in women with single, multiple, and atypical papilloma. *Am J Surg Pathol* 2006;30:665-672.

[16] Valdes EK, Feldman SM, Boolbol SK. Papillary lesions: a review of the literature. *Ann Surg Oncol* 2007;14:1009-1013.

[17] Mercado CL, Hamele-Bena D, Oken SM, et al. Papillary lesions

[18] Sydnor MK, Wilson JD, Hijaz TA, et al. Underestimation of the presence of breast carcinoma in papillary lesions initially diagnosed at core-needle biopsy. *Radiology* 2007;242:58-62.

[19] Ciatto S, Andreoli C, Cirillo A, et al. The risk of breast cancer subsequent to histologic diagnosis of benign intraductal papilloma follow-up study of 339 cases. *Tumori* 1991;77:41-43.

[20] Murad TM, Contesso G, Mouriesse H. Nipple discharge from the breast. *Ann Surg* 1982;195:259-264.

[21] Jardines L. Management of nipple discharge. *Am Surg* 1996;62:119-122.

[22] King TA, Carter KM, Bolton JS, Fuhrman GM. A simple approach to nipple discharge. *Am Surg* 2000;66:960-965.

[23] Seltzer MH, Perloff LJ, Kelley RI, Fitts WT Jr. The significance of age in patients with nipple discharge. *Surg Gynecol Obstet* 1970;131:519-522.

[24] Klimberg VS. Nipple discharge: more than pathologic. *Ann Surg Oncol* 2003;10:113-116.

[25] Simmons R, Adamovich T, Brennan M, et al. Nonsurgical evaluation of pathologic nipple discharge. *Ann Surg Oncol* 2003;10:113-116.

[26] Chen L, Zhou WB, Zhao Y, et al. Bloody nipple discharge is a predictor of breast cancer risk: a meta-analysis. *Breast Cancer Res Treat* 2012;132:9-14.

[27] Kline TS, Lash SR. The bleeding nipple of pregnancy and postpartum period; a cytologic and histologic study. *Acta Cytol* 1964;8:336-340.

[28] Lafreniere R. Bloody nipple discharge during pregnancy: a rationale for conservative treatment. *J Surg Oncol* 1990;43:228-230.

[29] Scott-Conner CE, Schorr SJ. The diagnosis and management of breast problems during pregnancy and lactation. *Am J Surg* 1995;170:401-405.

[30] Maier WP, Rosemond GP, Harasym EL Jr, et al. Pagets disease in the female breast. *Surg Gynecol Obstet* 1969;128:1253-1263.

[31] Gray RJ, Pockaj BA, Karstaedt PJ. Navigating murky waters: a modern treatment algorithm for nipple discharge. *Am J Surg* 2007;194:850-854.

[32] Sickles EA. Galactography and other imaging investigations of nipple discharge. *Lancet* 2000;356:1622-1623.

[33] Adepoju LJ, Chun J, El-Tamer M, et al. The value of clinical characteristics and breast-imaging studies in predicting a histopathologic diagnosis of cancer or high-risk lesion in patients with spontaneous nipple discharge. *Am J Surg* 2005;190:644-646.

[34] Ballesio L, Maggi C, Savelli S, et al. Adjunctive diagnostic value of ultrasonography evaluation in patients with suspected ductal breast disease. *Radiol Med* 2007;112:354-365.

[35] Cardenosa G, Doudna C, Eklund GW. Ductography of the breast: technique and findings. *AJR Am J Roentgenol* 1994;162:1081-1087.

[36] Morrogh M, Morris EA, Liberman L, et al. The predictive value of ductography and magnetic resonance imaging in the management of nipple discharge. *Ann Surg Oncol* 2007;14:3369-3377.

[37] Orel SG, Dougherty CS, Reynolds C, et al. MR imaging in patients with nipple discharge: initial experience. *Radiology* 2000;216:243-249.

[38] Hirose M, Nobusawa H, Gokan T. MR ductography: comparison with conventional ductography as a diagnostic method in patients with nipple discharge. *Radiographics* 2007;27(Suppl 1):S183-S196.

[39] Ciatto S, Bravetti P, Cariaggi P. Significance of nipple discharge clinical patterns in the selection of cases for cytologic examination. *Acta Cytol* 1986;30:17-20.

[40] Kooistra BW, Wauters C, van de Ven S, Strobbe L. The diagnostic value of nipple discharge cytology in 618 consecutive patients. *Eur J Surg Oncol* 2009;35:573-577.

[41] Golshan, M, Khan, S,. Role of breast epithelial sampling techniques in high risk women. Managing breast cancer risk. *Decker*, BC. London, UK, 2003. pp 138 -156.

[42] Escobar PF, Crowe JP, Matsunaga T, Mokbel K. The clinical applications of mammary ductoscopy. *Am J Surg* 2006;191:211-215.

[43] Kapenhas-Valdes E, Feldman SM, Cohen JM, Boolbol SK. Mammary ductoscopy for evaluation of nipple discharge. *Ann Surg Oncol* 2008;15:2720-2727.

[44] Moncrief RM, Nayar R, Díaz LK, et al. A comparison of ductoscopy-guided and conventional surgical excision in women with spontaneous nipple discharge. *Ann Surg* 2005;241:575-581.

[45] Uchida K, Fukushima H, Toriumi Y, et al. Mammary ductoscopy: current issues and perspectives. *Breast Cancer* 2009;16:93-96.

[46] Khan SA, Wolfman JA, Segal L, et al. Ductal lavage findings in women with mammographic microcalcifications undergoing biopsy. *Ann Surg Oncol* 2005;12:689-696.

[47] Alcock C, Layer GT. Predicting occult malignancy in nipple discharge. *ANZ J Surg* 2010;80:646-649.

[48] Dennis MA, Parker S, Kaske TI, et al. Incidental treatment of nipple discharge caused by benign intraductal papilloma through diagnostic Mammotome biopsy. *AJR Am J* Roentgenol 2000;174:1263-1268.

[49] Cabioglu N, Hunt KK, Singletary SE, et al. Surgical decision making and factors determining a diagnosis of breast carcinoma in women presenting with nipple discharge. *J Am Coll Surg* 2003;196:354-364.

[50] Woods ER, Helvie MA, Ikeda DM, et al. Solitary breast papilloma: comparison of mammographic, galactographic, and pathologic findings. *AJR Am J Roentgenol* 1992;159:487-491.

[51] Jaffer S, Bleiweiss IJ, Nagi C. Incidental intraductal papillomas (<2 mm) of the breast diagnosed on needle core biopsy do not need to be excised. *Breast J* 2013;19:130-133.

[52] Ciatto S, Andreoli C, Cirillo A, et al. The risk of breast cancer subsequent to histologic diagnosis of benign intraductal papilloma follow-up study of 339 cases. *Tumori* 1991;77:41-43.

[53] Lewis JT, Hartmann LC, Vierkant RA, et al. An analysis of breast cancer risk in women with single, multiple, and atypical papilloma. *Am J Surg Pathol* 2006;30:665-672.

[54] Valdes EK, Feldman SM, Boolbol SK. Papillary lesions: a review of the literature. *Ann Surg Oncol* 2007;14:1009-1013.

[55] Mercado CL, Hamele-Bena D, Oken SM, et al. Papillary lesions of the breast at percutaneous core-needle biopsy. *Radiology* 2006;238:801-808.

[56] Sydnor MK, Wilson JD, Hijaz TA, et al. Underestimation of the presence of breast carcinoma in papillary lesions initially diagnosed at core-needle biopsy. *Radiology* 2007;242:58-62.

[57] Ahmadiyeh N, Stoleru MA, Raza S, et al. Management of intraductal papillomas of the breast: an analysis of 129 cases and their outcome. *Ann Surg Oncol* 2009;16:2264-2269.

[58] Wen X, Cheng W. Nonmalignant breast papillary lesions at core-needle biopsy: a meta-analysis of underestimation and influencing factors. *Ann Surg Oncol* 2013;20:94-101.

[59] Jaffer S, Bleiweiss IJ, Nagi C. Incidental intraductal papillomas (<2 mm) of the breast diagnosed on needle core biopsy do not need to be excised. *Breast J* 2013;19:130-133.

[60] Mercado CL, Hamele-Bena D, Oken SM, et al. Papillary lesions of the breast at percutaneous core-needle biopsy. *Radiology* 2006;238:801-808.

[61] Ali-Fehmi R, Carolin K, Wallis T, Visscher DW. Clinicopathologic analysis of breast lesions associated with multiple papillomas. *Hum Pathol* 2003;34:234-239.

In: Benign Disease of the Breast
Editors: J. de la Garza Salazar, C. Arce Salinas et al.
ISBN: 978-1-63321-624-2

Chapter 6

Inflammatory Lesions

Diana Vilar-Compte[1], Consuelo Diaz[2], Patricia Cornejo-Juarez[1] and Martha Patricia Perez-Badillo[3]

[1]Infectious Diseases Department.
[2]Medical Oncology Division.
[3]Department of Radiology
Instituto Nacional Cancerologia-Mexico,
Mexico City, DF, Mexico

Abstract

Inflammatory diseases are observed in many different entities, ranging from benign self-limited processes to malignant neoplasms. Some of them are uncommon, and may look alike. Patients' age, race, lactation, and smoking are important risk factors that should always be addressed. Clinical and radiological characteristics of these lesions may allow an accurate differential diagnosis, and appropriate treatment. In this chapter, we address several breast inflammatory diseases. Acute and chronic mastitis (infectious and non-infectious causes), lactating and non-lactating abscess, ductal ectasia, fat necrosis and foreign-body related reactions are reviewed.

Inflammatory Diseases of the Breast

"Inflammatory" changes of the breast can be observed in many different entities, ranging from benign self-limited processes to highly aggressive malignant tumors. While clinically many of these "inflammatory" processes may look alike, there are some characteristics that allow accurate differential diagnosis and appropriate treatment [1].

Breast Infections in Lactating Women

Mastitis and Abscesses

Puerperal mastitis is a relatively common disease. The condition develops in 1-24% of breastfeeding women and is most often encountered in primiparous patients. [2]. A breast abscess develops as a complication of mastitis in 5–11% of cases and generally occurs during the first 12 weeks after childbirth or at the time of weaning [3].

The majority of abscesses result from secondary bacterial infection from skin contamination. Bacteria enter the skin by a small laceration or proliferate in a stagnant lactiferous duct. *Staphylococcus aureus* is by far the main pathogen, but *Staphylococcus epidermidis*, *Streptococcus pyogenes*, and anaerobes such as *Peptostreptococcus* and *Bacteroides* can also be encountered. Sterile cultures have been reported at between 21–45%, but this finding may be a false-negative result due to prior treatment with antibiotics [3, 4].

Differentiating between mastitis and an abscess can be difficult. Mastitis usually presents with a painful erythematous mass in the breast associated with local edema, leukocytosis, and fever. It tends to be a localized process that requires prompt treatment with empiric antibiotics with the aim of avoiding the possible complications of abscess and fistula formation. When there is suspicion of an abscess, the woman should be referred for Ultrasound (US), considered the first line of clinical workup because it is relatively painless and provides guidance for percutaneous drainage [1, 2].

In US, mastitis will appear as an ill-defined area of altered echotexture with increased echogenicity in the infiltrated and inflamed fat lobules. Diagnosis of an abscess requires identification of a hypoechoic collection, often with a thick echogenic periphery [1–3] (Figure 1).

Oral antibiotics should always be offered, and women must be encouraged to continue breastfeeding throughout the treatment to keep the ducts from becoming engorged. Cessation of breastfeeding is necessary only when antibiotics are contraindicated for the newborn, or if surgical drainage is performed.

First-choice antibiotics are those with appropriate coverage for *Staphylococci*; first-generation cephalosporins (e.g., Cefazolin or Cephalexin) are the preferred antibiotics. If *Streptococcus* is suspected, Amoxicillin should be considered. Clindamycin also offers excellent coverage for the most common organisms, including anaerobes. If an abscess is diagnosed, percutaneous drainage is required. A drain may be placed as needed for full evacuation of the cavity. Aspirates should be sent for culture and antimicrobial sensitivity testing; antibiotic therapy must be redirected accordingly [2, 3].

Open surgical drainage is reserved for patients with loculated collections or for those who failed conservative management with antibiotics and percutaneous drainage. Open surgical drainage is the last resource in lactating patients to avoid the potential for milk fistula development [2].

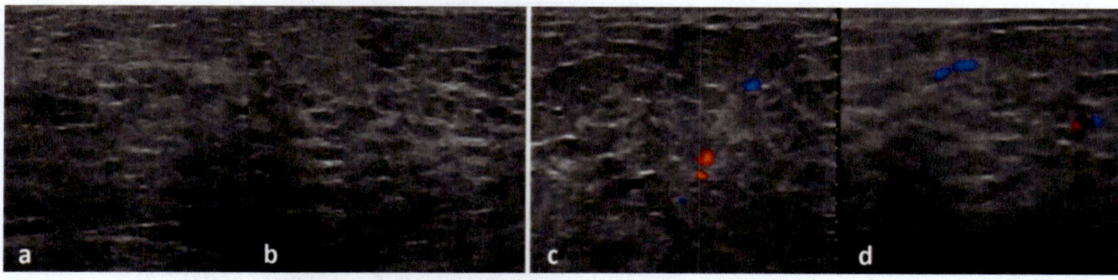

Figure 1. a-d. Mastitis and lactating abscess a, b) Echography of puerperal mastitis shows hyperechogenic subcuteneous fat, thickened skin, slightly hypoechogenic and slightly hypoechoic thickened fibrous elements. c, d) Hyperemia of all the elements (increased vascularity is shown on Doppler).

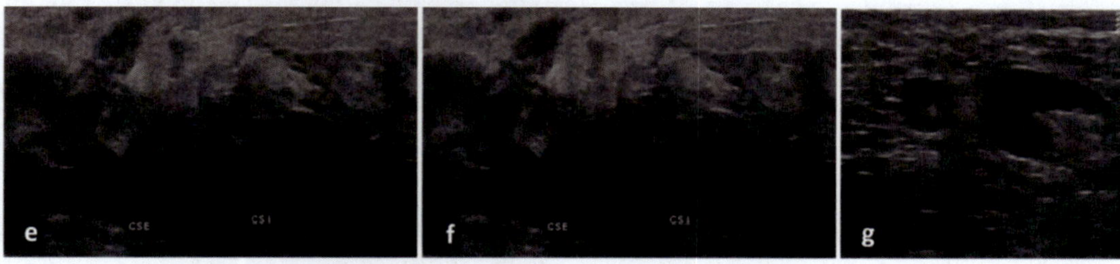

Figure 1.e-g. Mastitis and lactating abscess e) Echography of an abscess with a peripheral pattern. f) Echography of a galactocele. Infection localized in deep tissue tends to present with a central or peripheral pattern. The peripheral pattern tends to be due to an infected galactocele. Differentiation can be difficult g) Puerperal mastitis with an abscess. The cavity of the abscess tends to be oval, parallel to the periareolar ducts. It is usually unilocular.

Breast Infections in Nonlactating Individuals

Mastitis and Abscesses

Breast abscesses not associated with lactation are termed nonpuerperal and can be a challenging clinical problem that often recurs despite treatment in up to 25–40% of women.

Risk factors for the development of nonlactating breast abscesses include tobacco smoking, Black race, and obesity. More recently, nipple piercing appears to be associated with an increased risk and may be as high as 10–20% after the procedure. Patients with diabetes may also be at an increased risk for developing an abscess [3, 5].

Abscesses are classified according to location: either central (periareolar) or peripheral. Central nonpuerperal abscesses are the most common form and develop outside of the breastfeeding period. They usually affect young women, the majority of whom are smokers [3, 7, 8]. These abscesses form as a complication of periductal mastitis. Squamous metaplasia of the cuboidal epithelium is a first step and leads to formation of keratin plugs and central acute inflammatory infiltrates, and cellular debris distends and obstructs the lactiferous ducts, with ductal dilation as a consequence. Secondary infection occurs with stagnation, leading to abscess formation and the development of cutaneous fistulas that involve the periareolar region. In Figure 2, there is a sequence of an abscess observed by US and mammography. Bilateral abscess formation may occur in as many as 25% of these patients [2, 3].

Central nonpuerperal abscesses are the most difficult to treat, with a recurrence rate between 25 and 40%. Cutaneous fistulas occur in one third of patients. These abscesses are usually caused by mixed flora (*Staphylococcus* and *Streptococcus*), and anaerobes also may be involved [2, 3, 6]. Empiric broad-spectrum antibiotics against most common microorganisms should be started. To clear the infection, 2–3 weeks of treatment may be required, along with percutaneous drainage during or after a US evaluation. With the common use of US, treatment is typically percutaneous drainage with repeated aspirations as needed, and may include saline lavage of the cavity. In the majority of cases, this procedure will allow for appropriate treatment but occasionally, an indwelling catheter may be left in place for collections >3 cm, although this is seldom necessary [2]. Patients should be encouraged to stop smoking. In patients >35 years of age, a mammography is recommended after symptom resolution. If there is any doubt, a tissue sample should be sent for pathological evaluation.

Peripheral nonpuerperal abscesses are less common and occur at a slightly older age than central nonpuerperal abscesses. They usually occur in women with underlying medical conditions, such as diabetes or rheumatoid arthritis. Peripheral nonpuerperal abscesses have also been found in patients taking steroids, or with recent breast surgery or radiotherapy, although the majority has no associated medical conditions [3] (Figure 2).

As with any other breast abscesses, *S. aureus*, *Streptococcus*, and anaerobes are the most frequently isolated species, and treatment should consider the microbiologic profile of these infections. This form of abscess responds well to drainage and antibiotics. Recurrences are rare [2, 3].

Zuska's Disease

A mammillary fistula, also known as Zuska's disease, is a recurrent condition usually associated with a nonlactating subareolar abscess. It most commonly affects women aged between 20 and 50 years, and a history of subareolar abscess or spontaneous rupture of an inflammatory mass precedes the development of a mammillary fistula in the majority of patients [8, 9].

The cause of the disease is controversial, with multiple factors thought to contribute, including duct ectasia, squamous metaplasia with keratinization, or epidermization of the duct. The occlusion of hair follicles by keratinous plugging may also contribute to the development of these fistulas. Smoking has also been related with the disease [9].

Mammillary fistulas cause prolonged morbidity and are difficult to manage, with a negative impact on the patient's quality of life. Complete excision of the fistula tract and of the diseased duct is the preferred treatment for complex fistulas; unfortunately, recurrence remains a problem. Simple fistulas should be treated by fistulectomy and primary closure. More recently, sonographically guided percutaneous Triamcinolone injection has been reported as an option for fistula management. Because of the high recurrence rate and complex management, mammillary fistulas should be treated at specialized breast centers [8–11].

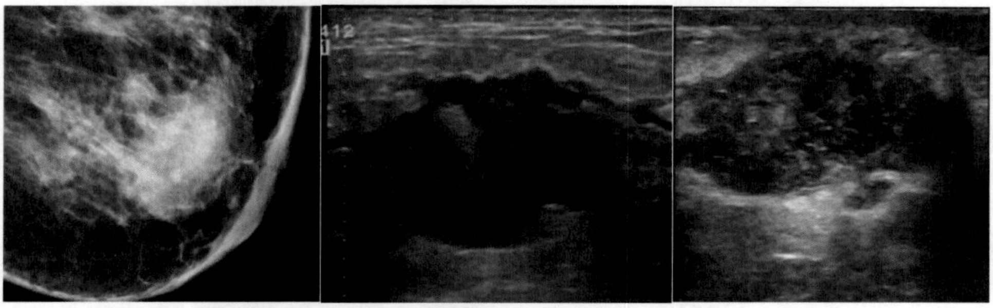

Figure 2. Peripheral nonlactating abscess Mammography (left) and echographic image of an abscess (right). A dense nodule with occult margins associated with inflammatory changes of the surrounding tissue are shown. By US (central), these tend to be seen as heterogenous lesions with internal echoes, indistinct margins, and posterior acoustic reinforcement, or even as complex lesions with inflammatory changes in the adjacent tissue. Abscesses that are not treated properly by surgery, percutaneous drainage, or antibiotics can become chronic, developing a solid aspect (right figure), difficult to distinguish from other lesions. In these cases, a confirmatory biopsy may be needed.

Chronic Mastitis

Chronic mastitis is a group of diseases characterized by chronic inflammation of the breast that mainly affect women of reproductive age. Histopathologically, it is defined as inflammation of the breast with microabscess formation and/or the presence of granulomas [12].

This disease generally involves the breast unilaterally. Cases mainly present with a breast mass, which may involve the overlying skin or penetrate into the underlying pectoralis muscle with nipple retraction, sinus formation, and axillary lymphadenopathy. The disease may be locally aggressive, with recurrence rates between 16 and 50% [12, 13].

Diagnosis of chronic mastitis should be performed after exclusion of other causes of infectious breast lesions, including tuberculosis, brucellosis, filariasis, histoplasmosis and actinomycosis, among others. Duct ectasia, fat necrosis, and breast cancer are also exclusion diagnoses. Immune-related diseases, such as sarcoidosis, Wegener's granulomatosis, and giant-cell arteritis, should also be considered in some cases. In the absence of a specific etiologic agent, the term granulomatous lobular mastitis or idiopathic granulomatous mastitis has been adopted for these lesions [1]. Due to the variable clinical presentation and similar symptoms to those of inflammatory breast cancer, diagnosis is difficult and must be confirmed histopathologically.

Idiopathic Granulomatous Mastitis

Idiopathic granulomatous mastitis (IGM) is a rare chronic inflammatory disease that was described by Kessler and Wolloch in 1972 [14]. The prevalence of IGM is unknown. It has been described worldwide in all races and has been associated with breastfeeding, hormonal contraception, and smoking. It mainly affects women of childbearing age [12, 15–18], but has also been described in men and in older women [15, 19, 20].

Certain etiologic factors that have been postulated comprise an autoimmune phenomenon, a chemical reaction associated with oral contraceptive pills, or an infection related with unidentified pathogens. [15] IGM can be idiopathic or secondary to other causes, including infectious and noninfectious granulomatous lesions in the breast, such as trauma, mammary duct ectasia, foreign body granulomas, sarcoidosis, Tuberculosis (TB), bacterial (*Corynebacteria* infection), and mycotic or parasitic infections [15, 17, 18, 21, 22].

Presentation is not different from other chronic mastitis, and symptoms vary from a few days to months. Lesions are of variable size ranging from 1 to 9cm, and are usually firm, tender, and well-defined [15, 19]. In mammograms and US, lesions are described as well-circumscribed, asymmetrical, or focally asymmetrical lumps [15, 16]. In (Figure 3), mastographic and ultrasonographic images are depicted.

Pathological findings include granulomatous inflammation centered in mammary lobules, frequently accompanied by multinucleated giant cells and microabscess formation [12, 15]. The presence of macrophages with intracytoplasmic, Periodic acid-Schiff (PAS)-positive hyaline globules, giant multinucleated cells, and clear lipoid-like spaces in areas of inflammation has also been reported. Treatment of IGM remains controversial. A number of therapeutic approaches have been reported, including clinical observation, antibiotics, immunosuppressant treatment (steroids ± Methotrexate), and surgery [15, 17]. For localized disease and mild symptoms, observation with close clinical and radiographic follow-up is warranted, considering that these lesions may resolve spontaneously [20]. Antimicrobial treatment is usually initiated in cases with purulent secretion through a skin sinus tract, local erythema or hyperthermia, ulceration, fever, or a positive culture. For patients with more extensive disease and severe symptoms, including pain or sinus formation, a trial of steroids is recommended. While the patient remains symptomatic, maintenance of Prednisone is recommended until resolution [15]. Steroids have been associated with long-term symptom control and a reduction in lesion size [17].

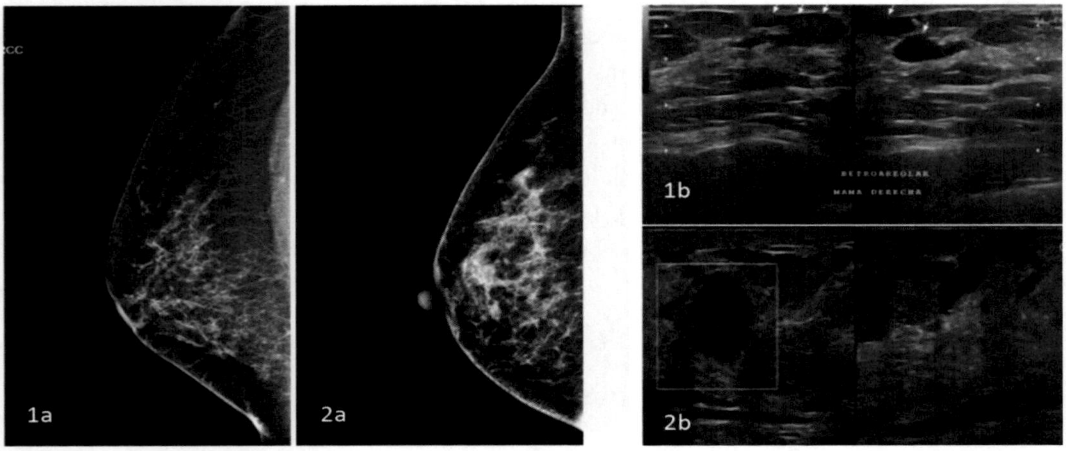

Figure 3. Granulomatous mastitis. Spectrum of images in granulomatous mastitis: 1. a) Mastographic and sonographic study with retroareolar dilated ducts, (b) dilated ducts with echogenic content, without changes in parenchyma. 2. a) Mammography with asymmetrical periareolar density, visualized echographically (b) as a rounded heterogeneous nodule of angulated margins and posterior acoustic reinforcement, associated with hypoechoic tubular trajectories with subareolar direction and hyperemia of the surrounding tissue.

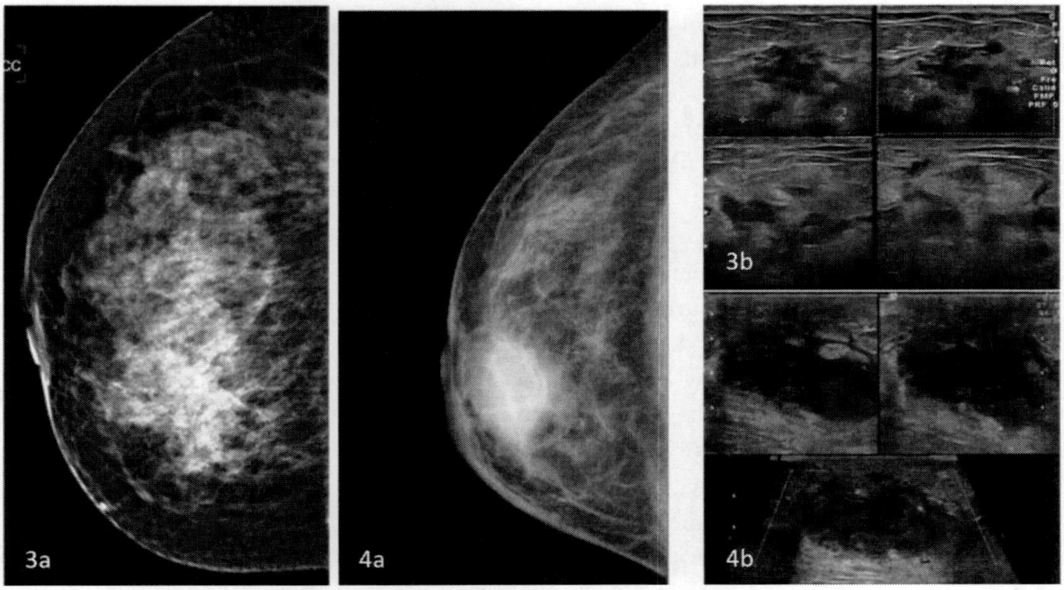

Figure 3. Granulomatous mastitis.3. a) Mammography with a dense spiculated image in internal quadrants and diffuse increase of the density of the parenchyma, b) ultrasonographically visualized as heterogeneous images of imprecise margins associated with diffuse increase of tissue echogenecity with hyperemia and multiple tortuous tubular trajectories of echogenic content. 4. a) Mammography shows a round dense nodule of obscured retroareolar margins with dermal thickening and an increase in preglandular fat density, b) ultrasound shows a heterogeneous nodule, of irregular morphology, and imprecise margins associated with hypoechoic trajectories that communicate to the nipple.

Surgical excision also comprises a treatment modality. It can additionally be useful in providing a precise diagnosis. Surgical excision should be considered in patients with treatment failure and non-response to more conservative treatment. Surgery has been reported as the most common treatment in various reports, but it is frequently complicated by a high rate of fistula formation, delayed wound healing, and anatomical breast disfigurement [12, 15].

In low- and middle-income countries, TB is an important differential diagnosis, particularly when the physician is considering treatment with steroids. In these cases, a chest x-ray film and a tuberculin test (Purified protein derivative, PPD) should be performed. It is also important to ascertain a history of contact with cases of TB or the ingestion of unpasteurized milk [19, 22].

Recurrence of granulomatous mastitis is a frequent complication regardless of the treatment modality, with a negative impact on the woman's QOL [15, 17, 23].

Tuberculous Mastitis

Breast tuberculosis is an uncommon form of TB and usually presents as a lump in the breast. Breast TB can masquerade as a variety of breast diseases, including malignancy and idiopathic granulomatous mastitis. The varied presentation poses a diagnostic and therapeutic dilemma for clinicians. Its presentation appears to be more frequent in low- and middle-income countries, where TB is more prevalent [24].

Presentation of breast TB may be protean. Unilateral breast mass, generalized breast edema and localized abscess with or without axillary involvement have all been described. The upper outer quadrant is the site most frequently involved. A persistent sinus discharge is common. Tenderness and erythema may also be present. One fifth of cases involve weight loss and low-grade fever, symptoms infrequently reported in IGM [24–26].

Breast TB has been classified into different types according to morphology: nodular (the most frequent presentation, characterized by a painless tumor), disseminated (multiple confluent nodules with fistulae), and sclerosing (older patients with extended fibrosis) [27].

The major routes of spread are lymphatic, contiguous, and hematogenous. Breast TB is denominated primary when no demonstrable tuberculous foci exist, and the disease may occur through a duct opening, by direct extension from contiguous structures (rib, sternum, costochondral cartilage, or shoulder joint), or from nipple and skin abrasions. It is classified as secondary when there is a tuberculous lesion elsewhere in the body and the breast is secondarily infected through hematogenous or lymphatic spread [26].

Diagnosis is established by the presence of granulomatous infiltrate and/or tubercle with central caseation on histology, or a positive *Mycobacterium* culture of the aspirate. Cultures are positive in 25–30% of cases, and Ziehl-Nielsen (ZN) stains are positive in 12%. It can also be reliably diagnosed by Fine-needle aspiration cytology (FNAC); epithelioid granulomas, Langhans giant cells, and lymphohistiocytic aggregates render the diagnosis. Failure to demonstrate necrosis on FNAC does not exclude TB in view of the small quantity of the sample harvested and examined. Demonstration of Acid-fast bacilli (AFB) is not mandatory, because in order for AFB to be observed microscopically, their number must be 10,000–100,000/mL of material [24, 25].

Polymerase chain reaction (PCR), developed for the diagnosis of TB, is highly sensitive, especially in culture-negative specimens from paucibacillary disease forms. PCR has positivity rates ranging from 40–90% in diagnosing tuberculous lymphadenitis [28].

Radiographic images are not different from those seen in granulomatous mastitis. Treatment for breast TB does not differ from that for pulmonary TB. Patients should be treated for 6 months, with 2 months of an intensive phase (a 4-drug combination: Isoniazid, Rifampin, Ethambutol, and Pyrazinamide), followed by a continuation phase of 4 months with two drugs (with Isoniazid and Rifampin). Patients treated with the previously mentioned first-line drugs usually achieve good response.

Duct Ectasia

Duct ectasia, also known as periductal mastitis, is a term that makes reference to the dilatation and inflammation of the terminal mammary ducts and to the presence of intraluminal secretions that cause rupture of the duct. Within benign breast pathologies, this occupies fifth place in frequency and, depending on the diagnostic method, its occurrence ranges between 1 and 75%. Duct ectasia presents most frequently in postmenopausal women aged between 40 and 60 years; it has also been described in young women, in girls, and in men [29–33].

In the literature diverse risk factors have been described, such as hormonal changes (especially those seen in older patients and during the premenstrual phase), nipple prolapse, vitamin A deficiency, multiple pregnancies, and smoking [33–36]. With regard to the latter, although the findings are controversial, a direct relationship has been observed between the smoking habit and the presence and recurrence of retroareolar abscesses and duct ectasia [36, 37].

The physiopathogenic mechanism of duct ectasia has been described as a dilatation of the retroareolar and subareolar ducts with segmentary centrifugal dissemination. The duct is distorted by alteration of the peripheral connective tissue, and within the lumen of the duct, there is an accumulation of fatty and serous material, or even fibrous tissue, causing tamponade [30, 31]. Some authors think that in addition to the dilatation and inflammation, bacterial contamination can play a relevant role. A chronic inflammation process can also be observed, with the presence of plasma cells. Histologically, the initial phase of ectasia is characterized by the presence of the dilatation of the main ducts in the subareolar region. The wall of the injured duct and the adjacent parenchyma present an intense inflammatory reaction, and can generate a granulomatous reaction to foreign body. Latter, the inflammatory process is substituted by fibrosis [31, 32].

Often, duct ectasia does not produce symptoms; however, many women can present miky galactorrhea from one or both nipples, as well as pain, erythema, a discrete increase in breast volume , nipple inversion or inflammation, especially when accompanied by infection.. Durring infancy [30], duct ectasia is usually manifested as a bloody discharge from the nipple; this condition usually resolves spontaneously after 6–9 months. While it is very rare in men, when it does present, nipple discharge may occur; less frequently, a retroareolar nodule may be palpated. A differential diagnosis of cancer is mandatory [32].

The diagnosis of ductal mammary ectasia is generally clinical; complementary examinations are recommended when there is diagnostic doubt. Mammograms can reveal asymmetrical findings, or can include calcifications that may mimic a carcinoma. Imagesare described as radiodense tubular structures that converge in the areolar-nipple complex [38].

By US, the duct appears as a smooth-walled thin anechoic image, with ramificating structures that narrow peripherally. The duct generally contains fluid or cellular residue; occasionally, it can contain calcifications [39]. These central findings trigger the diagnosis of a benign process, but duct ectasia can also be observed within a spectrum of malignant diseases. When localization of the duct ectasia is more toward the periphery and there is focal and irregular thickening in the wall of the duct, it is necessary to rule out a malignant process.

In the majority of cases, treatment is conservative. When pain is the prominent symptom, prescription of analgesics and anti-inflammatories is sufficient. Surgery is reserved for cases in which there is suspicion of malignancy and a biopsy is needed, as well as when required for the management of abscesses and fistulas [38, 39]. Resection is determined according to the extension, with selective resection of the affected duct performed through a periareolar incision in most cases. Alternately, resection may be performed en bloc for extensive areas of ductal ectasia, leaving a margin of healthy tissue at the periphery of the resected ducts [39]. In situations in which the symptoms are persistent, antimicrobial treatment can be initiated with coverage for anaerobic bacteria.

Fat Necrosis of the Breast

Fat necrosis of the breast is a benign inflammatory process. The first report in the literature was described by Hadfield in 1920 after the author reviewed the case of two patients whose histopathological findings revealed the presence of fat cells, excluding the preoperatory clinical diagnosis of breast cancer [40].

Fat necrosis is a rare disease. It is estimated to occur in between 0.6 and 2.75% of benign breast lesions. It has been observed in 0.8% of malignant mammary gland tumors and in up to 1% of patients who undergo reconstructive surgery [41]. Average age at presentation is 50 years.

In the literature, diverse risk factors have been described. Trauma is associated in up to 70% of cases. Radiotherapy, the use of anticoagulants, aspiration biopsies, conservative and reconstructive surgery, the placement of implants, duct ectasia, and breast infection have also been reported as associated risk factors [40]. In isolated cases, it has been associated with autoimmune diseases, such as polyarteritisnodosa, Weber-Christian disease, and granulomatous angiopanniculitis. It also can be idiopathic [41].

Fat necrosis is a sterile inflammatory process that results in the aseptic saponification of fat through the blood and the adipose tissue. It is recognized histologically by the presence of adipose tissue macrophages and foreign body giant cells surrounded by an interstitial infiltrate of plasma cells [42]. After trauma, hemorrhage extravasates to the parenchyma and the blood desiccates the fibrous planes of the breast, causing contusion. It can also occur as a consequence of capillary rupture, thrombophilia, allergic reaction, and thrombosis. Extravasation of blood into the parenchyma causes edema, inflammation, and ischemia, with the formation of intracellular vacuoles filled with necrotic lipid material. Later in the course of the disease, , calcifications adjacent to areas of fibrosis can be observed [43].

Fibroblasts and macrophages filled with lipid material accumulate in breast cystic areas. At a cellular level, there is apoptosis and necrosis, depending on the intensity of the interstitial lesion, which is a variable that determines whether apoptosis or necrosis predominates [42–44]. A major necrotic component results in more inflammation, a fact that translates into more clinical symptoms.

The symptomatic spectrum is variable. There are incidental, occult, and asymptomatic findings, or those found during a routine exploration. It can also present as a fixed nodule, simulating breast cancer. It generally appears as a mass of firm or hard consistency, often accompanied by skin or nipple retraction, cutaneous erythema, ecchymosis (an important findingsuggesting the diagnosis), and palpable axillary lymph nodes. Frequently, the lesion is superficial or subcutaneous. Hadfield et al. described 66% of lesions as petrous, up to 52% of lesions as adhering to the skin, and nipple retraction in approximately 10% [40]. Fat necrosis is more frequent in large breasts and atthe union of the upper quadrants. Occasionally it can be accompanied by nipple discharge. When it is related to surgery or trauma, it usually appears years later, at around 68.5 weeks[43, 44].

For the definitive diagnosis, a biopsy is required. Fine-needle aspiration cytology (FNAC) is a reliable and noninvasive method, with sensitivity and specificity of 87 and 99%, respectively. Use of this diagnostic tool can diminish the number of excisional biopsies; however, the diagnosis of fat necrosis can be limited by a sample with inadequate material. An incisional biopsy may be necessary when exclusion of a carcinoma is required as its diagnostic precision is superior to that of FNAC. From the radiological point of view, mastography and US are useful auxiliary studies. The appearance of fat necrosis in mastography images are afforded to a great extent by the degree of fibrosis. When there is no fibrosis or when there is a very small amount, the lesions tend to be benign in appearance, characterized by radiolucent images, dystrophic calcifications, and breast oil cysts. When there is fibrosis, the images are more irregular, and frequently, spiculated [45]. In approximately 4%, multiple pleomorphic calcifications suggestive of malignancy may be present(Figure 4).

US is also a useful tool in the diagnosis of fat necrosis, with hyperechogenic solid or cystic nodules of subcutaneous tissue and dim radiolucent posterior shadowing. US can diagnose breast oil cysts by defining an echogenic band that changes with the patient's orientation and position [45] (Figure 4).

Although less popular and more costly, magnetic resonance can be useful in the diagnosis of fat necrosis, with the advantage that there is high correlation of these images with histology. The images are described as hyperintense round or oval lesions in the T1 and T2 sequences, with fine capture of the contrast in the periphery surrounding an avascular center [46]. The presence and degree of enhancement depend on the intensity of the inflammatory process, being greater at initial stages when the inflammatory component is more vascularized. The lesions may or may not exhibit a poor fat component and predominance of granulation tissue, fibrosis, spiculated morphology and/or a thick and irregular peripheral uptake, indistinguishable from cancer.

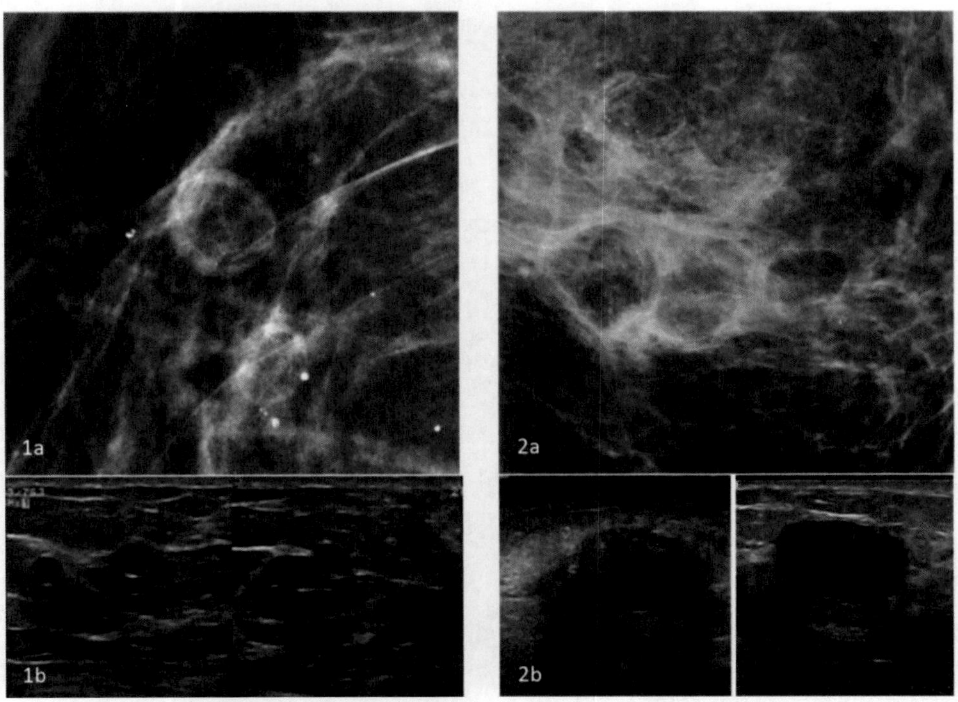

Figure 4. Fat necrosis: Mammogram of a patient with a previous contusion trauma in the right breast 1. a) In this mammography, breast oil cysts seen as radiolucent round lesions, with fine, dense walls are shown, b) echographic image characterized by cystic lesions with echogenic walls and posterior acoustic reinforcement. 2. a) Mammography with changes due to fat necrosis related to a previous image of abscess, showing multiple radiolucent images, circumscribed with a thin echogenic wall and ring or eggshell calcifications ; breast fat cysts, and b) echographic image characterized by complex cystic lesions.

Management is conservative at the beginning, including short-term follow-up with radiographic images and periodic physical examination. If there is any diagnostic doubt, an incisional biopsy is recommended along with radiolologic follow-up. Occasionally, surgical treatment is required. It is noteworthy that this is an exclusion diagnosis. [47].

Foreign Body-Related Reactions

The presence of a foreign body in the breast is an incidental finding during screening mammograms. Its incidence is low and, in the majority of cases, is associated with surgical interventions. Occasionally, there is a past history of foreign material injection or penetration of the breast and surrounding tissues by a foreign body [48].

These reactions are often the result of a prior cosmetic or esthetic surgical procedure. The voluntary injection of diverse materials to augment breast volume is common. Unfortunately, it can cause disease due to the injection of foreign materials, mainly, silicone.

Clinically, a reaction to a foreign body may manifest with enlarged axillary lymph nodes or granuloma formation [49]. In addition, breast prostheses may rupture causing their contents to migrate towards the skin, axillary region, arms, thorax or neck, with occasional fistula formation [49, 50].

Treatment is usually directed towards resolving complications, with poor results. The increased inflammatory response can be managed locally with steroids [51]. In (Figure 5)a sequence of images is shown.

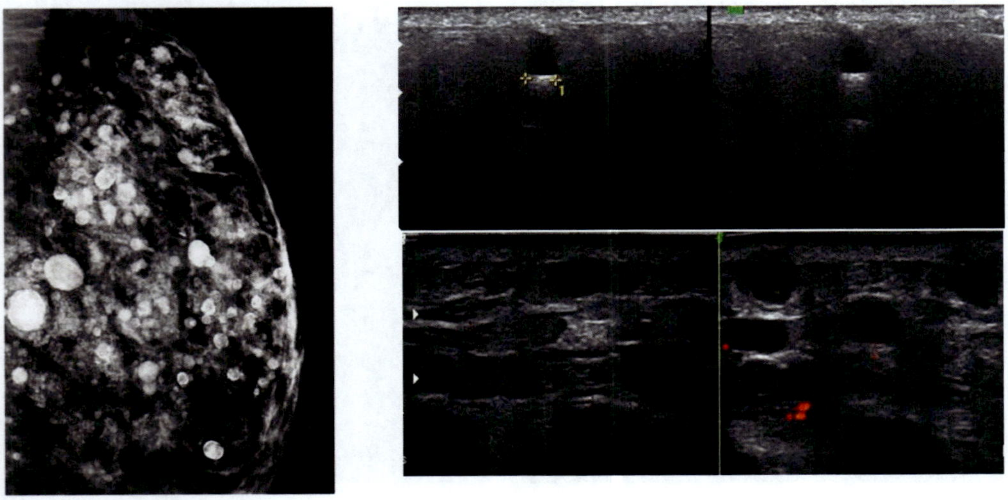

Figure 5. Breast injection of foreign materials (e.g., polyacrylamide) in a 47 year old female patient. In these images, diffuse increase of parenchymal density is shown, with nodules and breast cysts. By US, some disperse fat cysts are observed.

Acknowledgments

We are in debt to Dr. Robin Shaw for her review and valuable suggestions during the preparation of this chapter.

References

[1] Rosa, Marilin. "Inflammatory" changes in breast: how to provide a better care to our patients. *Arch GynecolObstet*, 2010, 281, 901-905.

[2] Amin, AL; Purdy, AC; Mattingly, JD; Kong, AL. Benign breast disease. *SurgClin North Am*, 2013, 93, 299-308.

[3] Trop, I; Dugas, A; David, J; ElKhoury, M; Jean-Francois, B; Larouche, NL. Breast abscesses: evidence-based algorithms for diagnosis, management, and follow-up. *Radiographic*, 2011, 31, 1683-1699.

[4] Bharat, A; Gao, F; Aft, RL; Gillanders, WE; Eberlein, TJ; Margenthaler, JA. Predictors of primary breast abscesses and recurrence. *World J Surg*, 2009, 33, 2582-2586.

[5] Gollapalli, V; Liao, J; Dudakovic, A; Sugg, SL; Scott-Conner, RJ; Weige, RJ. Risk factors for development and recurrence of primary breast abscesses. *J Am CollSurg*, 2010, 211,41-48.

[6] Imperiale, A; Zandrino, F; Calabrese, M; Parodi, G; et al. Abscesses of the breast: US-guided serial percutaneous aspiration and local antibiotic therapy after unsuccessful systemic antibiotic therapy. *ActaRadiol*, 2001, 42, 161-165.

[7] Bharat, A; Gao, F; Aft, RL; Gillanders, WE; et al. Predictors of primary breast abscesses and recurrence. *World J Surg*, 2009, 33, 2582-2586.

[8] Versluijs-Ossewaarde, FN; Roumen, RM; Goris, RJ. Subareolar breast abscesses: characteristics and results of surgical treatment. *Breast J*, 2005, 11, 179-182.

[9] Berná-Serna, JD; Berná-Mestre, JD; Piñero, A; Carrascosa, MC. Sonographically guided percutaneous intralesional triamcinolone injection: A new treatment for mammillary fistulas. Preliminary results. *J Ultrasound Med*, 2012, 31, 617-621.

[10] Hanavandi, S; Pereira, G; Mantel, RE. How mammillary fistulas should be treated. *Breast J*, 2005, 11, 254-256.

[11] Li, S; Grant, CS; Degnim, A; Donohue, J. Surgical management of recurrent subareolar breast abscesses: Mayo Clinic experience. *Am J Surg*, 2006, 192, 528-529.

[12] Kok, KY;Telisinghe, PU. Granulomatous mastitis: presentation, treatment and outcome in 43 patients. *Surgeon*, 2010, 8, 197-201.

[13] Oltean, HN; Soliman, AS; Omar, OS; Youssef, TF. Risk factors for chronic mastitis in Morocco and Egypt. (Abstract). *Int J Inflam*, 2013,184921. doi: 10.1155/2013/184921.

[14] Kessler, E;Wolloch, Y. Granulomatous mastitis: a lesion clinically simulating carcinoma. *Am J ClinPathol*, 1972, 58, 642-646.

[15] Patel, RA; Strickland, P; Sankara, IR; Pinkston, G; Many, W; Rodriguez, M. Idiopathic granulomatous mastitis: case reports and review of literature. *J Gen Intern Med*, *2009*, 25, 270-273.

[16] Hovanessian, Larsen, LJ; Peyvandi, B; Klipfel, N; Grant, E; Iyengar, G. Granulomatous lobular mastitis: imaging, diagnosis, and treatment. *AJR*, 2009, 193, 574-581.

[17] Wilson, JP; Massoll, N; Marshall, J; Foss, RM; Coopeland, M; Edward, M; Grobmyer, S. Idiopathic granulomatous mastitis: in search of a therapeutic paradigm. *Am Surg*, 2007,73, 798-802.
[18] Ozturk, E; Akin, M; Can, MF; Ozerhan, I; Kurt, B; Yagci, G; Tufan, T. Idiopathic granulomatous mastitis. *Saudi Med J*, 2009, 30, 45-49.
[19] Katz, U; Molad, Y; Ablin, J; Ben-David, D; Paran, D; Gutman, M; Langevitz. Chronic idiopathic granulomatous mastitis. *Ann N Y AcadSci*, 2007,1108, 603-608
[20] Erozgen, F; Erzoy, YE; Akaydin, M; Memmi, N; Celik, AS; Celebi, F; Guzey, Kaplan, F. Corticosteroid treatment and timing of surgery in idiopathic granulomatous mastitis confusing with breast carcinoma. *Breast CancerRes Treat*, 2010, 123, 447-452.
[21] Donn, W; Rebbeck, P; Wilson, C; Gilks, CB. Idiopathic granulomatous mastitis. A report of three cases and review of the literature. *Arch Pathol Lab Med*, 1994,118, 822-825.
[22] Mohammed, S; Statz, A; Lacross, JS; Lassinger, BK. Granulomatous mastitis, a 10 year experience from a large inner city county hospital. *J Surg Res*, 2013,184, 299-303.
[23] Baslaim, MM; Khayat, HA; Al-Amoudi, SA. Idiopathic granulomatous mastitis: a heterogeneous disease with variable clinical presentation. *World J Surg*, 2007, 31, 1677-1681.
[24] Mehmood, N; Zeeshan, HK; Khan, UA; Nawaz, A; Irfan, M; Khan, MI. Tuberculous mastitis- presentation and outcome in our setup. *Ann Pak Inst Med Sci*, 2009, 5, 245-250.
[25] Cuervo, SI; Bonilla, DA; Murcia, MI; Hernández, J; Gómez, JC. [Tuberculosis of the breast]. *Biomédica*, 2013, 33, 36-41.
[26] Gill, M; Chabbra, S; Sangwan, M; Singh, S; Praveen; Tanwar, P. Tuberculous mastitis- a great mimicker. *Asian Pac J Trop Dis*, 2012,2, 348-351.
[27] Soto, C; Vizcaíno, I; Isarria, S; Pastor, MR. [Tuberculosis of the breast: imaging findings in two patients]. *Radiología*, 2008, 50, 518-521.
[28] Tewari, M;Shukla, HS. Breast tuberculosis: diagnosis, clinical features and management. *Indian J Med Res*, 2005, 122, 103-110.
[29] Haagensen, CD. Mammary duct ectasia a disease that may simulate cancer. *Cancer*, 1951, 4, 749-761.
[30] Thomas, WG; Williamson, RC; Davies, JD; Webb, AJ. The clinical syndrome of mammary duct ectasia. *Br J Surg*, 1982, 69, 423-425.
[31] Dixon, JM; Ravisekar, O; Chetty, U; Anderson, TJ. Periductal mastitis and duct ectasia: different conditions with different aetiologies. *Br J Surg*, 1996, 83, 820-822.
[32] Chan, KW;Lau, WY. Duct ectasia in the male breast. *Aust N Z J Surg*, 1984,54, 173-176.
[33] Kelly, VM; Arif, K; Ralston, S; Greger, N; Scott, S. Bloody nipple discharge in an infant and a proposed diagnostic approach. *Pediatrics*, 2006, 117, 814-816.
[34] Peters, F;Schth, W. Hyperprolactinemia and non-puerperal mastitis (duct ectasia). *JAMA*, 1989,261,1618-1620.
[35] O'Brien, PH;Kreutner, AJr. Another cause of nipple discharge. Mammary duct ectasia with periductal mastitis. *Am Surg*, 1982, 48, 577-578.
[36] Rahal, RM; deFreitas-Junior, R; Paulinelli, RR. Risk factors for duct ectasia. *Breast J*, 2005, 11, 262-265.

[37] Bundred, NJ; Dover, MS; Aluwihare, N; Faragher, EB; Morrison, JM. Smoking and periductal mastitis. *BMJ*, 1993, 307, 772-773.

[38] Sweeney, DJ;Wylie, EJ. Mammographic appearances of mammary duct ectasia that mimic carcinoma in a screening programme. *AustralasRadiol*,995,39,18-23.

[39] Sakorafas, GH. Nipple discharge: current diagnostic and therapeutic approaches. *Cancer Treat Rev*, 2001, 27, 275-282.

[40] Hadfield, G. Fat necrosis of the breast. *Br J Surg*, 1930, 17, 673-682.

[41] Guray, M;Sahin, AA. Benign breast diseases: classification, diagnosis, and management. *Oncologist*, 2006,11, 435-449.

[42] Russo, AL;Taghian, AG. Fat necrosis of the breast in the accelerated partial breast irradiation era: the need for a universal grading system. *Breast Cancer Res*, 2013 Jul, 40,1-11.

[43] Rostom, AY;El-Sayed, ME. Fat necrosis of the breast: anunusual complication of lumpectomy and radiotherapy inbreast cancer. (Abstract). *ClinRadiol*, 1987,38, 31.

[44] Santen, RJ;Mansel, R. Benign breast disorders. *NEJM*, 2005, 353, 275-285.

[45] Bilgen, IG; Ustun, EE; Memis, A. Fat necrosis of the breast, clinical, mammographic and sonographic features. *Eur J Radiol*, 2001, 39, 92-99.

[46] Coady, AM; Mussurakis, S; Owen, AW; Turnbull, LW. Case report: MR imaging of fat necrosis of the breast associated with lipid cyst formation following conservative treatment for breast carcinoma. *ClinRadiol*, 1996,51,815-817.

[47] Tan, LM; Lai, EV; Carrington, AS; Opaluwa, AS; Ravikumar, KH; Chetty, N; Kaplan, V. Fat necrosis of the breast - a review. *Breast*, 2006, 15, 313-318.

[48] Caskey, CI; Berg, WA; Hamper, VM; Sheth, S; Chang, BW; Anderrson, ND. Imaging spectrum of extracapsular silicone: correlation of US, MR imaging, mammographic and histopathologic findings. *Radiographic*s, 1999, 19, S39-S51.

[49] Cho, N; Kimb, EK; Oh, KK; Son, EJ. Migrated foreign body granulomas on mammography after injection in the cervicofacial area. *ClinRadiol*, 2004, 59, 835-840.

[50] Bigata, X; Ribera, M; Bielsa, I; Ferrándiz, C. Adverse granulomatous reaction after cosmetic dermal silicone injection. *DermatolSurg*, 2001, 27, 198-200.

[51] Puckett, MA; DeFriend, D; Williams, MP; Roobottom, CA. A leaking breast prosthesis presenting as an abdominal mass. *Br J Radiol*, 2004, 77, 790-791.

In: Benign Disease of the Breast
Editors: J. de la Garza Salazar, C. Arce Salinas et al.
ISBN: 978-1-63321-624-2

Chapter 7

Fibrocystic Disease

Carlos Villegas-Cruz[1], Lesvia Olivia Aguilar-Cortazar[2] and David Cantu de Leon[3]

[1]Gynecology Oncology Department, Instituto Tecnólogico y de Estudios Superiores de Monterrey, Monterrey, NL, Mexico

[2]Radiology Department, Instituto Nacional Cancerologia-Mexico, Mexico City, DF, Mexico

[3]Clinical Research Department, Instituto Nacional Cancerologia-Mexico, Mexico City, DF, Mexico

Abstract

Benign lesions of the breast are a heterogeneous group of lesions that can present with a broad spectrum of symptoms, with fibrocystic changes the most common pathology of the breast, and these can be found in >50% of women. Cysts are considered a benign condition and analysis of the fluid is not necessary if it is citrine. Adenosis, either sclerosing or microglandular, could be found in around 5–7% of cancer-associated biopsies. Radial scar is a benign condition that in the majority of cases is an incidental finding in excisional biopsies of the breast, and it usually can be confounded with invasive disease because of the imaging characteristics. Intraductal papillomas are relatively infrequent and require a specific diagnostic process due to the broad spectrum of imaging characteristics. Among the proliferative breast lesions, epithelial hyperplasia is the most common entity, the atypical ones those associated with an increased risk for invasive carcinoma of the breast. Mammogram and ultrasound are very helpful in guiding the diagnostic process; nevertheless, core biopsy appears to be the most effective method in the diagnostic process of these conditions, and treatment must be individualized according to the patient's characteristics, familial history, and personal risk factors for developing an invasive neoplasm.

Introduction

Benign lesions of the breast are a heterogeneous group of lesions that can present with a broad spectrum of symptoms, as well as their high frequency in the general population, up to 30% of patients with these types of lesions will require some kind of treatment in their lives [1]. The importance of determining whether these lesions are a risk factor for the development of breast cancer is based on the classification proposed by Dupont and Page [2, 3], as nonproliferative lesions, proliferative lesions without atypia, and proliferative lesions with atypia. It is important to emphasize that up to 70% of the biopsies carried out due to a breast lesion will be reported as nonproliferative lesions.

The risk of cancer for each of the lesions depends on their histological characteristics, taking into account that nonproliferative lesions will not increase significantly the risk in comparison with the population not presenting these, while in proliferative lesions without atypia and in ductal or lobular hyperplasia, there is an increased risk of 1.3–1.9 and of 3.9–13 times, respectively, in comparison with general population [4]. In this respect, it is common to find discrepancies in terms of the results obtained in the different studies; because they tend to compare different groups of individuals as a reference (nonproliferative or proliferative lesions compared with the population without lesions), and that there are few cases of cancer associated with specific lesions [5].

Dupont and Page classification	
Nonproliferative lesions	Cysts, simple hyperplasia, simple, papillary apocrine changes
Proliferative lesions without atypia	Complex fibroadenoma, moderate or florid hyperplasia, florid sclerosing adenosis, radial scar, and intraductal papilloma
Proliferative lesions with atypia	Atypical lobular hyperplasia, atypical ductal hyperplasia

Adapted from: Dupont [6].

Fibrocystic Changes

Fibrocystic changes comprise the most common pathology of the breast, presenting with greatest frequency in women aged between 20 and 50 years, with highest incidence at the age of 40 years, when the hormonal function is at its maximal peak, and diminishing gradually when the women are in the menopause [7]. These changes tend to be multifocal and bilateral, causing breast pain and nodules that are very sensitive to the touch. The exact origin of these changes is unknown; however, a relationship has been found between alterations in the hormone balance with the predominance of estrogens. These changes are clinically present in more than 50% of women, and in the case that a breast biopsy is performed, this condition can be found in up to 90% of these and are associated with adenosis, epithelial ductal hyperplasia, apocrine metaplasia, radial scar, and papillomas. These pathologic findings are considered nonproliferative changes that entail three predominant morphological characteristics: the formation of cysts; fibrosis, and adenosis [8, 9], and have not been associated with an increase in the risk of cancer [2].

At present, with the studies that we now have, these type of lesion are frequently found in the population, diagnosis by fine-needle aspiration cytology is one of the most frequently utilized methods; however, it is noteworthy that among benign breast lesions, fibrocystic changes has the highest percentage of inadequate or indeterminate samples, this being as high as 38.6%, thus the importance of good sample-taking [10].

Mammary Cysts

These cysts are round or oval-shaped with liquid content that are found in one third of women between the ages of 35 and 50 years; clinically, only 20–25% of these cysts are palpable on physical exam and in the majority of cases, it presents as a unique cyst. Mammography and clinical examination cannot distinguish whether the palpable lesion is solid or cystic; thus, Ultrasound (US) of the breast and fine-needle aspiration are the most precise diagnostic tools [11, 12].

Simple cysts are circumscribed lesions with well-defined walls, anechoic, with posterior acoustic shadowing that lacks solid components on exploration by US (Figure 1). These are, by definition, benign and, if asymptomatic, only surveillance is recommended. On occasion, excessive growth can cause pain, which will be resolved with puncture of the lesion, which could be performed repeatedly if the lesion recurs. Analysis of the liquid is not recommended if it is clear or citrine; analysis should only be performed in cases in which the liquid aspirated is bloody. Due to that these do not raise the risk of cancer, only routine follow-up is recommended, depending on the patient's age and clinical and family history [13].

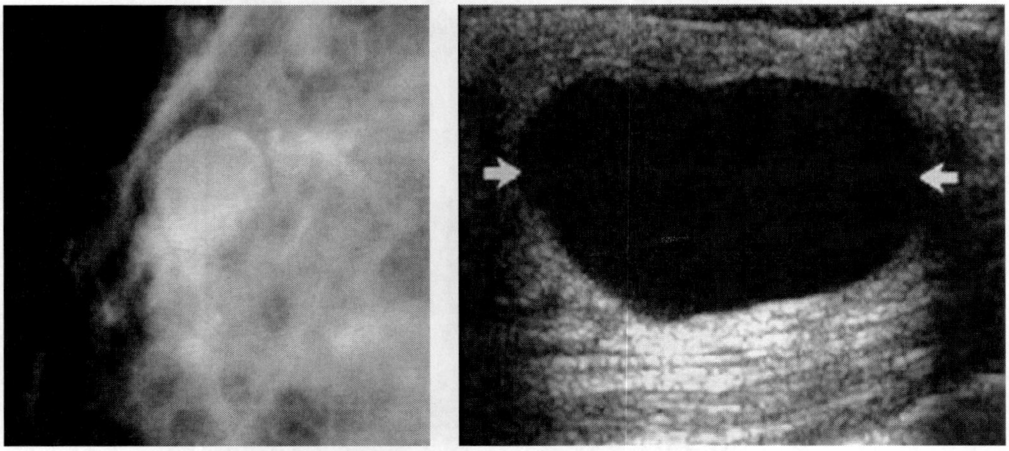

(A) (B)

Figure 1. (A) Mammographic magnification in Cranial to caudal view (CC) projection of the right breast in which a radiopaque nodule is identified, well defined, without calcifications. (B) Ultrasound (US) allows identification of the contents of the nodule, observing that it is anechoic with a thin wall and posterior acoustic reinforcement, in relation to a simple cyst.

Complicated cysts (Figure 2) are characterized by the presence of low-level internal echoes or detritus that change according to the position of the patient; they lack of thick walls, thick septae, or other discrete, solid components. Their risk for malignancy is less than 2%; therefore, these cysts can be followed by imaging in short time periods with aspiration of the content. However, if the cyst is symptomatic, of recent appearance, or is growing, it should be aspirated initially.

Complex cysts (Figure 3) are characterized by the presence of thick walls, thick septae, intracystic masses, or other solid components (Figure 3) [14]; a risk of malignancy has been reported as high as 21–31% [15, 16], thus indicating the performance of a percutaneous or an excisional biopsy.

Fibrocystic disease proceeds through distinct stages along time, such as dilatation of the ducts and acini to form cysts, proliferation and epithelial metaplasia, and the multiplication of ducts and acinar cells to give an image of adenosis, resulting in the obstruction of the terminal lobular duct unit [12].

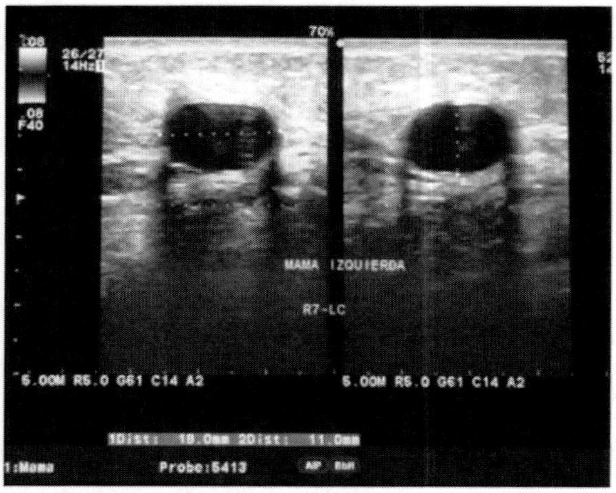

Figure 2. Complicated cyst: a ovoid image is identified in Ultrasound (US), predominantly hypoechoic, with a thin wall and some echoes in its interior that show movement in relation to debris.

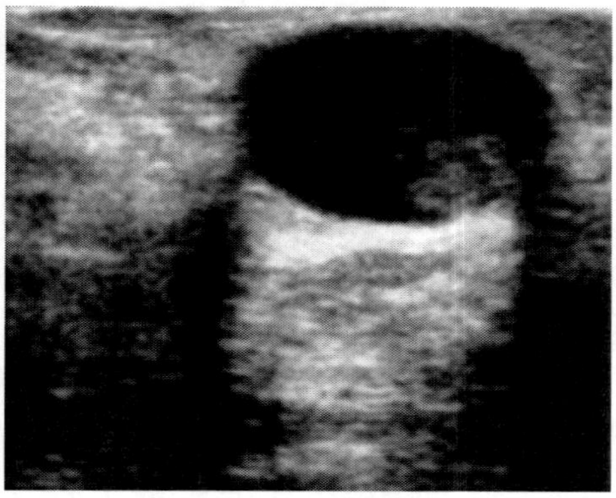

Figure 3. Complex cyst: an anechoic nodular image is identified, thin wall, with rounded hypoechoic image of lobulated cyst borders semidetached from the wall that does whose localization does not change with positioning of the patient in relation with a mural nodule.

After obstruction of the lobular duct unit, two types of cysts can be generated: Type 1 corresponds a secretory cyst that possesses active apocrine epithelial cells capable of producing a large amount of biocomponents that accumulate in the cyst, increasing cellular proliferation and promoting the development of atypia, hyperplasia, or preneoplastic alterations in the apocrine cyst, and Type 2 is a transudative cyst that only represents a retention cyst with a secretion similar to that of plasma and with a flat epithelium without hypertrophy; the difference between these types of cyst allows to explain their clinical behavior, because it is three times more probable that the unique cysts are flat epithelial cysts, and multiple cysts or those that appear repeatedly most probably correspond to apocrine cysts [17].

Adenosis

This is the increase in the number or size of the glandular components that form the lobular unit. Diverse types have been described, with sclerosing adenosis and microglandular adenosis being the most clinically important [11]. Sclerosing adenosis includes acinar cell, neoepithelial, and connective tissue elements that can mimic an infiltrating carcinoma. Histologically, it is characterized by an increase of fibrous tissue and intercalary glandular cells, with the characteristic of maintaining two cells lines along the basal membrane [18]. It presents in 12% of benign pathological samples and in 5–7% of cancer-associated samples [19]. Clinically, it can present as a palpable lesion or solely as a mastographic finding; it is related with other proliferative lesions, such as intraductal hyperplasia or sclerosing papilloma, complex sclerosing lesions, calcifications, and apocrine changes, in addition to being able to exist coexist with invasive cancer or *in situ* carcinoma [4, 20, 21]. Microglandular adenosis is characterized by the proliferation of small, rounded glands, irregularly distributed, with fibrous and dense adipose tissue. Its main histological characteristic is the lack of the external myoepithelial layer observed in other types of adenosis, which renders it difficult to differentiate it from tubular carcinoma. However, it can be differentiated from this carcinoma by the presence of the basal layer that surrounds the glandular structures and can also be demonstrated with the absence of staining of the epithelial membrane antigen in luminal epithelial cells [22]. Despite that is considered a benign lesion, in the case of not being completely resected it can recur, in addition that there is evidence of the potential of this lesion to become an invasive carcinoma (Figure 4) [23]. The apocrine adenosis, a variant of microglandular adenosis, is an apocrine change in deformed lobular units, sclerosing adenosis, radial scar, and complex sclerosing lesions. Tubular adenosis of the breast is another rare variant of microglandular adenosis that should be differentiated from tubular carcinoma, with the presence of an intact myoepithelial layer around the tubules the most useful characteristic [11].

Core biopsy appears to be the most effective method in the diagnostic process of these conditions; however, in the case of discrepancy among the clinics, imaging, or histological diagnoses, or in the case of existence cellular atypia, an excisional biopsy with hook localization should be the next step in the process of the diagnosis and treatment of these entities [19].

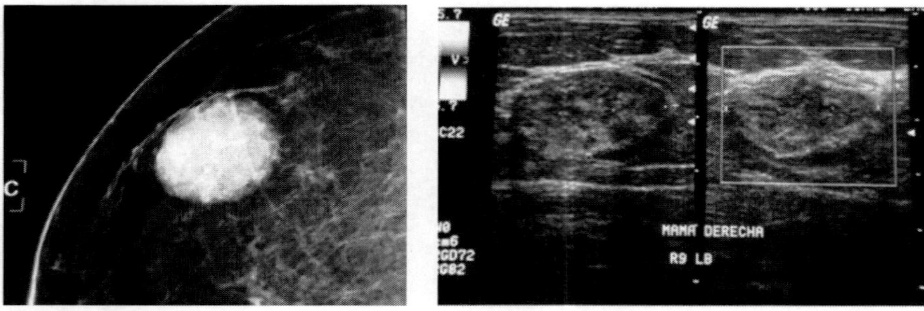

(A) (B)

Figure 4. Female aged 48 years who presented due to palpation of a nodule in her right breast. (A) Mammographic magnification in Cranial to Caudal view (CC) projection in which a microlobulated nodule was identified, partially defined, heterogeneous, and predominantly radiopaque with radiolucent areas in its interior. (B) Ultrasound (US) in which the presence was corroborated of a thin-walled, ovoid nodule, heterogeneous, predominantly hypoechoic with echogenic areas in its interior. A biopsy performed reported a microglandular adenosis.

Radial Scar

The radial scar is a benign lesion that consists of a fibroelastic nucleus surrounded by radial ducts and lobules with or without intraluminal proliferation that show epithelial hyperplasia, adenosis, ductal ectasia, and papillomatosis. This has also been denominated sclerosing papillomatosis, sclerosing ductal proliferation, indurate mastopathy, noncapulated sclerosing lesion, infiltrating epitheliosis, or radial sclerosing lesion (Figure 5) [24].

Some authors have suggested to name a radial scars to those lesions smaller than 1 cm, and complex sclerosing lesions to those larger than 1 cm, which are related to epithelial ductal hyperplasia.

In the majority of cases, this is an incidental finding in excisional biopsies of the breast, but its incidence has increased due to the greater number of mammograms performed in screening programs. Radiographic findings are unspecific and can simulate a carcinoma by the presence of spiculated lesions; performing a fine-needle biopsy is not useful and even with core needle biopsy, it is possible not to obtain the definitive diagnosis, because it is not possible to rule out malignancy when performing histological correlation with the radiographic image. Thus, if there is the suspicion that this is a radial scar, excisional biopsy of the lesion is recommended, depending on the size of the latter and amount of tissue obtained with the core needle biopsy, because in small lesions, the use of this latter model is acceptable with the desire of obtaining a precise diagnosis, therefore planning a resective procedure and not submitting the patient to treatment in two surgical procedures [25, 26, 27, 28].

Papilloma

Intraductal papilloma is a benign tumor originated from the epithelium of the mammary ducts, with greatest frequency in the terminal part of them. These lesions are relatively infrequent that require a specific diagnostic process due to the broad spectrum of imaging characteristics that they entertain, as well as the histopathological aspect and the potential risk of cancer, in which the Radiologist as well as the Pathologist play very important roles in determining these lesions [29]. Central papillomas tend to be unique, while peripheral papillomas can be multiple. Clinically, these are characterized by bloody discharge from the nipple (Figure 6).

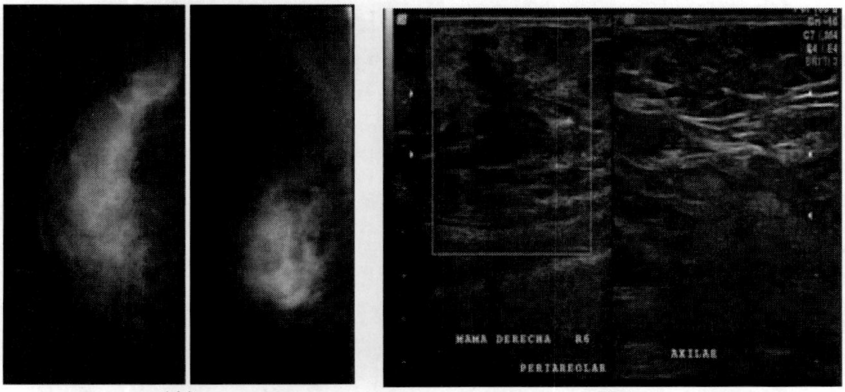

(A) (B)

Figure 5. Radial scar: Female 43 years of age, asymptomatic, who presents for a screening mammogram. (A) Right breast mammogram in which a dense, heterogeneously fibroglandular pattern is observed, a stellate lesion is identified in the middle third of the internal quadrants of the breast, a nearly retroareolar view in Cranial to Caudal (CC) projection that is modified in Mediolateral Oblique view (MLO). (B) In the Ultrasound (US), the presence is corroborated of a hypoechoic zone with spiculated borders, poorly defined in radial 6. Histopathological correlation is carried out with a hook marking. Radial scar was evidenced in the pathologic sample.

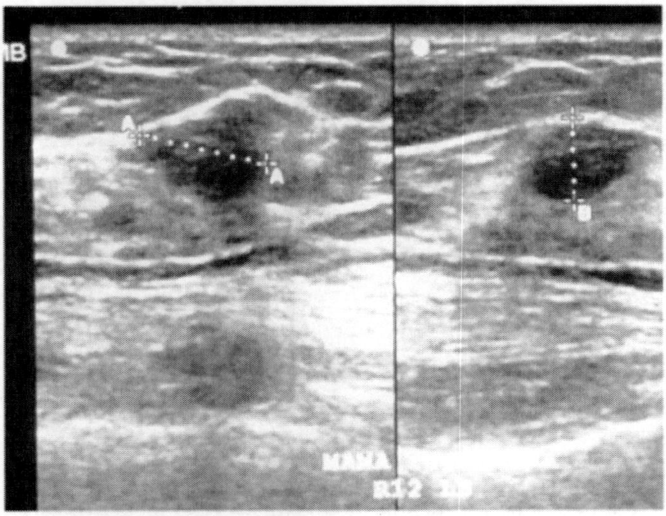

Figure 6. Breast Ultrasound (US) in which an ovoid nodule can be observed, partially defined, of heterogeneous echotexture predominantly hypoechoic, with cystic areas in its interior, of recent appearance. A biopsy was taken, corroborating the diagnosis of intraductal papilloma without atypia.

Papillomatosis is defined as the presence of at least five papillomas that are separated from each other but distributed in a localized segment of the breast, generally in the subareolar or peripheral region. It is common for these to present bilaterally; in case of being localized peripherally in the breast, they have a greater possibility of having a carcinoma *in situ* or an invasive carcinoma in comparison with the central papilloma. The diagnosis of these entities should be performed by excisional biopsy and, due to the increase in the risk of a malignant neoplasm, and the contralateral breast should be evaluated to discard this [30].

Histologically, these are characterized by the formation of epithelial ramifications that have a luminal epithelium and a layer of external myoepithelial cells, together with a fibrovascular stroma. In the epithelial component are found, in addition, changes ranging from metaplasia to hyperplasia, atypical ductal hyperplasia and, on occasion, carcinoma *in situ*.

Central papillomas are not considered as possessing a risk of malignancy, as long as atypia is not found in the surrounding tissue; some studies have shown a relationship between the presence of atypical ductal hyperplasia in papillary lesions in core needle biopsies and the presence of carcinoma *in situ* or invasive carcinoma when an excisional biopsy is performed [31, 32]. Thus, in case of finding atypia in an excisional biopsy, the surrounding tissue should be carefully checked; one must make sure that there is no malignant neoplasia in order to be able to continue with surveillance of the patient [33]. If the decision is made to conduct a core needle biopsy, it is preferable to use vacuum-assisted biopsy, because the latter entertains a much lesser risk of underestimating the presence of a malignant lesion, contrary to what happens when taking a biopsy with a core, 16-gauge and 18-gauge needles, which can by-pass a malignant neoplasm in up to 16 and 17.9%, respectively [34].

Epithelial Hyperplasia

Epithelial hyperplasia is the most common proliferative breast lesion and it is divided into lobular or ductal lesions. The ductal epithelium normally consists of two layers of cuboid cells. The increase in the number of layers is considered hyperplasia, which is classified according to the degree, the architecture, and the cytological characteristics of the cells. Usual or simple ductal hyperplasia is an increase in the number of cells without distorting the architecture and without distending the contour of the duct. Usual-type, mild hyperplasia presents 3–4 layers of epithelial cells that proliferate; in moderate hyperplasia, more than 4 layers are present, accompanied by septae of luminal space, while in florid hyperplasia, the lumen is distended and on occasion, obliterated. In each of these lesions, epithelial cells, myoepithelial cells, and apocrine metaplastic cells are found and tend to be combined, with morphologic differences in the characteristics of the epithelial cells and their nuclei; however, none of these increase the risk of breast cancer [11]. Proliferative lesions with atypia are divided into ductal or lobular hyperplasias with atypia and are characterized by the presence of ductal or lobular elements with the loss of uniform cells with loss of basal–apical cell orientation [4].

Currently, with the increased use of mammogram as the screening test for breast cancer and the detection of microcalcifications, the diagnosis of ductal hyperplasia with atypia is performed in up to 30% of percutaneous biopsies. The Relative risk (RR) of developing invasive breast cancer associated with atypical hyperplasia is 3–6 times higher; however, in patients with first-degree familial antecedents, this can rise up to 10 times [35].

The risk of developing invasive breast cancer will be present in both breasts, being greater in the affected breast. In cases of atypical ductal hyperplasia, cancer usually presents 10–15 years after the diagnosis of hyperplasia, and this risk diminishes after 15 years. After carrying out the diagnosis of this lesion by percutaneous biopsy, it is necessary to perform an excisional biopsy to confirm the diagnosis of the hyperplasia and to ensure not having found a ductal carcinoma *in situ*, which can present in 15–50% of cases [36].

In the case of lobular lesions, both atypical lobular hyperplasia as well as lobular carcinoma *in situ*, and in contrast with ductal lesions, these are grouped under the term lobular neoplasia due to that they exhibit histological characteristics that are very similar, and the only difference is the extension and degree of epithelial proliferation. Both lesions are considered more as a risk factor than as a precursor lesion of invasive cancer; clinically, it is rare for these to manifest themselves; it is more probable to come upon them as an incidental finding in excisional biopsies conducted for other lesions [11].

They are more common in perimenopausal women, with a greater probability of being a multifocal lesion and encompassing multiple quadrants of the breast. The RR of developing invasive cancer rises to 4 times in the case of lobular hyperplasia and up to 10 times in cases of lobular carcinoma *in situ*, its appearance being 3 times more probable in ipsilateral breast, where it can be found 15–20 years after the initial diagnosis [36].

In patients with these types of lesions, it is recommendable to consider the use of strict surveillance, as well as to consider the use of chemoprophylaxis with Tamoxifen or Raloxifene [37, 38].

Conclusion

Fibrocystic changes and associated conditions are very common abnormalities during the lifetime of women, several conditions do not increase the risk of cancer while others do; therefore, image studies as well as tissue sample might be essential in differentiating a lesion with the advantage of providing the specific diagnosis and propose a treatment.

References

[1] Sangma, MB; Panda, K; Dasiah, S. A clinico-pathological study on benign breast diseases. *J Clin Diagn Res*, 2013 Mar, 7(3), 503-506. doi: 10.7860/JCDR/2013/5355.2807

[2] Dupont, WD; Page, DL. Risk factors for breast cancer in women with proliferative breast disease. *NEJM*, 1985, 312(3), 146-151.

[3] Bernardi, S; Londero, AP; Bertozzi, S; Driul, L; Marchesoni, D; Petri, R. Breast-feeding and benign breast disease. *J Obstet Gynaecol*, 2012, 32(1), 58-61. doi:10.3109/01443615.2011.613496

[4] Rungruang, B; Kelley, JL; 3rd. Benign breast diseases: epidemiology, evaluation, and management. *Clin Obstet Gynecol*, 2011, 54(1), 110-124. doi: 10.1097/GRF.0b013e318208010e

[5] Kabat, GC; Jones, JG; Olson, N; Negassa, A; Duggan, C; Ginsberg, M; Kandel, RA; Glass, AG; Rohan, TE. A multi-center prospective cohort study of benign breast disease and risk of subsequent breast cancer. *Cancer Cause Control*, 2010, 21(6), 821-828. doi: 10.1007/s10552-010-9508-7

[6] Dupont, WD; Parl, FF; Hartmann, WH; Brinton, LA; Winfield, AC; Worrell, JA; Schuyler, PA; Plummer, WD. Breast cancer risk associated with proliferative breast disease and atypical hyperplasia. *Cancer*, 1993, 71(4), 1258-1265.

[7] Amin, AL; Purdy, AC; Mattingly, JD; Kong, AL; Termuhlen, PM. Benign breast disease. *Surg Clin North Am*, 2013, 93(2), 299-308. doi: 10.1016/j.suc.2013.01.001

[8] Schnitt, SJ; Connolly, JL. Pathology of benign breast disorders. In: Harris JR, Lippman ME, Morrow M, Osborne CK, Editors. Diseases of the Breast. 3rd ed. Philadelphia, PA, USA: Lippincott, Williams & Wilkins, 2004. 77-100.

[9] Tavassoli, FA. Intraepithelial neoplasia: risk factors for subsequent development of invasive carcinoma. In: Tavassoli FA. Pathology of the Breast. 2nd ed. Hong Kong: Appleton & Lange, 1999. 205-323.

[10] Yamaguchi, R; Tsuchiya, S; Koshikawa, T; Yokoyama, T; Mibuchi, K; Nonaka, Y; Ito, S; Higuchi, H; Nagao, M; Higaki, K; Watanabe, J; Kage, M; Yano, H. Evaluation of inadequate, indeterminate, false-negative and false-positive cases in cytological examination for breast cancer according to histological type. *Diagn Pathol*, 2012, 7, 53. doi: 10.1186/1746-1596-7-53

[11] Guray, M; Sahin, AA. Benign breast diseases: classification, diagnosis, and management. Oncologist, 2006, 11(5), 435-449.

[12] Rinaldi, P; Ierardi, C; Costantini, M; Magno, S; Giuliani, M; Belli, P; Bonomo, L. Cystic breast lesions: sonographic findings and clinical management. *J Ultrasound Med*, 2010, 29(11), 1617-1626.

[13] Hartmann, LC; Sellers, TA; Frost, MH; Lingle, WL; Degnim, AC; Ghosh, K; Vierkant, RA; Maloney, SD; Pankratz, VS; Hillman, DW; Suman, VJ; Johnson, J; Blake, C; Tlsty, T; Vachon, CM; Melton, LJ 3rd; Visscher, DW. Benign breast disease and the risk of breast cancer. *N Engl J Med*, 2005, 353(3), 229-237.

[14] American College of Radiology. ACR BI-RADS® Ultrasound. In: ACR Breast Imaging Reporting and Data System, Breast Imaging Atlas. Reston, VA, USA: *American College of Radiology*, 2003.

[15] Berg, WA; Campassi, CI; Ioffe, OB. Cystic lesions of the breast: sonographic-pathologic correlation. *Radiology*, 2003, 227(1), 183-191.

[16] Doshi, DJ; March, DE; Crisi, GM; Coughlin, BF. Complex cystic breast masses: diagnostic approach and imaging-pathologic correlation. *RadioGraphics*, 2007 Oct, 27(Suppl 1), S53-S64. doi: 10.1148/rg.27si075508

[17] Dixon, JM; Scott, WN; Miller, WR. Natural history of cystic disease: the importance of cyst type. *Br J Surg*, 1985, 72(3), 190-192.

[18] Yoshida, A; Hayashi, N; Akiyama, F; Yamauchi, H; Uruno, T; Kikuchi, M; Yagata, H; Tsugawa, K; Suzuki, K; Nakamura, S; Tsunoda, H. Ductal carcinoma *in situ* that involves sclerosing adenosis: high frequency of bilateral breast cancer occurrence. *Clin Breast Cancer*, 2012, 12(6), 398-403. doi: 10.1016/j.clbc.2012.08.002

[19] Taşkin, F; Köseoğlu, K; Unsal, A; Erkuş, M; Ozbaş, S; Karaman, C. Sclerosing adenosis of the breast: radiologic appearance and efficiency of core needle biopsy. *Diagn Interv Radiol*, 2011, 17(4), 311-316. doi: 10.4261/1305-3825.DIR.3785-10.2

[20] Jensen, RA; Page, DL; Dupont, WD; Rogers, LW. Invasive breast cancer risk in women with sclerosing adenosis. *Cancer*, 1989, 64(10), 1977-1983.

[21] Kundu, UR; Guo, M; Landon, G; Wu, Y; Sneige, N; Gong, Y. Fine-needle aspiration cytology of sclerosing adenosis of the breast: a retrospective review of cytologic features in conjunction with corresponding histologic features and radiologic findings. *Am J Clin Pathol*, 2012, 138(1), 96-102. doi: 10.1309/ AJCP8MN5GXFZULRD

[22] Eusebi, V; Foschini, MP; Betts, CM; Gherardi, G; Millis, RR; Bussolati, G; Azzopardi, JG. Microglandular adenosis, apocrine adenosis, and tubular carcinoma of the breast. An immunohistochemical comparison. *Am J Surg Pathol*, 1993, 17(2), 99-109.

[23] Acs, G; Simpson, JF; Bleiweiss, IJ; Hugh, J; Reynolds, C; Olson, S; Page, DL. Microglandular adenosis with transition into adenoid cystic carcinoma of the breast. *Am J Surg Pathol*, 2003, 27(8), 1052-1060.

[24] Farid, M. Essentials of Diagnostic Breast Pathology. A Practical Approach. Berlin, Germany: Springer-Verlag, 2007.

[25] Fasih, T; Jain, M; Shrimankar, J; Staunton, M; Hubbard, J; Griffith, CD. All radial scars/complex sclerosing lesions seen on breast screening mammograms should be excised. *Eur J Surg Oncol*, 2005, 31(10), 1125-1128.

[26] Jacobs, TW; Byrne, C; Colditz, G; Connolly, JL; Schnitt, SJ. Radial scars in benign breast-biopsy specimens and the risk of breast cancer. *NEJM*, 1999, 340(6), 430-436.

[27] Patterson, JA; Scott, M; Anderson, N; Kirk, SJ. Radial scar, complex sclerosing lesion and risk of breast cancer. Analysis of 175 cases in Northern Ireland. *Eur J Surg Oncol*, 2004, 30(10), 1065-1068.

[28] Tóth, D; Sebő, É; Sarkadi, L; Kovács, I; Kiss, C; Damjanovich L. Role of core needle biopsy in the treatment of radial scar. *Breast*, 2012, 21(6), 761-763. doi: 10.1016/j.breast.2012.02.009

[29] Jagmohan, P; Pool, FJ; Putti, TC; Wong, J. Papillary lesions of the breast: imaging findings and diagnostic challenges. *Diagn Interv Radiol*, 2013, 19(6), 471-478. doi: 10.5152/dir.2013.13041

[30] Ali-Fehmi, R; Carolin, K; Wallis, T; Visscher, DW. Clinicopathologic analysis of breast lesions associated with multiple papillomas. Hum Pathol, 2003, 34(3), 234-239.

[31] Agoff, SN; Lawton, TJ. Papillary lesions of the breast with and without atypical ductal hyperplasia: can we accurately predict benign behavior from core needle biopsy? *Am J Clin Pathol*, 2004, 122(3), 440-443.

[32] Ivan, D; Selinko, V; Sahin, AA; Sneige, N; Middleton, LP. Accuracy of core needle biopsy diagnosis in assessing papillary breast lesions: histologic predictors of malignancy. *Mod Pathol*, 2004, 17(2), 165-171.

[33] MacGrogan, G; Tavassoli, FA. Central atypical papillomas of the breast: a clinicopathological study of 119 cases. *Virchows Arch*, 2003, 443(5), 609-617.

[34] Jie-Ying, Z; Jie, T; Yu-Kun, L; Shuai, F; Qing, S; Qing-Hua, X. Underestimation of papillary breast lesions at ultrasound-guided breast biopsy. *Zhongguo Yi Xue Ke Xue Yuan Xue Bao*, 2013, 35(6), 662-666. doi: 10.3881/j.issn.1000-503X.2013.06.014

[35] Pinder, SE; Ellis, IO. The diagnosis and management of pre-invasive breast disease: ductal carcinoma *in situ* (DCIS) and atypical ductal hyperplasia (ADH)- current definitions and classification. *Breast Cancer Res*, 2003, 5(5), 254-257.

[36] Dupont, WD; Page, DL. Relative risk of breast cancer varies with time since diagnosis of atypical hyperplasia. *Hum Pathol*, 1989, 20(8), 723-725.

[37] Fisher, B; Costantino, JP; Wickerham, DL; Cecchini, RS; Cronin, WM; Robidoux, A; Bevers, TB; Kavanah, MT; Atkins, JN; Margolese, RG; Runowicz, CD; James, JM; Ford, LG; Wolmark, N. Tamoxifen for the prevention of breast cancer: current status of the National Surgical Adjuvant Breast and Bowel Project P-1 study. *J Natl Cancer Inst*, 2005 Nov 16, 97(22), 1652-1662.

[38] Hershman, D; Sundararajan, V; Jacobson, JS; Heitjan, DF; Neugut, AI; Grann, VR. Outcomes of tamoxifen chemoprevention for breast cancer in very high-risk women: a cost-effectiveness analysis. *J Clin Oncol*, 2002, 20(1), 9-16.

In: Benign Disease of the Breast
Editors: J. de la Garza Salazar, C. Arce Salinas et al.
ISBN: 978-1-63321-624-2

Chapter 8

Superficial and Deep Vascular Lesions

Flavia Morales-Vásquez, Horacio Noé Lopez-Basave, Kuauyama Luna-Ortiz, Dolores Gallardo-Rincón, Aura Rubi Espejo-Fonseca, Arturo Albrant-Salmeron, Eva Ruvalcaba-Limón, Antonio Maffuz-Aziz, Martin Granados-Garcia and Jaime G. de la Garza-Salazar
Medical Oncology Department,
Instituto Nacional Cancerologia-Mexico, Mexico City, DF. Mexico

Abstract

In this chapter, we describe different benign vascular lesions, including iatrogenic necrosis, spontaneous infarction, superficial migratory thrombophlebitis (Thrombophlebitis migrans), subclavian and axillary vein thrombosis, and Mondor's disease.

Fat necrosis or iatrogenic thrombosis is a benign inflammatory process that originates in adipose mammary tissue. Spontaneous infarction is a rare entity. Superficial migratory thrombosis is a disease in which phlebitis appears in small segments and that is characterized by multiple recurrences in a variety of localizations and at a variety of times. Upper limb thrombosis is a rare condition that has exhibited an increase in recent decades and that is, in many cases, due to lifestyle and to novel therapeutic modalities, while Mondor's disease or thrombophlebitis of the venous-thoracoepigastric system is localized, benign, and transitory.

All of these have in common that they should be differentiated from infection, inflammation and, rarely, from carcinoma.

Iatrogenic Necrosis

Fat necrosis or iatrogenic thrombosis is a benign inflammatory process that originates in adipose mammary tissue and was initially described in the breast in 1920 [1,2]. Hadfield described it as "an innocent breast lesion" that presents among women in the fourth or fifth decades of life, frequently with a history of recently resected fixed tumor [3]. Knowledge of the physiopathology of necrosis is fundamental for arriving at a correct diagnosis of this entity of very diverse appearance, in its clinical form, as well as in its different imaging modalities. It is excessively associated with malignant lesions.

Epidemiology

Incidence of the disease is estimated to be <0.6% in breast. It represents 2.75% of all benign lesions [1–4]. Fatty necrosis is found in 0.8% of breast tumors and in 1% of cases of surgical breast reduction [5]. Median age of patients is 50 years [4].

Etiology

Fat necrosis is a benign inflammatory process. It is very frequently considered idiopathic, but is generally cause by a trauma, and many cases considered idiopathic are due to microtraumas (21–70%) and other clinically associated conditions. The trauma that leads to fat necrosis of the breast can be the result of accidents or clinical treatments. Among accidental agents, the harm cause by automobile seat belts in traffic accidents is frequent, while iatrogenic agents, include breast surgeries (biopsies, lumpectomies, breast reductions, breast remodeling with implants or injection with silicone, paraffin, or other exogenous substances, and Transverse rectus abdominis [TRAM] or Deep inferior epigastricperformation [DIEP] flap breast reconstruction techniques, etc.) and, less frequently, percutaneous procedures (including excisional biopsy, imaging-assisted biopsy, or fine-needle aspiration cytology), radiotherapy[6–8], chemical irritation caused by anticoagulants[9] or the rupture of cysts or mammary duct ectasia, and some systemic diseases such as panniculitis (Weber-Christian disease), which come to have a pathogenesis and imaging manifestations similar to those of fat necrosis.

Pathogenesis

Fat necrosis is a sterile inflammatory process that results in the saponification of the fat by means of tissue lipase and the blood. Its appearance is varied depending on the state of the process. It is recognized histologically as a lesion with abundant macrophages filled with fat and surrounded by foreign giant cell bodies and plasma cells with interstitial infiltrate. After trauma to the breast, hemorrhage occurs within the surgical cavity, or it extravasates toward the parenchyma. The blood desiccates along the fibrous plane of the breast (contusion). Contusion can take place secondary to capillary rupture, thrombophilia, allergic reaction, and arterial or venous thrombosis.

At the cellular level, there is cell death, whether due to necrosis or to apoptosis; everything will depend on the severity of the insult, and a fine balance between apoptosis and necrosis will determine the clinical and radiological appearance of fat necrosis of the breast. A greater necrotic component will result in greater inflammation and a more sinister aspect.

Clinical Condition

The clinical presentation of fat necrosis entertains a clinical range that extends from an incidental and benign finding to a nodule that is highly suggestive of cancer. In the majority of cases, it is clinically occult; however, it can manifest as a nodule or various nodules: firm, round, and soft, or as an irregular mass, associated with ecchymosis, erythema, inflammation, pain, skin or nipple retraction, and even grown lymph glands, to the degree of simulating a carcinoma.

Hadfield[3] described 66% as a benign, petrous mass; 52% of the lesions were adhered to the skin, and 10% were associated with nipple retraction. Adair and Munzer described that 64% of patients had a skin affectation. Pullybank and colleagues[4] found signs suggestive of cancer in 45% of cases.

In the majority of those clearly related with trauma, the nodular mass appears at several weeks from the occurrence of damage due to trauma (within a range of 3–208 weeks) [4]. Fat necrosis is commonly found in superficial breast tissue and in the subareolar regions of obese women with pendulous breasts [10].

Diagnosis

The diagnosis is histopathological; however, it is necessary to consider the imaging studies prior to performing the biopsy.

Fine-needle aspiration biopsy (FNAB) is very limited, because it is sufficiently probable that it will be inadequate or that it will require being performed on repeated occasions.

Incisional biopsy is more adequate, with greater precision, but remains very limited. In the face of an incisional biopsy negative for malignancy, of an undetermined lesion, it is correct to carry out an excisional biopsy.

Imaging studies are very sensitive to the detection of alterations in this pathology, but poorly specific. Mastography [10] will show radiolucent, round, or oval cysts, with skin deformation, subcutaneous (s.c.) tissues, focal masses and, on occasion, speckled masses, and can even generate pleomorphic microcalcifications, multiple, and very suspicious of malignancy. Confusing the findings with images of fibrocystic mastopathy is most frequent.

Ultrasound (US) [11] reports a mass with intracystic lesions that modifies its aspect over time: these can look like complex cysts with echogenic internal bands. The solid mass is generally found well-circumscribed, with well-defined borders, despite distorting the mammary parenchyma. The most common US image in fat necrosis is the increase of s.c. tissue echogenicity and anechoic cysts with posterior acoustic shadowing.

Nuclear magnetic resonance (NMR) permits identification of an extensive gamma of changes originating due to fat necrosis, which can further orient the diagnosis, but in reality, the image obtained by means of this study is indistinguishable from that of a malignant. In conclusion, although the suspicion exists of fat necrosis by imaging, it is necessary to perform the excisional biopsy [12,13].

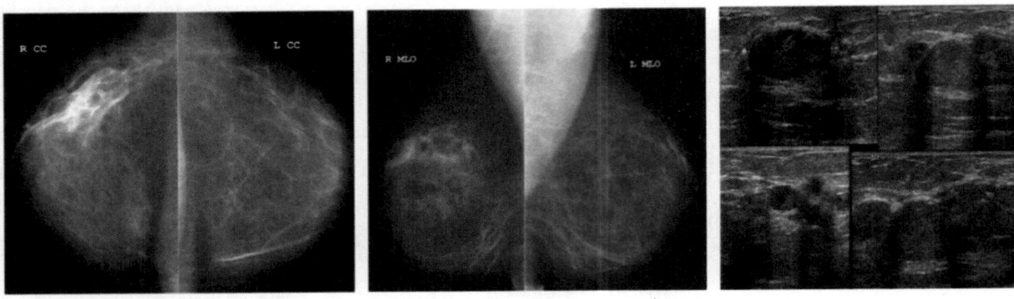

Figure 1. Iatrogenic necrosis post- biopsy.

Treatment

Management of fat necrosis continues to pose a challenge in clinical practice, from its diagnostic approach up to its management.

For example, in patients with a diagnosis of cancer submitted to conservative or reconstructive surgery, it is necessary to discard recurrent cancer, even by performing serial incisional biopsies, to confirm the diagnosis.

Even when there is a clear history of trauma, surgery, or biopsy, when faced with this presentation one must always suspect a subadjacent neoplasm, or discard it.

Management includes excisional biopsy, strict clinical follow-up, and frequent imaging studies every 3 or 6 months. Soo et al. [14] concluded that in terms of the sensitivity of current imaging studies, a lesion with sufficient benign characteristics could be managed with surveillance, as long as the lesion does not undergo changes that are suspicious of malignancy. The value of Positron emission mammography (PEM) [15] is not yet determined in this pathology.

Conclusions

The diagnosis of fat necrosis is only exclusion after discarding other possibilities, and the best option is excisional biopsy. After performing this, strict vigilance should be continued.

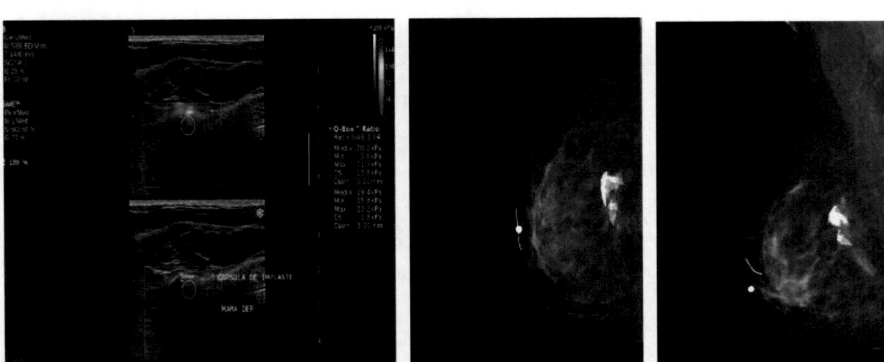

Figure 2. Iatrogenic necrosis post- prosthesis.

Spontaneous Infarction

This is a highly rare entity. It is described after performing biopsies for establishing the histopathological diagnosis in fibroadenomas, and with greater frequency in situations of pregnancy and lactancy, according to the cases and series reported. Infarction in a fibroadenoma of the breast was described by Delarue and Rendon in 1949 [16]. It should be differentiated from mastitis, mammary duct ectasia and, rarely, from carcinoma.

Epidemiology

Haagensen described the presence of spontaneous infarct of the breast in fibroadenomas in 0.5%, while other studies reported incidences of 0.9%, and a recent study of Al-Atrooshi reported the highest incidence, at 3.6%. On average, the literature suggests an index of 0.3% [16].

Etiology

In some cases, there is speculation concerning the physiological conditions of the increase in mammary metabolism as the triggering factor, especially in situations of pregnancy or lactancy [17]; other etiological factors are attributed to mechanical factors in fibroadenomas, where it is considered that the latter are very mobile, and torsion can be experienced, although it is surprising that its incidence should be so low. Some other conditions of the breast can be complicated with spontaneous infarct, such as intraductal papilloma, phyllodes tumor, and in some cases of patients under treatment with anticoagulants [18] and, in an even rarer form, with oral contraceptives.

Pathogenesis

The pathogenesis of spontaneous infarct has not been clearly established. Authors coincide in discarding preexisting vascular lesions for defining its diagnosis, and it has been proposed that the infarct occurs as a consequence of a relative vascular deficiency resulting from an increase in the metabolic demands of the mammary tissue, and that thrombosis takes place first and then the infarct is secondary, as proposed by Hasson and Pope in 1961 [18] and corroborated by other authors.

Clinical Condition

It generally presents in young women with a history of pregnancy or lactancy, with a rapidly growing nodule, mobile, and very painful. It is frequently the antecedent of performing a biopsy.

Diagnosis

US and Magnetic resonance imaging (MRI) are the auxiliary studies that can provide the greatest amount of data. They generally identify well-circumscribed tumors.

Aspiration biopsy reveals focal necrosis, on occasion hemorrhage, without evidence of malignant cells. Occasionally, there are areas of reassembled squamous metaplasia, sometimes called necrotizing syringometaplasia [16].

Treatment

Treatment is excisional biopsy, in view of the pain and the accelerated growth.

Conclusion

Spontaneous infarct is an extremely rare entity, without a clear etiological explanation and without defined risk factors.

Superficial Migratory Thrombphlebitis (Thrombophlebitis Migrans)

Superficial migratory thrombosis is a disease in which phlebitis appears in small segments in superficial veins and is characterized by superficial migratory thrombophlebitis. It is a disease in which phlebitis appears in small segments of the superficial veins and that is characterized by multiple recurrences in a variety of localizations and at a variety of times.

It is different from the thromboses, in which initially a vein is observed to be involved and there is a gradual extension of venous compromise. The first to employ the term “Thrombophlebitis migrans” was Hedblom in 1916, although cases had already been described within this category since 1845 by Jadioux, Frémy in 1864, and by Paget in 1866 [19]. In 1865, Trousseau described, for the first time, the association between thrombosis and cancer; the author originally described a very strange case of superficial migratory thrombosis, but afterward the name Trousseau syndrome was utilized to describe all cases of hypercoagulability associated with cancer.

Epidemiology

This is an entity that is probably much more frequent than reported in the literature. In the U.S., it occurs in 125,000 persons annually [20], in 1 of every 1,950 inhabitants; in France it occurs in 253,000: 1 of every 250 inhabitants is affected by superficial thrombosis. It has not been determined how many patients have affected mammary glands [21].

Etiology

It appears that varicose veins can be the risk factor that is most implicated. However, there is an extensive range of predisposing conditions, such as the following: immobilization; trauma; obesity; the hypercoagulability state; employment of oral hormones; hormone therapy; prior history of deep venous or superficial thrombosis; cancer, or autoimmune diseases [20].

There is superficial thrombosis of various veins and various sites, with previously described predisposing factors, in which there can be states of hypercoagulability in up to 35% of patients. Underlying diseases, such as neoplasias and vasculitis, must be eliminated with appropriate studies or tests[20].

Pathogenesis

These superficial throboses could be associated with the Factor V Leiden mutation, the mutation of the gene *20210* into an abnormal plasminogen, disorders of the activator factor of the tissular plasminogen, lupus anticoagulant, and the anticardiolipin syndrome, as well as with some primary hematological diseases such as polycythemia, thrombocythemia, and falciform cell disease [20,21].

Clinical Condition

The patient typically present erythematosus areas, along the superficial-vein trajectory, with heat and subadjacent swelling. The vein can be distended into a site proximal to the thrombosis. The pain can increase rapidly and become very intense.

Diagnosis

Diagnosis is established with the aid of Doppler US, when faced with a previously described clinical condition. The underlying disorder that can cause a state of hypercoagulability should be diagnosed [19–21].

It is important to ascertain the patient's clinical history, risk factors, and familial history. On occasion, thrombophilias, neoplasias, or vasculitis should be investigated.

Treatment

Treatment has as its basic objectives the control of pain, avoiding extension of the thrombus, complications, and recidivism, with medical and surgical treatment.

Within medical treatment: analgesics and anticoagulants, with the objective of reducing symptoms, with locally applied heat, anti-inflammatory agents and occasionally, compression measures [21].

Treatment is focused on diminishing pain, decreasing inflammation, and on preventing complications and recurrence. Much will depend on whether this is an initial event or a recurrent episode.

Surgical management is not an initial option, nor a preferred one, but should be opted for in very particular cases.

Anticoagulant therapy is not sustained in all patients, only in those presenting recurrent events, persistent symptoms, and progression of the thrombosis.

Conclusion

Superficial migratory thrombophlebitis is very frequent in general, although there isno precise data regarding its incidence. It is a phenomenon that in general comprises the superficial manifestation of diverse underlying diseases. Serious diseases such as neoplasias and vasculitis must be discarded with appropriate studies or tests.

Subclavian and Axillary Vein Thrombosis

Upper limb thrombosis is a rare condition that has exhibited an increase in recent decades and that is, in many cases, due to lifestyle and to novel therapeutic modalities. This does not affect the mammary gland directly or in terms of priority [20,21].

Epidemiology

According to the literature, only from 4–10% of all cases of venous thrombosis involve the veins, whether subclavian, axillary, or brachial [21].

Etiology

It is considered that in the absence of risk factors for the state of hypercoagulability, such as sedentarism, advanced age, coagulation disorders, trauma, or surgery, axillary or subclavian vein thrombosis is due to a mechanical condition of venous compression. This compression should be prolonged and asymptomatic [22,23,24].

Over recent decades, its incidence has increased due to the more frequent employment of central venous catheters and the implantation of cardiac pacemakers. In sum, the most common risk is cancer. This is considered primary and nearly one third of cases are classified as effort or idiopathic trombosis, or secondary if there are underlying risk factors [25].

Pathogenesis

Upper limb venous thrombosis can be classified as primary or secondary according to its pathogenesis [25]. Primary upper limb venous thrombosis is also known as Paget-Shrötter syndrome, which was described independently by Sir James Paget and at the same time by Leopold von Shrötter in the XIX century. Notwithstanding this, it is also called "effort thrombosis". It can occur spontaneously. What takes place, whether by exercise or previous physical effort, is a microtrauma at the level of the cap of the vessel, called theintima, by means of pressure of the clavicle, the first rib, or the dorsal muscle. This can present in women or men, in young and healthy persons, and has been found with greatest frequency on the right side [22,24].

Secondary venous trombosis is the more frequent presentation and can occur in patients with predisposing clinical situations such as catheter use for vascular access in patients requiring chemotherapy, transplantation, parenteral nutrition, or hemodialysis, or in states of hypercoagulability due to underlying diseases. The employment of defibrillators or pacemakers can also give rise to the risk of thrombosis in this trajectory. Affectation of mammary tissue will be due to contiguity.

Clinical Condition

It is usually characterized by pain and edema of the arm, occasionally with extension to the mammary gland; however, it can present asymptomatically, especially in patients with prolonged employment of a central venous catheter.

In the case of effort thrombosis, the clinical presentation is very dramatic; the presence of pain is important, with an increase of the latter, and this can have a fatal evolution, with secondary deaths due to that the risk of pulmonary thromboembolism is high and post-thrombotic syndrome and recurrence are present.

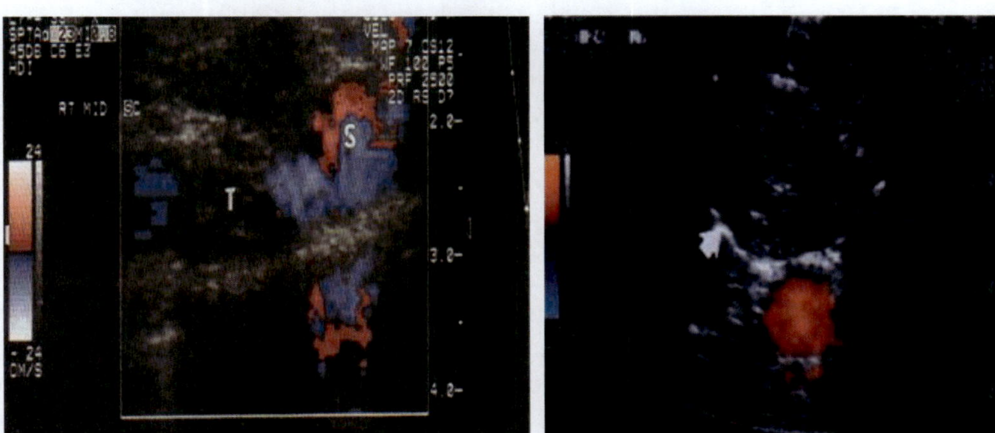

Figure 3. Subclavian vein thrombosis by Doppler ultrasound.

Diagnosis

The clinical condition in general is dramatic, as has been described previously and it requires rapid evaluation, especially when anticoagulation or thrombolysis treatment is being considered [25].

The best auxiliary imaging constitutes Doppler ultrasound.

Treatment

The basic objectives of treatment are pain control, avoiding extension of the thrombus, complications, and recurrence, with medical and surgical treatment.

Within medical treatment there are analgesics and anticoagulants, with the objective of reducing symptoms, with locally applied heat, anti-inflammatory agents and occasionally, compression measures [21].

Treatment focuses on diminishing pain, decreasing inflammation, and preventing complications and recurrence. This will depend greatly on whether this is an initial event or a recurrent episode.

Surgical management is not an initial option, nor a preferred one; the former should be opted for in very particular cases. Surgical management should be proposed very critically in cases with an antecedent of previous venous thromboembolism or medical conditions that contraindicate anticoagulation.

Anticoagulant therapy is not sustained for all patients, only for those presenting recurrent events, persistent symptoms, progression to thrombosis, or for those requiring prolonged employment of venous accesses.

Conclusions

In sum, on being confronted with the suspicion of axillary or subclavian vein trombosis, Doppler US should be carried out; the majority can be treated in ambulatory form, with analgesics, anti-inflammatories, topically applied heat and, in determined cases, anticoagulation.

Mondor's Disease

Mondor's disease, or thrombophlebitis of the venous-thoracoepigastric system, is localized, benign, and transitory. This condition was described in 1869 by Fagge [26], but did not become well-known until after the publication of Dr. Fránces Henri Mondor, who detailed its underlying pathology, its clinical course, and its resulting sequalae [27]. Thus, it is known as Mondor's disease.

Epidemiology

There is no adequate report of its incidence. A retrospective study in 9,675 patients with breast cancer demonstrated an incidence of 0.95% [28]. In a report of 2,052 mammoplasties, an incidence of 1.07% was described [28]. All reports describe populations of young women between the ages of 21 and 66 years, with a mean age of 43 years in one study and of 33 years in another [27–30].

Etiology

The process initiates in a superficial axillary vein of the thorax and is directed toward the right side, due to the presence of the unidirectional flow that prevents retrograde circulation at the level of the venous valves; this leads to ectasia and consequently, to the formation of thrombi or blood clots. There is a hypothesis that a protein S deficiency can favor the presence of Mondor's disease [31]. It is a disease that more frequently affects women than men, in a proportion of 3:1 [32].

Pathogenesis

Mondor's disease is frequently associated with breast cancer, but other numerous causes favor it, such as trauma, venous catheterization, and the use of intravenous (i.v.) drugs. In the absence of apparent causes, the physiopathological mechanism that would appear to be related is continuous compression of the venous walls, which can occur due to pectoral muscle contractions [33].

Johnson et al. describe its physiology as a phenomenon that initiates at a minimum and that is transitory, but with acute inflammation accompanied by trombosis and the organization of a clot in a superficial vein [29,34]. The fibrotic disease stage is characterized by the formation of a subcutaneous (s.c.) cord that leads to the formation of a fold in the skin.

Clinical Condition

The typical presentation is a cord in the thoracoabdominal wall, which is more visible when both arms are raised. The cord is firm, hard, and painful.

Diagnosis

The disease can affect one or more veins: the lateral thoracic vein, and the superior epigastric vein. US imaging gives the appearance of a slender cord through the dense and hyperechoic thoracic wall [33].

Treatment

This is basically focused on pain management; symptoms persist for 5–8 weeks [35,36] Anti-inflammatories and analgesics can provide help; invasive management is not recommended.

Conclusion

Mondor's disease is a process that is generally infrequent, benign, and transitory, whose diagnosis is clinical and whose treatment is symptomatic. Disease evolution is slow, but self-limiting.

References

[1] Lee, BJ; Adair, F. Traumatic fat necrosis of the female breast. *Ann Surg*, 1920, 72, 188-195.

[2] Adair, FE; Munzer, JT. Fat necrosis of the female breast: report of one hundred test cases. *Am J Surg*, 1947, 74, 117-128.

[3] Hadfield, G. Fat necrosis of the breast. *Br J Surg*, 1930, 17, 673-682.

[4] Pullyblank, AM; Davis, JD; Basten, J; Rayter, Z. Fat necrosis of the female breast-Hadfield re-visited. *Breast*, 2001, 10(5), 388-391.

[5] Pui, MH; Movson, IJ. Fatty tissue breast lesions. *Clin Imag*, 2003, 27(3),150-155.

[6] Stefanik, DF; Brereton, HD; Lee, TC; Chun, BK; Citgay, O; Dritschilo, A. Fat necrosis following breast irradiation for carcinoma, clinical presentation and diagnosis. *Breast*, 1982, 8, 4-6.

[7] Clarke, D; Curtis, JL; Martínez, A; Fajardo, L; Goffinet, D. Fat necrosis of the breast simulating recurrent carcinoma after primary radiotherapy in the management of early stage breast carcinoma. *Cancer*, 1983, 52(3), 442-445.

[8] Rostom, AY; El Sayed, ME. Fat necrosis of the breast: an unusual complication of lumpectomy and radiotherapy in breast cancer. (Abstract). *Clin Radiol*, 1987, 38, 31.

[9] López Valle, CA; Herbert, G. Warfarin-induced complete bilateral breast necrosis. *Br J PlastSurg*, 1992, 45, 606-609.

[10] Hogge, JP; Robinson, RE; Magnant, CM; Zuurbier, RA. The mammographic spectrum of fat necrosis of the breast. *RadioGraphics*, 1995,15(6),1347-1356.

[11] Atasoy, MM; Oren, NC; Ilica, AT; Güvenç, İ; Günal, A; Mossa-Basha, M. Sonography of fat necrosis of the breast: correlation with mamography and MR imaging. *J Clin Ultrasound*, 2013, 41(7), 415-423.

[12] Parker, SH; Burbank, F; Jackman, RJ; Aucreman, CJ; Cardenosa, G; Cink, TM; et al. Percutaneous large-core breast biopsy: a multi-institutional study. *Radiology*, 1994, 193(2), 359-364.

[13] Tan, PH; Lai, LM; Carrington, EV; Opaluwa, AS; et al. Fat necrosis of the breast. A review. *Breast*, 2006, 15, 313-318.

[14] Soo, MS; Kornguth, PJ; Hertzberg, BS. Fat necrosis in the breast: sonographic features. *Radiology*, 1998, 206(1), 261-269.

[15] Akkas, BE; UcmakVural, G. Fat necrosis may mimic local recurrence of breast cancer in FDG PET/CT. *Rev Esp Med Nucl Imagen Mol*, 2013, 32(2), 105-106

[16] Skenderi, F; Krakonja, F; Vranic, S. Infarcted fibroadenoma of the breast: report of two new cases with review of literature. *Diagn Pathol*, 2013, 8, 38.

[17] Hasson, J; Pope, H. Mammary infarcts associated with pregnancy presenting as breast tumor. *Surgery*, 1961, 49, 313-316.

[18] Deshpande, KM; Deshpande, AH; Raut, WK; Lele, VR; Bobhate, SK. Diagnostic difficulties in spontaneous infartaction of a fibroadenoma in an adolescent: case report. *Diagn Cytopathol*, 2002, 26, 26-28.

[19] Sullivan, JM; Walske, BR. Thrombophlebitis migrans. *Ann Surg*, 1950,132(2), 260-267.

[20] Litzendorf, ME; Satiani, B. Superficial venous thrombosis: disease progression and evolving treatment approaches. *Vasc Health Risk Manag*, 2011, 7, 569-575.

[21] Czarnevicz, D. Trombosisvenosa superficial. *Biomedica*, 2006, 2(3), 229-238.

[22] Allana, AM; Teo, LL; Chuah, BY; Liu, TC; Cheah, WK. Effort thrombosis in a young triathlete: an unusual presentation of painless neck swelling secondary to right brachiocephalic vein thrombosis. *Singapore Med J*, 2011, 52(3), e37-e39.

[23] Spiezia, L; Simioni, P. Upper extremity deep vein thrombosis. *Int J Emerg Med*, 2010, 2, 103-109.

[24] Thompson, RW. Comprehensive management of subclavian vein effort thrombosis. *Semin Intervent Radiol*, 2012, 29, 44-51.

[25] Rosen, T; Chang, B; Kaufman, M; Soderman, M; Riley, DC. Emergency department diagnosis of upper extremity deep venous thrombosis using bedside ultrasonography. *Crit Ultrasound J*, 2012, 4,1-5.

[26] Fagge, CH. Remarks on certain cutaneous affections. (Abstract). *Guy's Hosp Rep*, 1870, 15, 302.

[27] Mondor, H. Tronculite sous-cutanéesubaiguë de la paroithoracigueantéro-latérale. *Mem Acad Chir*, 1939, 65,1271-1278.

[28] Hou, MF; Huang, CJ; Huang, YS; et al. Mondor's disease in the breast. *Kaohsiung J Med Sci*, 1999, 15, 632-639.

[29] Bejanga, BI. Mondor's disease: analysis of 30 cases. *J Royal Coll Surg Edinb*, 1992, 37, 322-324.

[30] Cox, E; Siegel, D. Mondor disease: an unusual consideration in a young woman with a breast mass. *J Adolesc Health*,199721(3),183-185.

[31] De Godoy, JM; Godoy, MF; Batigália, F; Braile, DM. The association of Mondor'sdisease with protein S deficiency: case report and review of literature. *J Thromb Thrombolys*, 2002, Jun13(3),187-189

[32] Kikano, GE; Cáceres, VM; Sebas, JA. Superficial thrombophlebitisof the anterior chest wall (Mondor's disease). *J Fam Pract*, 1991, 33, 643-644.

[33] Draghi, F; Tarantino, CC; Madonia, L; Ferrozzi, G. Ultrasonography of the male breast. *J Ultras Med*, 2011,14, 122-129.

[34] Farrow, JH. Thrombophlebitis of the superficial veins of the breast and anterior chest wall (Mondor's disease). *Surg Gynecol Obstet*, 1955,101, 63-68.

[35] Sivula, A; Somer, T. Mondor's disease- observation on 14 patients and survey of literature. *Ann ChirGynaecolFenn*, 1973, 63, 361-369.

[36] Dirschka, T; Winter, K; Bierhoff E. Mondor's disease: a rare cause of anterior chest pain. *J Am Acad Dermatol*, 2003, 49, 905-906.

In: Benign Disease of the Breast
Editors: J. de la Garza Salazar, C. Arce Salinas et al.
ISBN: 978-1-63321-624-2

Chapter 9

Proliferative Stromal Lesions

Heriberto Medina-Franco and Adrian Mauricio Garza-Gangemi
Surgical Oncology Department, Instituto Nacional Ciencias Medicas y Nutricion Salvador Zubiran-Mexico, Mexico City, DF, Mexico

Abstract

Proliferative stromal lesions include Diabetic fibrous mastopathy (DFM), Pseudoangiomatous stromal hyperplasia (PASH), and Complex sclerosing lesion (CSL) or Radial scar (RS). The main interest in these lesions is that they are commonly diagnosed as malignant breast lesions. DFM is a fibrous fibroinflammatory lesion that represents <1% of benign breast lesions. It occurs predominantly in premenopausal women with long-standing insulin-dependent Diabetes mellitus (DM), although it has also been observed in patients with type 2 diabetes. Clinical findings included single or multiple ill-defined, nontender, palpable, firm-to-hard masses in one or both breasts that raise suspicion of carcinoma. Microscopically, they are characterized by keloid fibrosis and variable periductal, perilobular, or perivascular lymphocytic infiltration that consists primarily of B cells. DM has not been linked with subsequent development of breast carcinoma or stromal neoplasia. If core biopsy is sufficient for diagnosis, a surgical excision can be avoided, because there are reports that surgery may exacerbate the condition. PASH is an even more uncommon lesion with approximately 300 cases described in the literature. It may present in a broad clinicopathologic spectrum ranging from an incidental histological finding to a clinically palpable breast mass, typically unilateral. On histological examination, the typical lesion is composed of complex anastomosing, slit-like empty spaces in a dense fibrous stroma. Core needle biopsy is warranted in suspicious cases to exclude malignancy. The treatment of PASH depends on its clinical presentation. No additional specific treatment is required if PASH is an incidental finding in specimens excised for other lesions. An excision with adequate but close margins is the recommended treatment for tumorous PASH; the lesion is not considered a premalignant lesion or a risk factor for malignancy. RS is a rare benign breast lesion of unknown etiology commonly identified by screening mammography. RS are by definition <1 cm and CSL, which are considered part of the same disease continuum, are described as their larger counterpart (>1 cm). The incidence of this condition has increased significantly due to the implementation of national breast cancer screening programs and is considered to be from 0.03–0.09%. These lesions are usually nonpalpable and have radiological and gross pathological characteristics that mimic breast carcinoma. Classical findings of an RS on mammograms include a stellate lesion with the presence of a radiolucent center with long, fine radiodense spicules, which create a "black star" appearance. Currently, diagnostic procedures are unreliable and due to the inherent risk of RS for underlying malignancy, the safest and most recommended approach for treatment of a suspicious stellate lesion is surgical excision.

Diabetic Fibrous Mastopathy

Diabetic fibrous mastopathy (DFM) is an uncommon mastopathy associated with diabetes mellitus that can mimic a malignant neoplasm on physical examination. Diabetic mastopathy [1], also called diabetic fibrous breast disease [2], was first described by Soler and Khardori in 1984 as a dense, fibrous stromal proliferation that occurred in women with long-standing type I diabetes mellitus and multiple microvascular complications. Since that time, further studies have elucidated the histopathologic features of this unusual fibroinflammatory lesion that represents <1% of benign breast lesions.

Table 1. Clinical findings in diabetic mastopathy

Author, Year (Y)	Cases	DM, complications	Other endocrine disease	Age of onset (Y)	Duration of DM (Y, average)	Multiple or bilateral
Soler NG [1], 1984	12	11	5	32.2	20.3	10
Byrd BF [10], 1987	8	8	NS	33.9	6.0–37.0	NS
Logan WW [11], 1989	36	NS	NS	38.0	13.0	24
Tomaszewski JE [6], 1992	8	6	2	40.0	22.6	3
Seidman JD [7], 1994	5	3	NS	47.0	>13.0	NS
Morgan MC1 [12], 1995	20	7	NS	62.0	4.0–43.0	NS
Camuto PM [13], 2000	5	4	1	34.0	20.4	3
Andrews-Tan, 2000 [14]	11	9	NS	39.0	24.2	4
Valdez R [15], 2003	11	7	2	43.8	NS	NS
Martínez-Ramos [16], 2007	4	4	NS	39.0	14.5	NS
Chan [17], 2013	10	7	NS	61.5	10.0–40.0	0

DM = Diabetes mellitus; Y = Years; NS = Not stated.

Clinical Characteristics

The mean age of patients at diagnosis of the initial breast lesion ranged from 32.2–62 years, with duration of diabetes mellitus ranging from 4–43 years. The condition has also been observed in patients with type 2 diabetes mellitus who were insulin-dependent [6,7] and in patients with other endocrine disorders, especially thyroid diseases [1, 6, 7]. There have been rare reports of this condition in men [6, 8, 9]. A summary of the clinical features reported in the literature is presented in Table 1.

Clinical findings included single or multiple ill-defined, nontender, palpable, firm-to-hard masses in one or both breasts that raise the suspicion of carcinoma. About 60% of DFM tend to be bilateral and have a predilection for the subareolar region [18]. These lesions tend to recur after surgical excision [13].

Radiologic Findings

Mammographical features are usually unremarkable in DFM due to the presence of dense breast tissue (Figure 1).

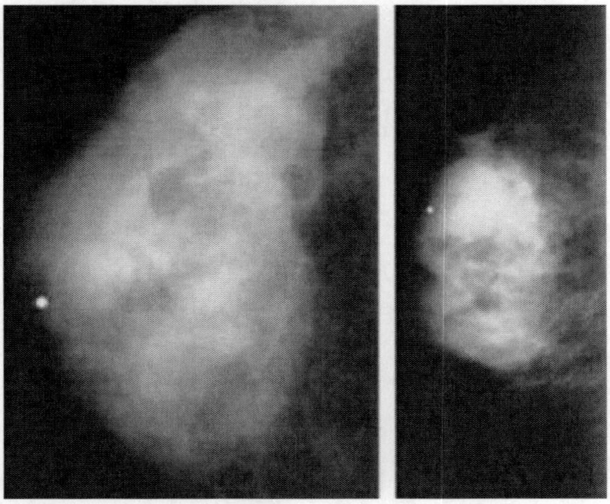

Figure 1. Left craniocaudal and mediolateral views of a mammogram obtained in a 40-year old patient with type 1 diabetes mellitus and a palpable mass in the subareolar area of the left breast, showing very dense breast parenchyma with a focal area of higher density at the site of the palpable mass (dot).

Ultrasonography (US) shows an irregular hypoechoic mass with posterior acoustic shadowing [11] (Figure 2).

Attenuation increases in proportion to the percentage of fibrous tissue [19], and the finding of strong acoustic shadowing is in keeping with the diagnosis of DFM. It is noteworthy that these US features are also characteristically observed in malignant breast disease.

Recent literature proposes that Magnetic resonance imaging (MRI) features of DFM show the absence of enhancing mass with nonspecific stromal enhancement as opposed to carcinoma, where there is a presence of an avidly enhancing focal mass with irregular margins [20]. One study states that MRI reveals homogeneous low enhancement with a gradual and progressive course without a washout. A corresponding time-intensity curve is related with benign lesions of low vascularity, the latter a potential criterion for differentiating between DFM and malignant processes [21] (Figure 3).

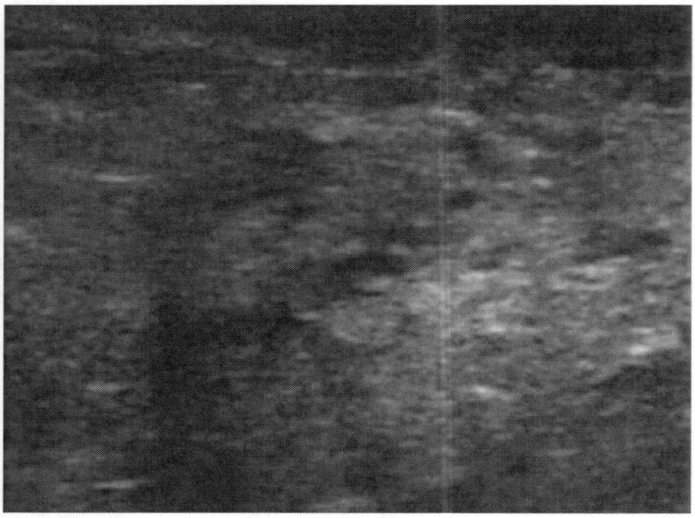

Figure 2. Ultrasound image of the left breast from the same patient showing irregular, mixed-echogenicity lesion with posterior acoustic shadowing.

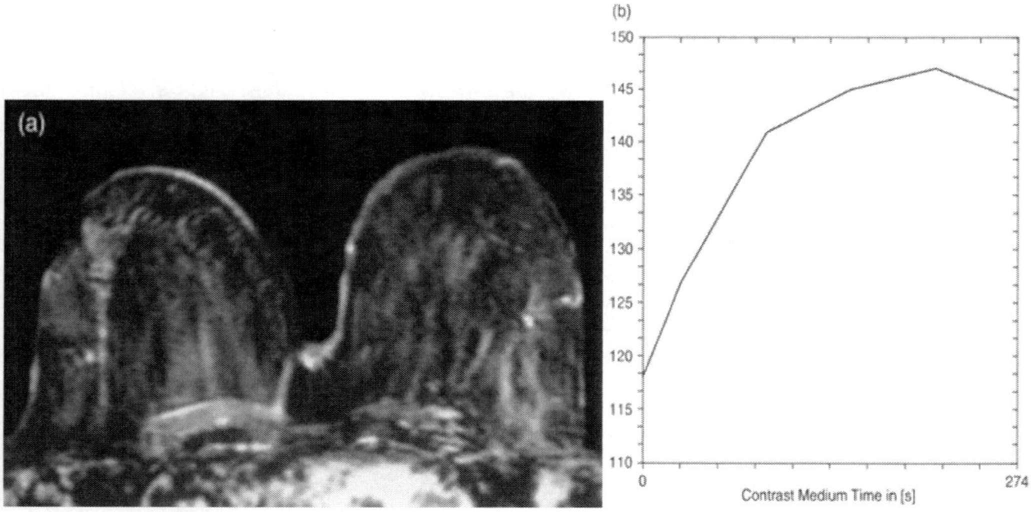

Figure 3. Postcontrast dynamic Magnetic resonance imaging (MRI) study of a patient with Diabetic fibrous mastopathy (DFM). A) Subtraction imaging shows homogeneous low-enhancement in the subareolar region and upper outer quadrant. B) Time intensity curve: gradual and progressive enhancement followed by washout in the delayed phase.

However, MRI features are not specific for DFM and may be difficult to differentiate from breast carcinomaa [22]. The surgeon would require a histological diagnosis to rule out malignancy.

Pathology

On Fine needle aspiration (FNA), the needle characteristically encounters unusually firm, hard resistance [11, 23]. Cytology frequently yields benign ductal epithelium with a moderate amount of peculiar-appearing, dense, hyalinized fibrous tissue [23]. A report of "insufficient cellular material" for evaluation is common, given the characteristic paucity of cellular material in DFM [24]. Histopathologic examination of these lesions have shown firm, homogeneous masses ranging in diameter from 2–6 cm. Microscopically, they are characterized by keloid fibrosis (Figure 4) and variable periductal, perilobular, or perivascular lymphocytic infiltration that consists primarily of B cells (Figure 5).

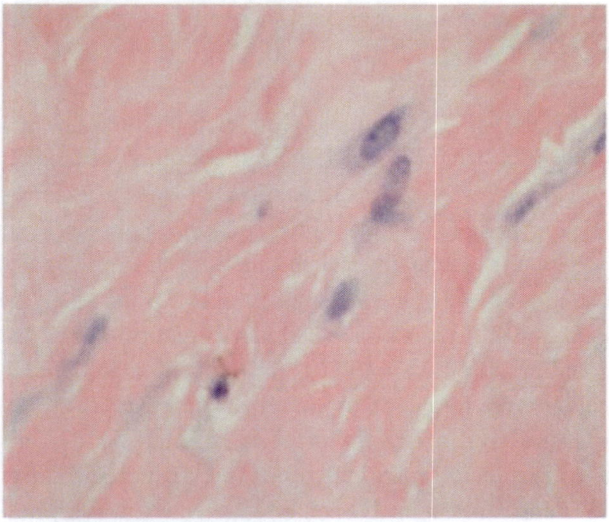

Figure 4. Photomicrograph of Diabetic fibrous mastopathy (DFM) shows epithelioid myofibroblasts (Hematoxylin & eosin, x400).

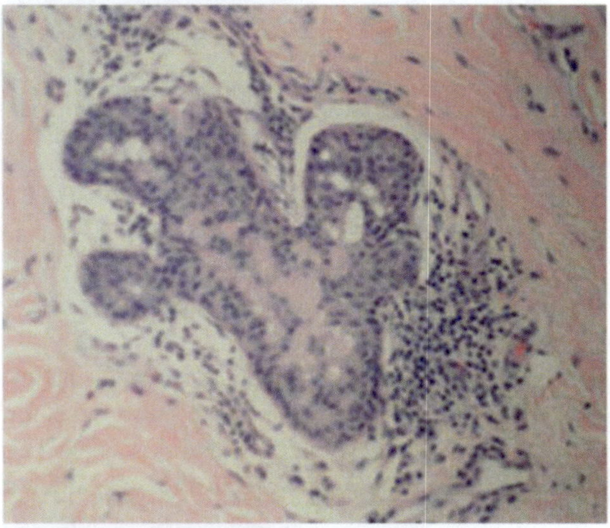

Figure 5. Photomicrograph of Diabetic fibrous mastopathy (DFM) shows perilobular lymphocytic infiltration (Hematoxylin & eosin, x200).

These features are unique to DFM, in contrast to patients with mastitis and fibrosis associated with other processes, where T-cell infiltrates predominate [6,7]. In some cases, epithelioid fibroblasts, characterized as rounded cells with abundant cytoplasm and oval nuclei embedded in dense collagen, have been described [6].

An association among autoimmune diseases, such as insulin-dependent diabetes, thyroid disease, and connective tissue abnormalities, has been reported [25]. It is also interesting to note that while normal non-lactating breast epithelium lacks major histocompatibility complex class II products, these are observed in the epithelium of inflamed lobules [11]. These inflamed lobules resemble the lymphoepithelial lesions observed in other autoimmune diseases.

Pathogenesis

The pathogenesis of DFM is not completely understood and is most likely multifactorial. Many researchers suggest a role of a secondary autoimmune reaction to an abnormal extracellular matrix accumulation, a manifestation of the effects of hyperglycemia in connective tissue. Hyperglycemia induces glycosylation, increased intermolecular cross-linkage, and matrix expansion that is altered in quantity and quality and that is resistant to degradation. The accumulation of abnormal matrix and advanced glycosylated endproducts creates a "neoantigen" that triggers a secondary autoimmune reaction, with B-cell proliferation and autoantibody formation [26]. Subsequent macrophage-mediated advanced glycosylation endproduct removal and cytokine release may act as growth factors and induce additional matrix expansion and proliferation of collagen [6,7]. Given the resemblance of lymphocytic infiltrate to extranodal marginal zone B-cell/Mucosa-associated lymphoid tissue (MALT) lymphomas, clonal studies have been conducted. However, no evidence of B-clone has been found and no increased risk of breast lymphoma has been documented [15].

Clinical Management

Diabetic mastopathy has not been linked with subsequent development of breast carcinoma or with that of stromal neoplasia. For lesions that are unilateral, treatment with excisional biopsy is sufficient. However, a summary of the data in the literature demonstrates that approximately 63% of lesions are bilateral, recurrent, or both. This suggests that the natural history of this condition involves a multicentric field effect of diabetes on mammary tissue. Because recurrences tend to be in the same location and involve more breast tissue than the preceding lesion, it may be that this mastopathy affects breast tissue healing processes and that surgery itself could exacerbate this condition.

To properly counsel and manage these patients, surgeons need to be aware of the association of long-standing diabetes mellitus with the development of distinctive fibroinflammatory breast lesions in premenopausal women. Diagnosis can be made, avoiding surgical excision in a premenopausal woman with type I long-standing diabetes mellitus that is usually associated with microvascular complications. The patient may or may not have a history of other autoimmune diseases. A palpable breast mass, identified on physical examination, is hard, nontender, and clinically suspicious of carcinoma. Mammographic studies show increased density but do not confirm the presence of a localized mass. US also fails to identify a solid or cystic mass; contrast-enhanced MRI could further aid diagnosis. FNA is not adequate for diagnosis. Finally, core biopsy shows dense, keloid fibrosis associated with a perivascular, periductal, or perilobular lymphocytic infiltrate; epithelioid fibroblasts may or may not be present. Given these clinical characteristics, surgical excision can be avoided. Minimal routine annual follow-up of patients with DFM is recommended. A diabetic woman with a suspicious breast mass or mammogram that does not have pathologic findings consistent with DFM on core biopsy requires an excisional biopsy to rule out neoplasia. However, with a high index of suspicion in the proper clinical setting, the diagnosis of DFM can usually be made on core biopsy, with the avoidance of unnecessary surgical procedures that may exacerbate the condition.

PseudoAngiomatous Stromal Hyperplasia (PASH)

PASH was first described by Vuitch et al. in 1986 [27]. The authors described histologic and ultrastructural features of tumorous PASH in nine premenopausal women. Each of them presented with a palpable, unilateral breast mass. Approximately 300 cases of tumorous PASH have been described in the literature. In a recent review of excisional biopsies from the Pathology Department of the University of Ann Arbor (MI, USA), PASH was identified in 579/9,065 biopsies (6.4%). Women with PASH were younger, more likely to have a palpable mass as indication for biopsy, and had less lobular involution compared with those without PASH, but they did not differ by familial history of BC or degree of epithelial proliferation [28]. The largest series reported to date comprises 79 cases diagnosed at Loyola University Medical Center (Chicago, IL, USA) that includes 76 females and three males [29].

Clinical Characteristics

PASH can affect persons in any age group, ranging from 12–75 years, but it occurs more commonly in premenopausal women [28–31]. It was originally described in females; later, it was documented in males in association with gynecomastia [32], but has been described in the normal male breast [29,33]. Isolated cases have been reported involving anogenital mammary-like glands [34].

PASH may present in a wide clinicopathologic spectrum, ranging from an incidental histologic finding to a clinically palpable breast mass. The patients with tumorous PASH present with a slow-growing breast mass. On physical examination, tumorous PASH is a solitary, firm, painless, well-circumscribed and freely mobile mass simulating a fibroadenoma. Sometimes, the mass may enlarge rapidly and mimic a malignant tumor [35]. Rarely, the patient may present with diffuse massive enlargement of the breast [36]. Tumorous PASH is typically unilateral, but there are rare documented reports of asymmetric diffuse enlargement of both breasts [35]. It can also arise in the axillary tail of the breast and, very rarely, tumorous PASH may involve the nipple-areola complex and accessory breast tissue in the axilla [30,37,38].

Pathogenesis

The exact etiology and pathogenesis of PASH is not clearly understood. In the past, some authors considered it to be a hamartomatous lesion and classified it with the mammary hamartomas. However, the World Health Organization (WHO) classified PASH as distinctive from mammary hamartomas [39]. The most widely accepted hypothesis in the literature is that the stromal hyperplasia in PASH results from an exaggerated, aberrant response of mammary myofibroblasts to hormonal stimuli. The hormonal influence may be endo- or exogenous. The main hormone implicated in the stimulation of the fibroblasts is progesterone. The nuclei of myofibroblasts in PASH have been shown to express Progesterone receptors (PR) [40]. Powell et al. [41] found the expression of PR in 36% (5 of 14) and that of Estrogen receptors (ER) in 12% (2 of 14) of PASH cases. These authors found stronger expression of PR, similar to the previous study. These studies indicate that progesterone probably stimulates the stromal cells in estrogen-primed breast tissue. The epithelial nuclei of the ducts and lobules are frequently positive for ER as well as for PR [40,41]. The hormonal base is further supported by the similarity of histologic changes observed in PASH and in normal breast tissue during the luteal phase [42]. The fact that more than one half of postmenopausal women with tumorous PASH described in the literature were receiving hormone replacement therapy further supports the role of the hormonal influence in its pathogenesis [29,30,41]. PASH has been described in immunosuppressed patients in whom it presented as a rapidly growing breast lesion; however, the role of immunosuppression in PASH is not clear [43].

There is no consensus on the origin of the slit-like spaces in PASH (Figure 6).

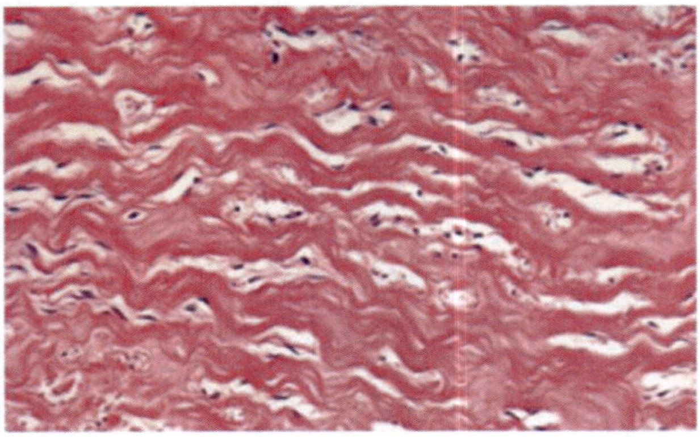

Figure 6. Slit-like spaces lined with benign spindle cells with no cytologic atypia characteristic of Pseudoangiomatous stromal hyperplasia (PASH).

Initially, the spaces were considered to be artifacts, but their presence in frozen, as well as in permanent, sections confirmed their true nature. Immunohistochemical staining and ultrastructural studies have supported the myofibroblastic origin of stromal spindle cells. In immunohistochemistry, the spindle cells exhibit the expression of myofibroblastic markers, such as vimentin, CD34, and Smooth muscle actin (SMA) [41]. In addition, the spindle cells have been shown to be positive for BCL-2 [44]. Damiani et al. [45] reported carcinoma infiltrating the slit-like spaces in PASH. The authors proposed that this could be an unrecognized pathway of tumor spread. Furthermore, they suggested that these spaces may represent prelymphatic channels described in the breast stroma by Hartveit [46]. This prelymphatic origin of spaces in PASH has not been supported by any other study. Moreover, Damiani et al. [45] showed that the spindle cells lining the spaces were positive for CD34 and SMA and negative for CD31, which is consistent with the immunophenotype of myofibroblasts. On electron microscopy, the slit-like spaces are lined by an incomplete layer of spindle cells joined together by rudimentary cell junctions or, occasionally, by tight cell junctions. The cells show cytoplasmic processes extending along and around the spaces. The cytoplasm contains abundant endoplasmic reticulum, well-developed Golgi apparatus, and small bundles of intermediate filaments [27]. Collagen fibrils are observed in the stroma present between spaces.

Radiologic Findings

The mammographic findings consist of a well-circumscribed, round-to-oval density without calcification. A study conducted by Celliers et al. [47] described the mammographic and sonographic features of 73 cases of PASH. The most common appearance in the mammograms was a solid, noncalcified mass or one of localized increased stroma. Stromal distortion and stellate opacities were rare. On US, PASH presented most commonly as a well-defined hypoechoic mass [47,48]. Mercado et al. [49] described the spectrum of sonographic findings in 13 cases of tumorous PASH. The authors described a solid, well-circumscribed, homogenous, hypoechoic mass as the most common appearance of tumorous PASH on US. Less commonly, the mass may be ill- defined or hyperechoic. Rarely, it may have a cystic component. Wieman et al. [31] studied the US findings in 22 patients with tumorous PASH and found hypoechogenicity in 83% of cases and ill-defined borders in 62%. These radiographic findings lead to an initial diagnosis of fibroadenoma in a large percentage of cases, or to an overall benign diagnosis (Figure 7).

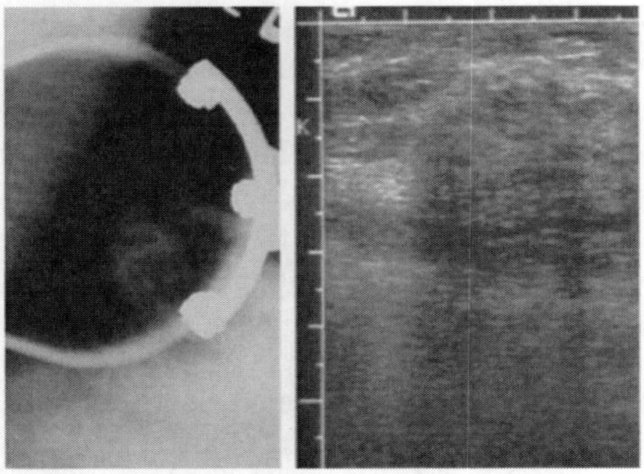

Figure 7. Right mediolateral oblique spot magnification view obtained on routine mammography in a 61-year-old woman shows a focal area of asymmetric density not observed at previous mammographic screening examinations. Ultrasound (US) image shows a hypoechoic area with unhomogeneous echogenicity. Core biopsy was diagnostic of Pseudoanginomatous stromal hyperplasia (PASH).

In the largest study of PASH to date [29], 59.8% of patients presented with a palpable breast mass, and in the remaining 40.2% of patients, the lesion was an incidental radiological finding. MRI revealed isointense mass on T1-weighted gradient echoic images and may show a linear, reticular, "lacelike" pattern on axial T2-weighed images, indicative of slit-like spaces within the lesion [35]. The presence of these linear reticular lines may potentially be a helpful feature in diagnosing PASH. However, tumorous PASH does not show any unique features in imaging studies, and histologic examination of the lesion is necessary to make a definitive diagnosis and to rule out malignancy.

Pathology

The size of tumorous PASH ranges from 0.6–12 cm [29,41]. The largest size of tumorous PASH documented in the literature is 20 cm, found in a 36-year-old woman [50]. Grossly, the excised mass is round-to-oval, well-circumscribed, and rubbery. The outer surface is usually smooth and unencapsulated. The cut surface reveals a homogeneous solid lesion with gray-white color and occasional cysts [49]. Necrosis and hemorrhage are rare except when induced by previous FNA or Needle core biopsy (NCB) [51].

PASH can occur as an isolated mass or may coexist with any breast lesion ranging from benign to malignant, including proliferative and nonproliferative benign breast lesions, fibroadenoma, phyllodes tumor, and carcinoma. Ibrahim et al. [52] demonstrated at least one microscopic focus of PASH in 23% (46 of 200) of consecutive breast biopsies and mastectomy specimens. PASH has been described in breast stroma in association with gynecomastia in males. Milanezi et al. [32] described the presence of PASH in 23.8% of breast biopsies from men with gynecomastia.

On histologic examination, PASH exhibits a wide spectrum of morphological changes, ranging from atypical appearance to being more proliferative. The typical lesion is composed of complex anastomosing, slit-like empty spaces in dense fibrous stroma (Figure 6). These spaces are lined with a discontinuous layer of flat, benign spindle cells. No mitosis or nuclear atypia is observed. The stromal hyperplasia may involve peri- as well as intralobular stroma. Expansion of intralobular stroma may cause effacement of Terminal duct lobular units (TDLU). Isolated involvement of perilobular stroma is more common than that of intralobular stroma [30]. The epithelium of lobules and ducts may be unremarkable or may show ductal hyperplasia and/or apocrine metaplasia. Sometimes, the hyperplasia may also involve myoepithelial cells. The ducts may show gynecomastia-like changes, including nuclear overlapping, nuclear hyperchromasia, and nucleoli with hyperplastic myoepithelial cells. The presence of gynecomastia-like changes has been shown as strongly associated with the involvement of intralobular stroma [30].

Proliferative lesions show variable cellularity, ranging from increased stromal cellularity to the formation of cellular bundles in a dense, collagenous background, and these lesions show a lobulocentric growth pattern. In proliferative lesions, the stromal cells may be larger and have conspicuous nuclei, but cytologic atypia is rare [41].

Core needle biopsy is warranted in suspicious cases to exclude malignancy. Wieman et al. [31] attempted to characterize PASH preoperatively on the basis of imaging studies and core needle biopsies. They found that core biopsies had a sensitivity of 83% for diagnosing the lesion. However, careful correlation of histologic features with clinical and radiologic findings is required to ensure that the target lesion has been appropriately and adequately sampled. FNA and cytologic examination is not very helpful in making a definitive diagnosis [53]. Tumorous PASH does not have any unique features on cytology that can aid in making an accurate diagnosis. Differential diagnosis on cytologic examination includes fibroadenoma, phyllodes tumor, or fibrocystic changes due to overlapping cytologic features. The major usefulness of cytologic examination lies in ruling out a malignant lesion rather than in providing a definitive diagnosis.

On immunohistochemistry, the spindle cells lining the slit-like spaces are positive for myofibroblastic markers including CD34 (Figure 8), vimentin, and SMA [27,41]. They are negative for cytokeratin, S100, and endothelial markers such as von Willebrand factor antigen and CD31. SMA expression is observed more conspicuously in lesions with plump spindle cells and fascicular foci. Fascicular areas may show expression of desmin. Stromal cells show nuclear positivity for PR. ER expression is focal and faintly positive when present. Epithelial nuclei are frequently positive for ER as well as PR [41]. Spindle cells show myofibroblastic features in ultrastructural studies. The spaces are lined with an incomplete layer of spindle cells with elongated cytoplasmic processes [27]. The cytoplasm contains well-developed Golgi apparatus and abundant endoplasmic reticulum. The cells are joined together by rudimentary cell junctions or, very occasionally, tight junctions. Differential diagnoses of PASH include low-grade angiosarcoma, myofibroblastoma, phyllodes tumor, and breast hamartoma; however, the most common differential diagnosis is fibroadenoma.

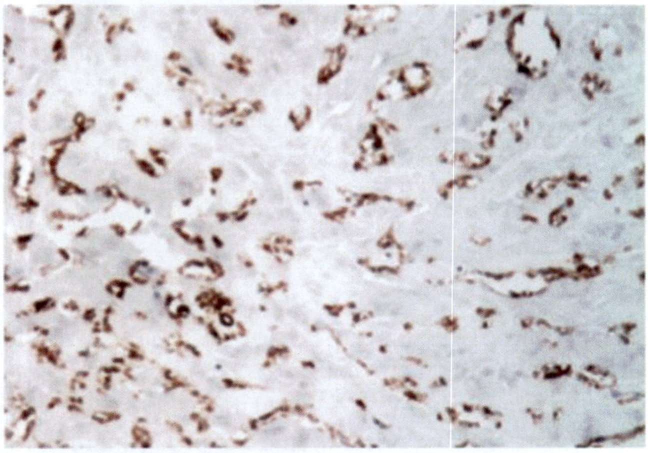

Figure 8. CD34 shows strong and diffuse cytoplasmic reactivity in spindle cells in Pseudoangiomatous stromal hyperplasia (PASH).

Clinical Management

Treatment of PASH depends on its clinical presentation. No additional specific treatment is required if PASH is an incidental finding in specimens excised for other lesions. An excision, with adequate but close margins, is the recommended treatment for tumorous PASH. Sometimes, diffuse PASH may require wide excision of breast tissue or mastectomy, for cosmetic reasons, or due to persistent pain and patient discomfort. The recurrence rate after excision ranges from 0–22% [30, 31, 41]. Recurrence is more likely if the lesion is not completely excised. Recurrent PASH occurs in the ipsilateral breast but can also occur in the contralateral breast [41]. Recurrent lesions behave in a benign fashion and can be managed with re-excision. A conservative approach with close clinical follow-up for selected patients with PASH (with benign features on pathology and imaging studies) has been reported [31]. In a large series of 80 patients with PASH, lesions were palpable in 56% and the remainder was found on imaging studies. CNB was performed in 81% of patients and PASH was confirmed in 65%; authors reported a progression rate of 26% in the observation arm vs. 13% in the excisional arm [54]. The authors suggest that a patient with a diagnosis of PASH on core biopsy in the absence of suspicious radiologic features may be managed with routine follow-up and imaging at a 6-month interval.

There is no well-established medical treatment for tumorous PASH. One case report by Pruthi et al. [55] documented successful treatment with Tamoxifen of bilateral tumorous PASH in a 39-year-old woman. The patient presented with progressive enlargement of both breasts and cyclic pain. The tumors disappeared completely after 6 months of medical treatment. However, this report is the one of a kind and further studies are needed to establish the role of medical treatment in this condition.

Tumorous PASH is slow-growing and is known to recur after excision [27,41]. Overall, the prognosis for PASH is excellent. Pseudoangiomatous stromal hyperplasia is not considered a premalignant lesion or a risk factor for malignancy. Only a single instance has been reported in which invasive ductal carcinoma was present within tumorous PASH, and the authors considered that to be an incidental finding rather than a true malignant transformation [30]. In another study of 76 patients with PASH, nine cases of invasive carcinoma were reported; however, the authors emphasize that no malignant pathology was within the bulk of the PASH lesion and that therefore, it was not related [29].

The current recommendation for clinical management of a tumorous PASH lesion is surgical excision. A conservative approach may be considered in selected patients with histological diagnosis in the absence of clinical or radiological features suggestive of breast carcinoma.

Radial Scar (RS)/Complex Sclerosing Lesion (CSL)

Radial scar is a rare benign breast lesion of unknown etiology commonly identified by screening mammography. Historically, it has been described with different names by diverse authors, but RS is the most common nomenclature employed by the international community. Radial scars (RS) are by definition <1 cm and Complex sclerosing lesions (CSL), which are considered part of the same disease continuum, are described as their larger counterpart (>1 cm) [56]. The incidence of this condition has increased significantly due to the implementation of national breast cancer screening programs and is at present considered to be 0.03–0.09% [57].

RS/CSL and Breast Cancer

The relationship between the RS/CSL complex and breast cancer is controversial. Some authors state that this entity is considered a premalignant lesion [58], while others postulate that there is no evidence that this lesion serves as a precursor or promoter for neoplastic changes [59]. Mokbel et al. propose that RS are linked with breast cancer because they are associated with all stages of mammary carcinogenesis (epithelial hyperplasia, ductal carcinoma *in situ*, and early invasive malignancy) [58]. Malignancy involving RS frequently arises at the periphery of the lesion and tends to be low-to-intermediate grade [60].

Historic evidence of the Nurses' Health Studies suggests that RS are an independent histologic risk factor for Breast cancer (BC) (Relative risk [RR], 1.8; 95% Confidence interval (95% CI), 1.1–2.1) [61]. In a recent updated analysis of the Nurses' Health Study, there was a two-fold increased risk of BC in patients with RS (Odds ratio [OR] = 2.0; 95% CI, 1.4–2.8) [62]. This remains controversial because some authors believe that this increased risk is due to the atypical ductal hyperplasia/lobular carcinoma-*in situ* association with RS [63]. Berg et al. acknowledge this risk; however, the authors state that RS convey no increased breast cancer risk above that of other proliferative lesions, including atypical hyperplasia [64].

Some authors think that increasing age and lesion size can increase the probability of malignancy [64,65]; however, additional studies have failed to validate this association and state that increasing lesion size is not associated with greater risk [63,66]. On the other hand, the presence of multiple lesions (≥2 RS) has been found to confer a greater risk for BC (OR = 2.7; 95% CI, 1.5–5.0) [62].

Clinical Characteristics

Due to the fact that these lesions are usually identified by routine mammograms, the majority of studies have a mean patient age of 55 years. These lesions are usually nonpalpable and have radiological and gross pathological characteristics that mimic breast carcinoma. In a Swedish study of nearly 19,000 women, the incidence of RS was 0.06%, and 64% of these lesions were located in the upper outer quadrants [67].

Radiological Findings

Classical findings of a RS in mammograms are a stellate lesion with the presence of a radiolucent center with long, fine radiodense spicules, which create a "black star" appearance (Figure 9) [60]. Other typical mammographic findings include asymmetric density, architectural distortion with central translucent areas, microcalcifications, the absence of a central mass, and speculated, irregular opacities [68].

Traditionally, US has played a limited role in the diagnostic approach of RS/CSL, because their radiological characteristics mimic carcinoma of the breast [68]. The classic sonographic features of RS, when this is visible, include heterogeneous internal echoic texture, irregular hypoechoic masses with irregular borders, and diminished posterior sound transmission [69]. A more recent study revealed that specific US findings may aid in discriminating RS and carcinoma of the breast. These findings include the following: RS are less sonopositive than BC (43 vs. 93%; $p<0.001$); there is less sound attenuation (55 vs. 86%, $p<0.005$) and there is less breast architecture disruption (43 vs. 91%; $p<0.001$) [70]. However, we think that these findings possess limited clinical usefulness.

Pediconi et al. observed, in a series of 30 patients, that every lesion with presence of carcinoma revealed postcontrast enhancement, and that the reported specificity, sensitivity, and accuracy for Contrast-enhanced-Magnetic resonance mammogram (CE-MRM) in the diagnosis of RS is 89, 83, and 87%, respectively [71]. A possible explanation for the absence of enhancement in RS is due to the histological nature of this lesion and their lack of vascular supply. These authors recommend that CE-MRM be performed in every mammographic lesion suspicious for RS [71]. (Figure 10) demonstrates a time-intensity curve with typical malignant characteristics.

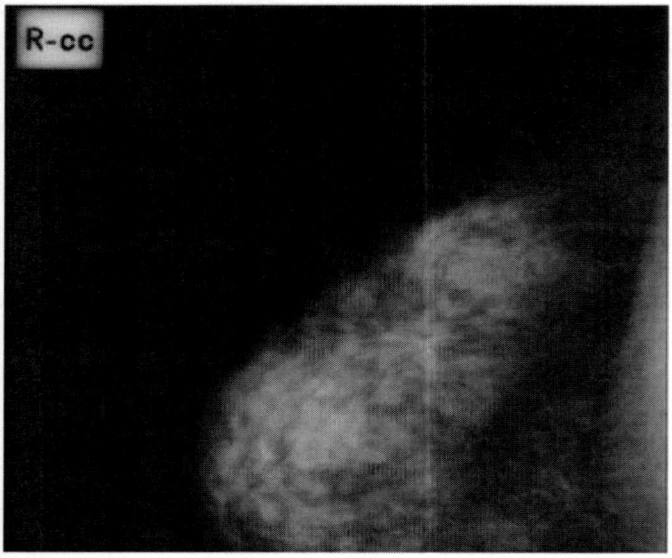

Figure 9. Right mammogram, craniocaudal view:Stellate/spiculated appearance of radial scar, with long, thin spicules radiating from a low-dense/lucent central area. Reproduced with permission from Bianchi et al. [60].

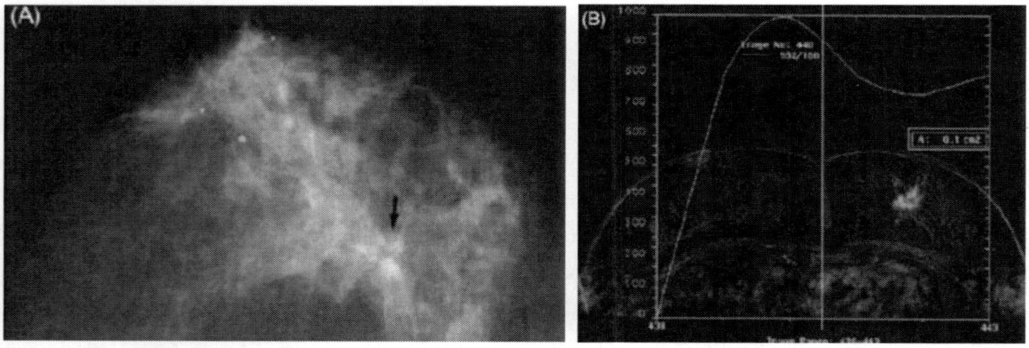

Figure 10. A 53-year-old asymptomatic woman who underwent screening mammography. Invasive ductal carcinoma diagnosed on pathology. (A) Screening mammogram, craniocaudal view, shows a region of stromal distortion without a central mass (arrow). (B) T_1-weighted axial subtracted image after injection of gadolinium shows an enhancing lesion with ill-defined borders in the left breast. Time-intensity curve has typical malignant characteristics. Reproduced with permission from Pediconi et al. [71].

Pathology

RS are pseudo-infiltrative stellate lesions that are characterized by a fibroelastotic core surrounded by a corona of radiating tubular structures that have a double layer of epithelial and myoepithelial cells (See Figure 11). CSL are larger lesions (>1 cm) that exhibit greater architectural distortion of architecture and that are often accompanied by nodular masses around the periphery [56]. Calcification can be present and is often associated with areas of epithelial hyperplasia with or without atypia. Occasionally, lesions may be multifocal, clustered, or bilateral [57].

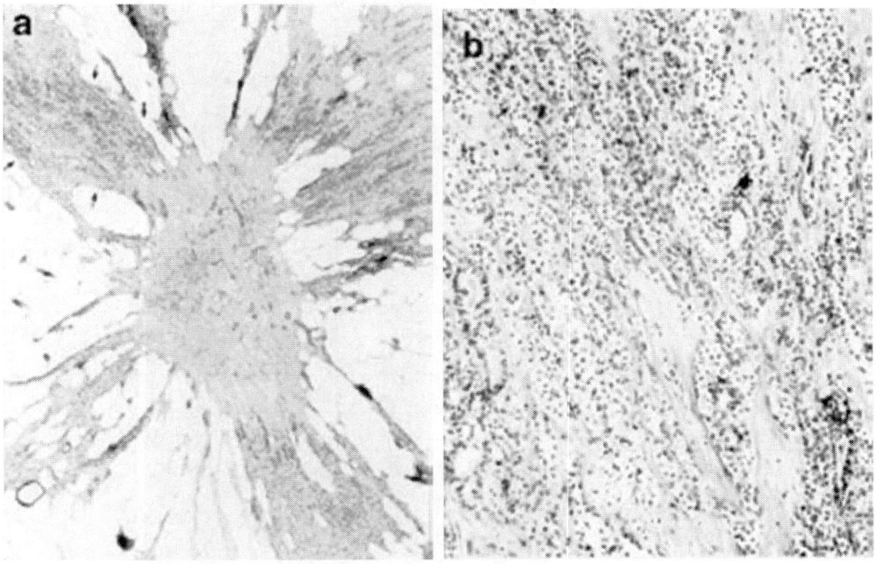

Figure 11. (a) Stellate appearance of a Radial scar (RS) involved by lobular neoplasia; arrow points to the area magnified in (b). (Hematoxylin & eosin; magnification x312.) (b) Higher magnification shows LN cells within compressed tubules around the RS. Some of the LN cells contain barely visible intracytoplasmic lumens (arrows). (Hematoxylin & eosin; magnification x3200) [59].

Clinical Management

Several authors advocate the use of FNA [72,73]or CNB [74] in the diagnostic approach of stellate lesions detected on screening mammography. Table 2 describes common cytological features observed in the FNA of RS/CSL. Mak & Field observed a positive predictive value of 0.63 in the cytological diagnosis of these lesions. We think that the diagnostic yield of this technique is inferior to CNB for the majority of breast lesions [75–77]and do not recommend its routine use.

An acceptable diagnostic yield for CNB is achieved by an experienced operator utilizing image-guidance and 14-G needles [78]. However, a diagnosis of RS on a CNB does not rule out underlying malignancy, and further tissue sampling is frequently warranted [60]. A reasonable substitute is mammotome excision utilizing 8-G to 11-G needles, avoiding surgical excision in selected patients [79].

Currently, diagnostic procedures are unreliable [66] and, due to the inherent risk of RS for underlying malignancy, the safest and most recommended approach in the treatment of a suspicious stellate lesion is surgical excision [57,58,68,74,80–83].

Table 2. Fine needle aspiration (FNA) characteristics commonly observed in Radial scars/Complex sclerosing lesions (RS/CSL)

Category of feature	Criterion	RS/CSL
Cellularity	Cellularity	Moderate-to-marked in all cases
Pattern	Size of Tissue fragments (TF)	Mix of small and large TF
Background	Background material	Proteinaceous background with macrophages ± siderophages
	Bare bipolar nuclei (BBN)	BBN present in all cases
Dispersed epithelial cells	Dispersed cells and Columnar cells (CL)	Scant-to-moderate dispersed epithelial cells and single CL
Stromal fragments	Stellate TF	Present in small number in a small number of cases
Specific architectural features of epithelial TF	"Meshwork"	Present occasionally in some of the cases in small numbers
	Myoepithelial cells	Present in the majority of cases
	Tubular structures	Commonly observed

Modified and permission to reproduce received from Field & Mak [73].

References

[1] Soler NG, Khardori R. Fibrous disease of the breast, thyroiditis and cheiroarthropathy in type I diabetes mellitus. *Lancet* 1984;1:193–195.

[2] Pluchinotta AM, Talenti F, Lodovichetti G, et al. Diabetic fibrous breast disease: a clinical entity that mimics cancer. *Eur. J. Surg. Oncol.* 1995;21:207–209.

[3] Honda M, Mori Y, Nishi T, et al. Diabetic mastopathy of bilateral breasts in an elderly Japanese woman with type 2 diabetes: a case report and a review of the literature in Japan. *Intern. Med.* 2007;46:1573–1576.

[4] Sotome K, Ohnishi T, Miyoshi R, et al. An uncommon case of diabetic mastopathy in type II non-insulin dependent diabetes mellitus. *Breast Cancer* 2006;13:205–209.

[5] Gump FE, McDermott J. Fibrous disease of the breast in juvenile diabetes. *N. Y. State J. Med.* 1990;90:356–357.

[6] Tomaszewski JE, Brooks JSJ, Hicks D, LiVolsi VA. Diabetic mastopathy: a distinctive clinicopathologic entity. *Hum. Pathol.* 1992;23:780–706.

[7] Seidman JD, Schnaper LA, Phillips LE. Mastopathy in insulin-requiring diabetes mellitus. *Hum. Pathol.* 1994;25:819–824.

[8] Akahori H, Kaneko M, Kiyohara K, et al. A rare case of diabetic mastopathy in a Japanese man with type 2 diabetes mellitus. *Intern. Med.* 2009;48: 915–919.

[9] Weinstein SP, Conant EF, Orel SG, et al. Diabetic mastopathy in men: findings in two patients. *Radiology* 2001;219:797–799.

[10] Byrd BF, Hartmann WH, Graham LS, Hogle HH. Mastopathy in insulin-dependent diabetics. *Ann. Surg*. 1987;205:529–532.

[11] Logan WW, Hoffman NY. Diabetic fibrous breast disease. *Radiology* 1989;172: 667–670.

[12] Morgan MC, Weaver MG, Crowe JP, Abdul-Karim FW. Diabetic mastopathy: a clinicopathologic study in palpable and non palpable breast lesions. *Mod. Pathol.* 1995;8:349–354.

[13] Camuto PM, Zetrenne E, Ponn T. Diabetic mastopathy: a report of 5 cases and a review of the literature. *Arch. Surg.* 2000;135:1190–1093.

[14] Andrews-Tang D, Diamond AB, Rogers L, Butler D. Diabetic mastopathy: adjunctive use of ultrasound and utility of core biopsy on diagnosis. *Breast J.* 2000;6:183–188.

[15] Valdez R, Thorson J, Finn WG, Schnitzer B, Kleer CG. Lymphocytic mastitis and diabetic mastopathy: a molecular, immunophenotypic and clinicopathologic evaluation of 11 cases. *Mod. Pathol.* 2003;16:223–228.

[16] Martínez-Ramos D, Alcalde-Sánchez M, Laguna-Sastre M, et al. Diabetic mastopathy. Features in four patients. *Cir. Esp.* 2007;81:224–226.

[17] Chan CLR, Ho RSL, Shek TWH, Kwong A. Diabetic mastopathy. *Breast J.* 2013;19:533–538.

[18] Rollins SD. Fine-needle aspiration cytology of diabetic fibrous mastopathy. *Diagn. Cytopathol.* 1993;9:687–690.

[19] Cole-Beuglet C, Soriano RZ, Kurtz AB, Goldberg BB. Ultrasound analysis of 104 primary breast carcinomas classified according to histopathologic type. *Radiology* 1983;147:191–196.

[20] Wong KT, Tse GMK, Yang WT. Ultrasound and MR imaging of diabetic mastopathy. *Clin. Radiol.* 2002;57:730–735.

[21] Tuncbilek N, Karakas HM, Okten O. Diabetic fibrous mastopathy: dynamic contrast-enhanced magnetic resonance imaging findings. *Breast J.* 2004;10:359–362.

[22] Sakuhara Y, Shinozaki T, Hozumi Y, et al. MR imaging of diabetic mastopathy. *AJR Am. J. Roentgenol*. 2002;179:1201–1203.

[23] Rollins SD. Fine-needle aspiration cytology of diabetic fibrous mastopathy. *Diagn. Cytopathol* 1993;9:687–690.

[24] Lakshmanan R, Clarke MJ, Putti TC. Diabetic fibrous mastopathy. *Singapore Med. J.* 2007;48:579–581.

[25] Lammie GA, Bobrow LG, Staunton MD, et al. Sclerosing lymphocytic lobulitis of the breast- evidence for an autoimmune pathogenesis. *Histopathology* 1991;19:13–20.

[26] Schwartz IS, Strauchen JA. Lymphocytic mastopathy: an autoimmune disease of the breast? *Am. J. Clin. Pathol*. 1990;93:725–730.

[27] Vuitch MF, Rosen PP, Erlandson RA. Pseudoangiomatous hyperplasia of mammary stroma. *Hum. Pathol*. 1986;17:185–191.

[28] Degnim AC, Frost M, Radisky D, et al. Pseudoangiomatous stromal hyperplasia and breast cancer risk. *Ann. Surg. Oncol*. 2010;17:3269–3277.

[29] Drinka EK, Bargaje A, Ersahin CH, et al. Pseudoangiomatous stromal hyperplasia (PASH) of the breast: a clinicopathological study of 79 cases. *Int. J. Surg. Pathol.* 2012;20:54–58.

[30] Ferreira M, Albarracin CT, Resetkova E. Pseudoangiomatous stromal hyperplasia tumor: a clinical, radiologic and pathologic study of 26 cases. *Mod. Pathol.* 2008;21:201–207.
[31] Wieman SM, Landercasper J, Johnson JM, et al. Tumoral pseudoangiomatous stromal hyperplasia of the breast. *Am. Surg.* 2008;74:1211–1214.
[32] Milanezi MF, Saggioro FP, Zanati SG, Bazan R, Scmitt FC. Pseudoangiomatous hyperplasia of mammary stroma associated with gynaecomastia. *J. Clin. Pathol.* 1998;51:204–206.
[33] Bolla D, Wiedemann N, Öhlschlegel C, et al. Pseudoangiomatous stromal hyperplasia of breast in a man: a case report. *Breast J.* 2011;17:311–312.
[34] Kazakhov DV, Bisceglia M, Mukensnabl P, Michal M. Pseudoangiomatous stromal hyperplasia in lesions involving anogenital mammary-like glands. *Am. J. Surg. Pathol.* 2005;29:1243–1346.
[35] Yoo K, Woo OH, Yong HS, et al. Fast-growing pseudoangiomatous stromal hyperplasia of the breast: report of a case. *Surg. Today* 2007;37:967–970.
[36] Baskin H, Layfield L, Morrell G. MRI appearance of pseudoangiomatous stromal hyperplasia causing asymmetric breast enlargement. *Breast J.* 2007;13:203–210.
[37] Iancu D, Nochomovitz LE. Pseudoangiomatous stromal hyperplasia: presentation as a mass in the female nipple. *Breast J.* 2001;7:263–265.
[38] Lee JS, Oh HS, Min KW. Mammary pseudoangiomatous stromal hyperplasia presenting as an axillary mass. *Breast* 2005;14:61–64.
[39] Virk RK, Khan A. Pseudoangiomatous stromal hyperplasia. An overview. *Arch. Pathol. Lab. Med.* 2010;134:1070–1074.
[40] Zanella M, Falconieri G, Lamovec J, Bittesini L. Pseudoangiomatous hyperplasia of the mammary stroma: true entity or phenotype? *Pathol. Res. Pract.* 1998;194:535–540.
[41] Powell CM, Cranor ML, Rosen PP. Pseudoangiomatous stromal hyperplasia (PASH): a mammary stromal tumor with myofibroblastic differentiation. *Am. J. Surg. Pathol.* 2008;21:201—207.
[42] Vogel PM, Georgiade NG, Fetter BF, Vogel FS, McCarty KS Jr. The correlation of the histologic changes in the human breast with the menstrual cycle. *Am. J. Pathol.* 1981;104:23–34.
[43] Seidman JD, Borkowski A, Aisner SC, Sun CC. Rapid growth of pseudoangiomatous hyperplasia of mammary stroma in axillary gynecomastia in an immunosuppressed patient. *Arch. Pathol. Lab. Med.* 1993;117:736–738.
[44] Moore T, Lee AH. Expression of CD34 and bcl-2 in phyllodes tumours, fibroadenomas and spindle cell lesions of the breast. *Histopathology* 2001;38:62–67.
[45] Damiani S, Peterse L, Eusebi V. Malignant neoplasms infiltrating pseudoangiomatous stromal hyperplasia of the breast: an unrecognized pathway of tumor spread. *Histopathology* 2002;41:208–215.
[46] Hartveit F. Attenuated cells in breast stroma: the missing lymphatic system of the breast. *Histopathology* 1990;16:533–543.
[47] Celliers L, Wong DD, Bourke A. Pseudoangiomatous stromal hyperplasia: a study of the mammographic and sonographic features. *Clin. Radiol.* 2009;65:145–149.
[48] Yoon JC, Eun YK, Shinho K. Diagnosis of pseudoangiomatous stromal hyperplasia of the breast: ultrasonographic findings and different biopsy methods. *Yonsei Med. J.* 2008;49:757–764.

[49] Mercado CL, Naidrich SA, Hamele-Bena D, Fineberg SA, Buchbinder SS. Pseudoangiomatous stromal hyperplasia of the breast: sonographic features with histopathologic correlation. *Breast J.* 2004;10:427–432.

[50] Sasaki Y, Kamata S, Saito K, Nishikawa Y, Ogawa J. Pseudoangiomatous stromal hyperplasia (PASH) of the mammary gland: report of a case. *Surg. Today* 2008;38:340–343.

[51] Abdull Gaffar B. Pseudoangiomatous stromal hyperplasia of the breast. *Arch. Pathol. Lab. Med.* 2009;133:1335–1338.

[52] Ibrahim RE, Sciotto CG, Weidner N. Pseudoangiomatous hyperplasia of mammary stroma: some observations regarding its clinicopathologic spectrum. *Cancer* 1989;63:1154–1160.

[53] Levine PH, Nimeh D, Guth AA, Cangiarella JF. Aspiration biopsy of nodular pseudoangiomatous stromal hyperplasia of the breast: clinicopathologic correlates in 10 cases. *Diagn. Cytopathol* 2005;32:345–350.

[54] Gresik CM, Godellas C, Aranha GV, Rajan P, Shoup M. Pseudoangiomatous stromal hyperplasia of the breast: a contemporary approach to its clinical and radiologic features and ideal management. *Surgery* 2010;148:752–757.

[55] Pruthi S, Reynolds C, Johnson RE, Gisvold JJ. Tamoxifen in the management of pseudoangiomatous stromal hyperplasia. *Breast J.* 2001;7:434–439.

[56] Group RC of PW. Pathology reporting in breast cancer screening. *J. Clin. Pathol.* 1991;44:710–725.

[57] Kennedy M, Masterson A, Kerin M, Flanagan F. Pathology and clinical relevance of radial scars: a review. *J. Clin. Pathol.* 2003;56:721–724.

[58] Mokbel K, Price RK, Mostafa A, et al. Radial scar and carcinoma of the breast: microscopic findings in 32 cases. *Breast* 1999;8:339–342.

[59] Alvarado-Cabrero I, Tavassoli F. Neoplastic and malignant lesions involving or arising in a radial scar: a clinicopathologic analysis of 17 cases. *Breast J.* 2000;6:96–102.

[60] Bianchi S, Giannotti E, Vanzi E, et al. Radial scar without associated atypical epithelial proliferation on image-guided 14-gauge needle core biopsy: analysis of 49 cases from a single-centre and review of the literature. *Breast* 2012;21:159–164.

[61] Jacobs T, Byrne C, Colditz G, Connolly J, Schnitt S. Radial scars in benign breast-biopsy specimens and the risk of breast cancer. *NEJM* 1999;11:430–436.

[62] Aroner S, Collins L, Connolly J, et al. Radial scars and subsequent breast cancer risk: results from the Nurses' *Health Studies. Breast Cancer Res. Treat.* 2013;139:277–285.

[63] Bunting D, Steel J, Holgate C, Watkins R. Long term follow-up and risk of breast cancer after a radial scar or complex sclerosing lesion has been identified in a benign open breast biopsy. *Eur. J. Surg. Oncol.* 2011;37:709–713.

[64] Berg J, Visscher D, Vierkant R, et al. Breast cancer risk in women with radial scars in benign breast biopsies. *Breast Cancer Res. Treat.* 2008;108:167–174.

[65] Krishnamurthy S, Bevers T, Kuerer H, Yang WT. Multidisciplinary considerations in the management of high-risk breast lesions. *AJR Am. J. Roentgenol.* 2012;198:W132–W140.

[66] Patterson J, Scott M, Anderson N, Kirk S. Radial scar, complex sclerosing lesion and risk of breast cancer. Analysis of 175 cases in Northern Ireland. *Eur. J. Surg. Oncol.* 2004;30:1065–1068.

[67] Azavedo E, Svane G. Radial scars detected mammographically in a breast cancer screening programme. *Eur. J. Radiol.* 1992;15:18–21.
[68] Dinakara Babu E, Power D, Powis S. Radial scar. *Breast* 2000;9:66–71.
[69] Cohen MA, Sferlazza SJ. Role of sonography in evaluation of radial scars of the breast. *AJR Am. J. Roentegenol.* 2000;174:1075–1078.
[70] Cawson J. Can sonography be used to help differentiate between radial scars and breast cancers? *Breast* 2005;14:352–359.
[71] Pediconi F, Occhiato R, Venditti F, et al. Radial scars of the breast: contrast-enhanced magnetic resonance mammography appearance. *Breast J.* 2005;11:23–28.
[72] Field A, Mak A. The fine needle aspiration biopsy diagnostic criteria of proliferative breast lesions: a retrospective statistical analysis of criteria for papillomas and radial scar lesions. *Diagn. Cytopathol.* 2007;35:386–397.
[73] Mak A, Field AS. Positive predictive value of the breast FNAB diagnoses of epithelial hyperplasia with atypia, papilloma, and radial scar. *Diagn. Cytopathol.* 2006;34:818–823.
[74] Farshid G, Rush G. Assessment of 142 stellate lesions with imaging features suggestive of radial scar discovered during population-based screening for breast cancer. *Am. J. Surg. Pathol.* 2004;28:1626–1631.
[75] Usami S, Moriya T, Kasajima A, Suzuki A, Ishida T, Sasano H. Pathological aspects of core needle biopsy for non-palpable breast lesions. *Breast Cancer* 2005;12:272–278.
[76] Joulaee A, Kalantari M, Kadivar M, et al. Trucut biopsy of breast lesions: the first step toward international standards in developing countries. *Eur. J. Cancer* 2012;48:648–654.
[77] Britton PD. Fine needle aspiration or core biopsy. *Breast* 1999;44:1–4.
[78] Bilous M. Breast core needle biopsy: issues and controversies. *Mod. Pathol.* 2010;23:S36–S45.
[79] Rajan S, Wason A-M, Carder PJ. Conservative management of screen-detected radial scars: role of mammotome excision. *J. Clin. Pathol.* 2011;64:65–68.
[80] Corben A, Edelweiss M, Brogi E. Challenges in the interpretation of breast core biopsies. Breast J. 2010;16:S5–S9.
[81] Osborn G, Wilton F, Stevens G, Vaughan-Williams E, Gower-Thomas K. A review of needle core biopsy diagnosed radial scars in the Welsh Breast Screening Programme. *Ann. R. Coll. Surg. Engl.* 2011;93:123–126.
[82] Douglas-Jones AG, Denson JL, Cox AC, Harries IB, Stevens G. Radial scar lesions of the breast diagnosed by needle core biopsy: analysis of cases containing occult malignancy. *J. Clin. Pathol.* 2007;60:295–298.
[83] Fasih T, Jain M, Shrimankar J, Staunton M, Hubbard J, Griffith CDM. All radial scars/complex sclerosing lesions seen on breast screening mammograms should be excised. *Eur. J. Surg. Oncol.* 2005;31:1125–1128.

In: Benign Disease of the Breast ISBN: 978-1-63321-624-2
Editors: J. de la Garza Salazar, C. Arce Salinas et al.

Chapter 10

Benign Tumors of the Breast

Rafael Vazquez-Romo, Silvia Patricia Villarreal-Colin and Yolanda Villaseñor Navarro
Surgical Oncology Department, Instituto Nacional Cancerologia-Mexico,
Mexico City, DF, Mexico

Abstract

Benign neoplasms of the breast are frequent entities, constituting a heterogeneous group of lesions that may either present as a palpable mass, as a nonpalpable lesion detected in an imaging study or as a fortuitous finding in the report of a biopsy performed for another reason. Although benign tumors represent nearly 90% of breast pathology, they are often underdiagnosed and poorly understood due to the diverse clinical presentations they exhibit. The importance of correct diagnosis lies mainly in the exclusion of malignant neoplasms of the breast and the identification of lesions which may have the potential to evolve into cancer.

Physicians who treat breast pathology should have a full understanding of benign tumors in order to correctly evaluate and manage each patient. Often, it may be necessary to dissipate the patient´s anxiety in relation to the finding a breast lesion and the possibility of its degenerating into cancer.

In this chapter, we present the most relevant aspects with regard to epidemiology, clinical presentation, diagnosis, and treatment of six specific benign neoplasms, including fibroadenoma, hamartoma, granular cell tumor, phyllodes tumor, lipoma, and adenomas of the breast.

Fibroadenoma

Fibroadenoma (FA) is the most common of benign breast tumors, occurring most commonly in women in their second and third decades of life. Population prevalence in this age group is reported to be 2.2% [1]. Fibroadenomas are usually solitary tumors, however, they may be multiple in 15% and bilateral in 10% of cases [2].

In adolescents, FA account for up to 30–50% of breast tumors in medical series and 44–94% in surgical series. Because the FA is the most common surgically treated or biopsied breast lesion in adolescents, it is important that healthcare providers be familiar with this condition [3].

FAs are benign tumors that arise from the epithelium and the stroma of the terminal ductolobular unit and can be comprised of stromal and epithelial cells [4]. Variants of FA include juvenile FA, giant FA, and complex FA. Conventional, typical or simple FAs are the most common types observed in young women. A giant FA is defined as any FA >500 g, or >5–10 cm, or as those replacing at least four fifths of the breast. Giant FA account for <4% of all FA and are typically observed in adolescents [3]. The term juvenile FA is sometimes employed interchangeably with cellular FA. Cellular fibroadenomas are characterized by a dense spindle cell stroma. They account for up to 10% of all FAs in adolescents, grow rapidly, and are more likely to become giant, to be multiple, or to be recurrent [3].

Pathological Features

Macroscopically, FAs are typically observed as well defined masses; the outer surface has a smooth, lobular contour. The cut surface is composed of bulging, firm, and gray, white, or tan tissue. A minority has a myxoid or gelatinous appearance. Some tumors appear to be composed of multiple aggregated nodules divided by septa. Discrete round cysts are sometimes present, measuring 1 mm–1.0 cm or more in diameter [4].

Microscopically, the histological hallmark of a FA comprises a concurrent proliferation of glandular and stromal elements with growth patterns that have been referred to as either intra- or peri canalicular. In the majority of instances, microscopic diagnosis of a FA is accomplished without difficulty when the tumor has a sharply defined border or the peri- or intra canalicular growth pattern. The microscopic characteristics of the stroma vary from one FA to another, but are usually homogeneous in any given lesion. Women <20 years of age tend to have more cellular stroma and more proliferative epithelium as a group than tumors from older women [4]. Stromal cells are variably CD34-positive, and inmunoreactivity for actin is observed when there is myofibroblastic proliferation. Stromal cells are variably reactive for progesterone receptors, and at most, weakly positive for estrogen receptors. In a minority of FAs, uncommon forms of stromal differentiation are encountered, including smooth muscle (myoid) metaplasia and adipose differentiation. Alterations in the epithelial component include foci of squamous metaplasia, cyst formation, and the spectrum of proliferation termed fibrocystic changes, including apocrine metaplasia [4].

Complex fibroadenomas are those with sclerosing adenosis, papillary apocrine hyperplasia, cysts measuring >3 mm, or epithelial calcifications. At least one of these features must be present for the lesion to be classified as complex [5]. Complex FA account for 15% of all fibroadenomas in patients aged 20 years and over. The median age at diagnosis for these lesions is 47 years. Complex FA are rarely observed in adolescence. Women with complex FA have an increased risk of developing breast cancer as opposed to those with simple FA, although the rate is low (1.6% over 2 years) [5].

The fine needle aspiration biopsy (FNA) specimen obtained from a FA typically presents a characteristic combination of epithelial and stromal components. Findings considered to be diagnostic include abundant bipolar stromal cells (usually observed with bare nuclei), irregular flat sheets of epithelium composed of uniform, evenly spaced polygonal cells, the so-called "antler horn" clusters, and fenestrated or "honeycomb" sheets made up of similar cells [4, 6].

The mechanisms involved in the development of FAs are poorly understood [7]. In addition to the role of estrogen and progesterone receptors expressed by epithelial cells, growth factors and their receptors may play a role in the pathogenesis of benign breast diseases, including FA, suggesting that multiple signaling routes may be involved in the growth and differentiation of benign breast disorders [8]. Fibroadenomas present higher levels of progesterone receptors which suggests an involvement in the development of these tumors. However, unlike what has been observed in breast cancer, alpha estrogen receptors appear not to be involved in the tumor formation process [9]. Schneider et al. compared p53 and p21 mRNA and protein levels between FA and the adjacent normal mammary tissue of women in reproductive age. These authors found higher gene expression of p53 and p21 and higher protein expression of p53 in FA as compared with normal breast tissue. p21 protein expression was not different between FA and the normal adjacent mammary tissue samples, which suggests the participation of p53 in the formation of FA. The role of p21 in FA development remains to be defined [10].

Genetic alterations, which are most frequently involved in malignant breast carcinomas, are not present in FA, regardless of their association with breast cancer or their histological complexity, suggesting that FAs are not associated with breast carcinogenesis [11]. Chromosomes involved in cases with clonal chromosomal alterations include 1, 4, 6, 12, and 20 in structural rearrangements and 5, 11, 17, and 18 in numerical changes. Although some of these alterations are common in FA, they are not specific for these lesions, because many have also been detected in other benign histological entities of the breast and in breast cancer specimens [12]. Amiel et al. reported two new aberrations, 15q+ and 16p-, however, the significance of this finding is yet to be determined [13].

Environmental risk factors for FA have not yet been identified and the role of long-term estrogen exposure in their incidence remains controversial. The incidence and development of FA could be associated with reproductive risk factors such as no history of breast feeding, nulliparity and hormonal dysfunction. Adiposity and excessive weight gain after the age of 18 could be considered a major background factor that induces FA and that may contribute to the level of endogenous estrogen. Lower age at first oral contraceptive pill consumption and living near polycyclic aromatic hydrocarbon-producing factories are sources of exposure to xenoestrogens in patients with FA. An inverse association has been shown between FA and cigarette smoking due to the antiestrogenic activities of cigarette smoking [14]. Some rare cancer syndromes are associated with the development of multiple FA; these include Mafucci syndrome, Cowden syndrome, and the Carney complex [15].

The natural history of FA is variable. They tend to grow slowly, reaching 2–3 cm in size before remaining static for months or years. However, they may enlarge as much as 16% per month in premenopausal women. FA often lose their cellularity with age, degenerating and becoming smaller over time. Regression may occur due to infarction, with resulting calcification and hyalinization.

The overall rate of complete regression of a clinically detectable breast mass in an adolescent is between 10 and 40% [3, 16]. FA may rarely occur synchronously with phyllodes tumors. Phyllodes tumors are closely related to FA, yet display greater stromal cellularity and a distinct "leaf-like" pattern histologically.

FAs show polyclonality of both epithelial and stromal components, whereas phyllodes tumors exhibit monoclonality of the stromal component and may represent FA that have undergone somatic mutation, resulting in stromal monoclonality [17, 18]. FA and phyllodes tumor are clonally related and allelic loss at TP53 and D22S264 may be implicated in the progression of FA to phyllodes tumor [19]. Fibroadenomas carry a small risk for breast cancer (0.3% or less) although lobular and ductal carcinomas may arise within FA. Primary carcinoma arising within an FA was described in 1931 by Cheatle and Cutler; since that time, >200 cases have been reported in the scientific literature [20].

Clinical Presentation

Fibroadenomas usually occur in young women <35 years of age. They present without symptoms in 25% of cases. FAs are multiple in 13–20% of cases and bilateral in 10% [2, 16]. In relation to race, FAs are more common in African-American than in Caucasian women. They most frequently present as a self-detected mass, which may have been present for months or years [3]. FAs are most often located in the left breast and in the upper external quadrant. FA may range in size from small lesions of <1 cm to lesions of huge dimensions, such as 10–15 cm [16]. The characteristic clinical features of FA include smooth, round or lobulated lesions firm with discrete swelling, and high mobility [3, 7, 21]. This latter feature is due to encapsulation and to the softness of the breast in young women. In older women, the clinical presentation is much less characteristic because of glandular involution and fibrotic changes, therefore, cancer must be excluded unequivocally [7]. Sometimes, the breast may feel warm on palpation and surface veins may exhibit dilation. There is usually no axillary lymphadenopathy appreciated on physical examination. Immobility or nipple and skin changes are not common; thus, their presence should trigger further evaluation to exclude a possible malignant neoplasm [3]. Spontaneous infarction is a very rare occurrence [22].

The imaging modality of choice is the ultrasound (US) using grey scale and color Doppler. Ultrasonographic characteristics include an oval shape, a horizontal axis, a smooth or lobulated border, and the occasional identification of a thin, hyperechoic pseudocapsule. The internal echo pattern is hypoechoic and often homogeneous. The surrounding tissue is mostly displaced and demonstrates no architectural distortion. Enhancement or shadowing can sometimes be observed in the posterior areas of the tumor [23]. Ultrasonography is more specific than mammography when breast density, patient age, size on ultrasonography, and palpability are taken into account. Ultrasonography should, therefore, be favored, especially in younger patients.

One must be aware of the effects of palpability and the patient's age regarding ultrasonographic differentiation of "malignant" vs. "benign". In some cases, mammography should be considered as complementary [24] (Figures 1A and B; Figures 2A and B).

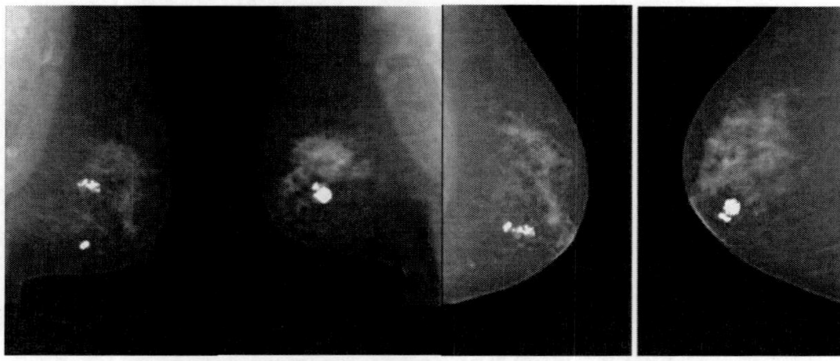

Figure 1A. Female aged 66 years with screening mastography that shows bilateral nodules associated with the “popcorn calcifications” characteristic of fibroadenomas.

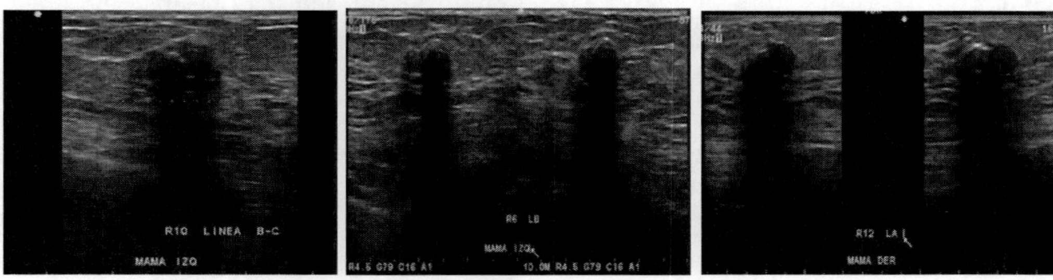

Figure 1B. On Ultrasound (US), these images are observed as hypoechoic lobulated nodules associated with coarse calcifications that project posterior sonic shadowing.

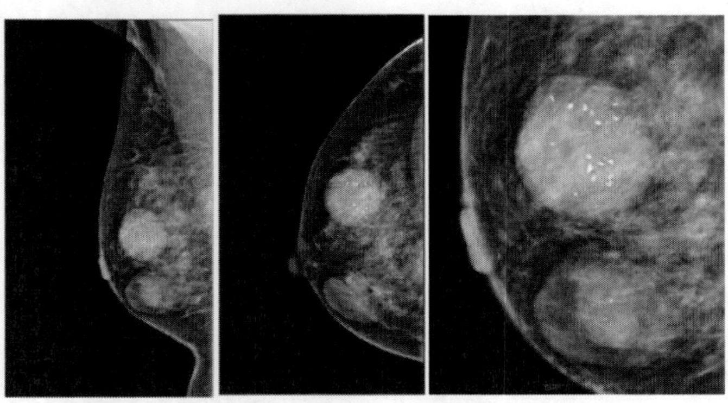

Figure 2A. Female aged 54 years with digital mastography that shows lobular nodules with circumscribed margins, mixed density associated with thick calcium deposits, affecting the central and posterior region of the right mammary gland.

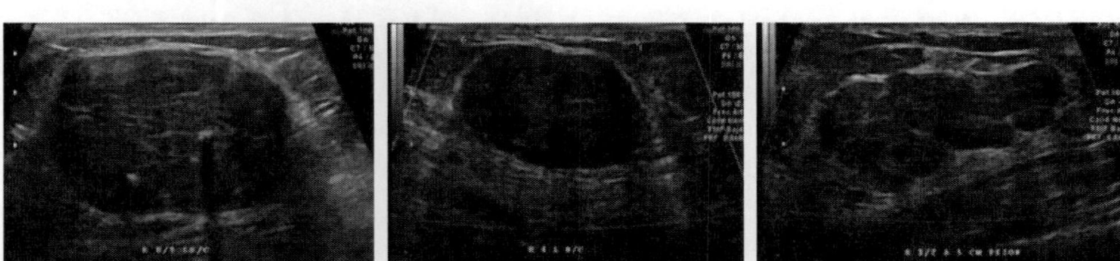

Figure 2B. In the echographic correlation, these are observed as hypoechoic nodules, circumscribed and lobulated, with echogenic images in their interior that correspond to calcifications.

Diagnosis and Management

The triple test comprising clinical examination, US imaging, and tissue sampling is considered the gold standard for the diagnosis of breast masses in young adult women <30 years of age [25–27]. The decision of whether to biopsy these breast lesions is often based on Breast Imaging-Reporting and Data System (BI-RADS) criteria in the U.S. [28], or on the Stavros criteria in the U.K. [29]. However, a palpable lump that has US characteristics that are entirely consistent with an FA need not be biopsied unless there is overriding clinical concern [26, 30, 31]. The use of fine needle aspiration biopsy (FNA), interpreted by an experienced cytologist, means that short-term follow-up of FA can be avoided [32]. The most important differential diagnosis of FA are phyllodes tumors and hamartomas.

Treatment for breast FA is heterogeneous. Tumors of <1cm may undergo partial or total regression in up to one third of cases. A wait-and-see approach may be the best option, particularly for small tumors in females <25 years of age, or <35 years of age without familial risk for breast cancer [16, 33]. Criteria for excision include size >2–3 cm, symptomatic tumors, or imaging findings of increased vascularity or irregular borders on US leading to uncertain diagnosis. Additionally, an increase in size documented by serial US measurements or clinical examination increases the potential for an alternative diagnosis and warrants removal of the lesion. When performed, excision is focused on removing the tumor without additional surrounding breast tissue. Because these lesions are not infiltrative, they usually do not cause deformities of the breast after removal [34].

Recently, an alternative to excision has been developed. Lesions that have undergone the triple test of clinical examination, US imaging, and tissue sampling with benign findings are candidates for cryoablation. Cryoablation is performed percutaneously and destroys the lesion by freezing. Excellent long-term cosmetic results are possible with the use of cryoablation, however, its performance requires specialized training and equipment [35–37]. Radiofrequency ablation is a novel approach to percutaneous eradication of benign breast lumps. Percutaneous ultrasonographically or stereotactic-guided radiofrequency-assisted excision of FA of the breast may be performed in an ambulatory setting under local anesthesia. The procedure provides treatment for intact specimens that, in the majority of cases, appear to be completely removed after a 4–6-month follow-up. The procedure is well tolerated by patients and is associated with minimal complications [38].

Patients nearing menopause with FA should be educated as to the likely involution of these lesions with aging and a changing hormonal environment, which would argue against the consideration of either excision or ablation for the majority of patients.

Hamartoma of the Breast (HB)

The hamartoma is a benign tumor-like lesion that can affect various organs of the body, including lungs, kidneys, skin and rarely the breast. The term mammary hamartoma was introduced by Arrigoni et al. in 1971 to describe well circumscribed lesions in the breast characterized by varying amounts of benign epithelial elements, fibrous tissue, and fat. Such lesions have been known by various names, including lipofibroadenoma, adenolipoma, and fibroadenolipoma, a composite term reflecting the histological features [39]. Mammary hamartoma is not a well recognized entity. This is probably because it can be diagnosed with certainty only by employing a combination of clinical, radiological, gross, and microscopic pathological features [39]. This rare clinicopathologic entity of the breast has a reported incidence of 0.1–0.7% and comprises 0.7–4.8% of all benign breast tumors [39, 40]. HB are probably more common than anticipated in the literature and are important because they may be confused with other well circumscribed tumors, such as phyllodes tumor and fibroadenoma [41].

The pathogenesis of the hamartoma remains unclear; the histological structure and immunohistochemical profile suggest that the hamartoma probably results from a dysgenesis more than from a true tumorous process. The fact that mammary hamartoma is observed in other dysgenetic disorders such as Cowden's syndrome, favors this hypothesis [41]. Hamartomas may originate as developmental anomalies. A mass of breast tissue becomes separated during fetal development and continues its development as a "breast within a breast" [42].

The clinical presentation is that of a painless breast lump or an enlarged or slowly enlarging breast. The well circumscribed, smooth, mobile, round mass of soft-to-firm consistency feels similar to normal breast tissue [39, 40, 42]. Mammary hamartomas have been reported at all ages [39].

Average age at presentation is about 45 years, nearly 2 decades after that for fibroadenoma [42, 43]. There is usually no predilection for any specific location [41, 42]. The vast majority of patients have a single mass, with only few cases of multiple hamartomas reported [41, 44]. There is no cycle-related size fluctuation in adolescent females [44]. The size of hamartomas varies greatly, but most commonly measure between 1 and 4 cm in diameter, with an average diameter of 6–20 cm. The weight of hamartomas ranges from 5–1,500 gr [43]. The lesion can grow to a large size and become a giant hamartomas, producing marked asymmetry of the breast [43, 45–47].

The mammographic appearance of the hamartoma is fairly characteristic (Figures 3A and B); it is referred to as a "breast-in-breast" lesion and is observed as a well circumscribed mass containing both fat and soft-tissue density. A thin radio-opaque line (pseudocapsule) is often observed surrounding at least a portion of the mass. Mammographic diagnosis can be made when the lesion has a classic appearance [48–50]. The mass is surrounded by a thin radio-opaque pseudocapsule, and the degree of opacity depends on the constituents of the hamartomatous tissue [51, 52]. The lobulated densities scattered within the encapsulated fat are termed "slices of salami". These densities may be accompanied by benign amorphous or round microcalcifications [48, 49]. The mass may replace the subcutaneous fatty tissue without altering the skin [49]. There is a wide spectrum of ultrasonographic appearance. The most frequent finding is a well circumscribed solid and oval tumor, without intratumor microcalcifications [52–54] (Figures 3C and D). There may be complete, partial, or no posterior acoustic shadowing [48]. The internal echotexture may be hyperechoic, isoechoic, or heterogeneous with mixed echogenicity. Harmatoma echotexture varies across studies, but heterogeneous echotexture is the most typical feature of hamartomas [51, 54]. Cystic areas have been described within hamartomas in 24% of cases. The hamartoma may present compressibility, which indicates a benign lesion [54]. Because of their variable appearance, US plays a minimal role in diagnosing hamartomas [48, 53]. However, it is noteworthy that for these masses, which comply with benign sonographic criteria for solid breast masses, histological sampling by core biopsy may be considered optional by those who think that there is sufficient evidence in the literature for sonographic surveillance of solid masses when these specific criteria are fulfilled [55].

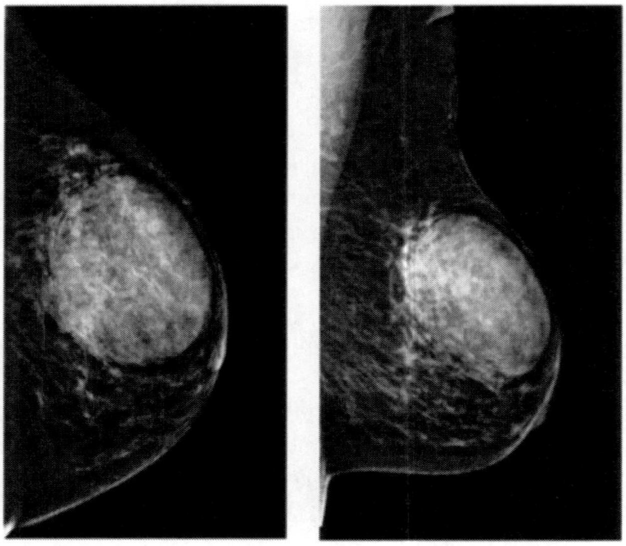

A B

Figures 3A, B. 63 year old female with an ovoid nodule in the left upper outer quadrant of the left breast. The nodule is well circumscribed with heterogeneous density and a dense halo.

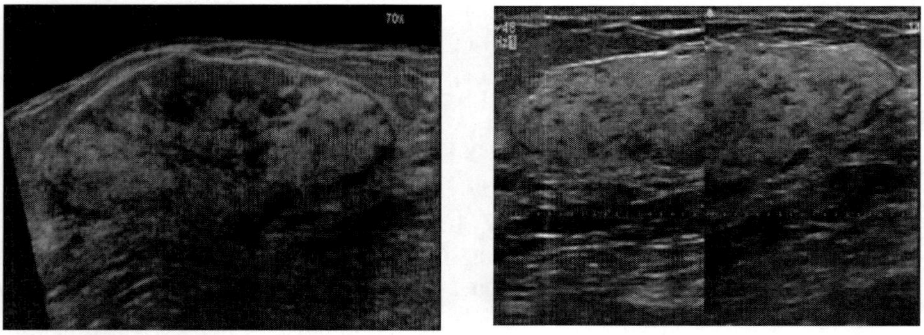

C D

Figure 3C, D. On Ultrasound (US), it is observed as an ovoid nodule of heterogeneous echogenicity, with margins circumscribed by fine echogenic line (pseudocapsule). *US image in extended scan.

Pathological Features

Macroscopically, these tumors are well defined round masses with a rubbery, fleshy cut surface and gray or yellow in color, depending on the relative proportions of the components. Microscopically, hamartomas are well circumscribed, unencapsulated lesions composed of a variety of normal breast constituents, with stroma surrounding the duct and lobular structures. Adipose tissue and smooth muscle may be present [62]. Differential diagnosis of hamartoma includes fibroadenoma and phyllodes tumor [55, 62, 63]. The immunohistochemical profile of hamartomas is generally similar to that of normal breast tissue or breast tissue with fibrocystic changes [41]. It is important to realize that hamartomas do not possess specific diagnostic histological features, and that the role of FNAB and Core needle biopsy (CNB) in arriving at a diagnosis is limited [51]. Clinical and radiological correlation is required to avoid making an incorrect diagnosis [64]. The low risk of discovering a carcinoma within a hamartoma and typical mammographic findings are sufficient reasons for counseling against systematic surgical removal or biopsy. Such an attitude must depend on other considerations related with the classical aspects of breast cancer diagnosis [60]. Excisional biopsy is diagnostic and can only exclude the possibility of malignancy [44, 65]. Surgical excision may be avoided when such a typical appearance of breast hamartoma is observed in the mammogram [64] and if this diagnosis is determined after CNB [55]. Surgical excision should be considered for large masses and those with rapid growth, because more serious lesions, such as phyllodes tumors, cannot be excluded, even if limited sampling appears benign [44]. Surgical treatment is the curative method when hamartomas present as giant breast masses [65].

In sum, breast hamartomas are rare breast masses. Diagnosis of these lesions depends on mammographic and US findings in combination with clinical, gross, and microscopic pathological features. Because of the low risk of discovering a carcinoma within the hamartoma and its typical mammographic findings, systematic surgical removal or biopsy is not recommended.

Granular Cell Tumor of the Breast

Granular cell tumor (GCT) is a soft tissue neoplasm defined as a neoplastic proliferation of cells derived from peripheral nerve Schwann cells [62]. It arises at virtually any body site but is mainly found in the skin, oral cavity and digestive tract. About 5–8% of all GCT occurs in the breast [66]. This tumor was first described by Abrikossoff in 1926 as ''granular cell myoblastoma'', assuming it to be of myogenic origin. Further immunohistochemical analysis has shown that these lesions have a perineural or Schwann cell origin, apparently due to the positivity of the tumor for the S-100 protein and to the similarities exhibited in the structural features of the tumor cells and those of Schwann cells [67, 68]. Although there are a limited number of cases reported in the literature, the frequency of GTC is estimated as 1 in every 1,000 breast cancers [68, 69].

Breast GCT occur more commonly in middle aged, premenopausal women with a slight preponderance in African-American women [67–70]. GCT of the breast have also been described in men [71, 72]. The preponderance of these tumors in women, especially in premenopausal females, has led to the hypothesis that hormones are implicated in the pathogenesis of this breast tumor; however, to date, no estrogen or progesterone receptors have been found in the tumor cells of any of these tumors reported in the literature [73, 74].

GTC arises from interlobular breast stroma. In contrast with the majority of other breast tumors, which occur predominantly in the upper outer quadrant, GCT are most frequently found in the upper inner quadrant, corresponding to the cutaneous sensory territory of the supraclavicular nerve [67, 69, 73]. GCT usually appears as a solitary unilateral lump, but multicentricity has been reported in 5.4–17.5% of cases. Multicentricity includes other lesions both within the breast and external to it. The multicentricity of lesions does not appear to affect prognosis adversely [67, 68, 72]. Cases of multifocal GCT involving the breast are not well described in the literature. A multiplicity of lesions can narrow the differential diagnosis and point the breast imager in the right direction, as the only other significant diagnostic considerations would be metastatic disease and lymphoma. This unique feature of granular cell tumors should be considered when evaluating for multifocal disease involving the breast [71].

GCT usually present as a firm and painless mass; however, elastic consistency and breast pain have been reported [72]. They are generally mobile, but may be adhered to the pectoral muscle or to the skin, thus mimicking a malignant lesion [73–77]. They can range from well defined, regular, and round to ill defined and irregular. Skin involvement includes thickening, tethering, dimpling, and retraction [78]. Associated lymphadenopathy is rare, but two cases were identified with nodal enlargement. Examination of these lymph nodes revealed marginal reactive change but no evidence of disease in either case [79].

GCT are usually solitary. Approximately 10% coexist with malignancy. Coexistence and co localization with ductal carcinoma has been previously described. The existence of co localization and the predominant relationship with ductal carcinoma raises the question of whether there is a causal or coincidental relationship between GCT and ductal carcinoma [80].

Malignant granular cell tumors (MGCT) are extremely rare neoplasms, representing only 1–2% of all GCT. Since the first reported case of an MGCT by Ravich et al., >100 cases have been reported in the English-language literature [81]. Features of malignant GCTB include large, rapidly growing masses, which are associated with lymphadenopathy, aggressive local invasion, and poor circumscription. However, these factors should not be utilized to assess malignant character in isolation [82]. It appears that best management for a malignant GCT is wide, local excision with axillary lymph node dissection [81].

Traditional imaging techniques including mammography and US scanning are widely employed when investigating the presence of a breast mass. However, the issue with these modalities in cases of GCT is that the radiological findings are often indistinguishable from those of breast malignancies [72, 80].

The mammographic features of GCT of the breast are indeterminate in the majority of patients; their appearance on mammography is widely variable, ranging from well circumscribed, benign appearing nodules to highly suspicious spiculated masses associated with skin retraction and thickening. These tumors are known to evoke a desmoplastic reaction, leading to retraction of surrounding tissue and skin. Thus, spiculations are common mammographic findings and some lesions may show subtle or partial spiculations. Some tumors appear as vague densities, whereas others may have a lobulated appearance. Granular cell tumor-associated calcifications have not been reported in the literature. The tumors occurred at various depths from the skin, ranging from very superficial, mimicking a sebaceous cyst, to deep and close to the thoracic wall [69, 71, 83].

Ultrasonography characteristics for GCT generally infer a suspicion of malignancy. Common features include solid, heterogeneous, poorly defined masses with a high depth:width ratio. They may show hypervascular echotexture, particularly peripherally, although this is not consistent. GCT could be higher than wide. They are generally hypoechoic and display posterior shadowing with a coarse internal echo and high boundary echo. There may also be disrupted fascial planes associated with dimpling. On Doppler sonography, a GCT may show variable vascularity, whereas another exhibits prominent arterial flow within the tumor. The range of USG findings is as wide as those of mammography; they are often suggestive of malignancy and most importantly, there are no specific recognized features for GCT [69, 71, 80, 83].

Magnetic resonance imaging (MRI) could be performed to evaluate disease extent and the presence or absence of the aggressive features observed in other breast malignancies. MRI findings of GCT of the breast reported in the literature include isointensity on T1- and T2-weighted images and non homogeneous rim enhancement after gadolinium injection [82, 84].

Clinically and radiographically, it is impossible to establish a definitive diagnosis of GCT of the breast without a biopsy. Sonograph-guided percutaneous biopsy of the lesion is well established as the diagnostic procedure-of-choice for histopathological sampling.

Pathological Features

Macroscopically, granular cell tumors form a yellowish- white solid mass with irregular or well defined borders, usually <2 cm in their maximal dimension.

Microscopic Findings

The tumor is composed of sheets, nests, or cords of large oval or polygonal cells with abundant granular eosinophilic cytoplasm. Nuclei are small with inconspicuous nucleoli. The cellular aggregates are separated by prominent fibrous septa and may appear to infiltrate irregularly into the adjacent breast parenchyma. Mitoses are rare and pleomorphism, unusual [62, 69].

The most accepted histological criteria for diagnosing malignant GCT were established by Fanburg-Smith et al. in 1998. These criteria include the following: necrosis; spindling of the tumor cells; vesicular nuclei with large nucleoli; an increased mitotic rate (>2 mitoses/10 high-power fields at 200X magnification); a high nuclear-to-cytoplasmic ratio, and pleomorphism. A granular tumor cell was classified as ''malignant'' if it had 3 or more of these features, ''atypical'' if it had only 1–2, and ''benign'' if none of these features or if a focal nuclear pleomorphism were present [85]. Recently, Nasser et al. [86] proposed criteria for tumors with necrosis detected in histological specimens to be classified as ''GCT with uncertain malignant potential'' and for tumors with metastases to be classified as ''MGCT". Nesser considered that metastasis was the sole denominator of a malignant case. It is necessary for proper treatment to evaluate the malignant disease before it spreads distally [81, 86].

Ancillary Studies

Cytoplasmic granules are positive for Periodic Acid Schiff (PAS) and are diastase-resistant.

Immunohistochemistry

Tumor cells stain positively for S100 protein, Neuron-specific enolase (NSE), and vimentin; CD68 and Carcinoembryonic antigen (CEA) positivity is variable. Estrogen and progesterone receptors and cytokeratins are negative.

Ultrastructural Features

Granular cells contain abundant secondary lysosomes in the cytoplasm and replicated basal lamina around the granular cells. Some cells may contain triangular membrane-bounded structures composed of microtubules and microfibrils [62, 69, 71, 82].

FNA cytological features of GCT are cellular with cohesive groups of cells exhibiting a syncytial appearance, as well as dispersed single cells. The cells contain abundant, finely eosinophilic granular cytoplasm and small, round-to-slightly oval nuclei. Bare bipolar cells of stromal or myoepithelial type are absent. This, combined with the increased cellularity, may be confused with malignancy. Cytological features of GCT are not pathognomonic. Differential diagnoses include inflammatory, benign, and malignant lesions and most notably, inflammatory fat necrosis, apocrine carcinoma, secretory carcinoma, the alveolar variant of lobular carcinoma, alveolar soft part sarcoma, malignant melanoma, and metastatic renal cell carcinoma. Another lesion of the breast that can mimic GCT on cytological analysis is apocrine metaplasia [62, 72, 80, 87]. Markers that could help differentiate GCT from granular histiocytes include NSE and CD57. The use of a panel of markers may not always be feasible on fine needle aspirates because of the limited material available. Percutaneous core biopsy may be necessary to provide more adequate sampling [87].

Diagnostic work-up or follow-up should be conducted in accordance with the clinical presentation and the level of radiographical suspicion. Therefore, histological assessment of a breast lesion is mandatory [82].

Management of benign breast GCT is largely dependent on clinical presentation and includes conservative follow-up or wide excision. Resection with adequate margins is necessary because the tumor has no capsule and is proliferative and invasive. Llocal recurrence after adequate excision, although rare, has been reported [66, 79, 82, 88]. Axillary clearance or sentinel lymph node biopsy is not indicated except in the cases of malignant GTC [73, 80]. Further adjuvant chemotherapy or radiotherapy is not required [66, 76]. The definitive diagnosis is arrived at with histopathological assessment and confirmed by immunohistochemical examination; this should be kept in mind while dealing with breast masses to prevent overtreatment [88, 89]. Malignant GCT should be treated similarly to other breast malignant neoplasms [73, 81]. Treatment should be associated with annual follow-up, although it is not specified whether this should be by examination or imaging [90].

The prognosis for benign GCT of the breast is excellent. Recurrence occurs in 2–8% of individuals after excision with wide margins. However, even in these cases, prognosis is favorable [80, 90, 91].

Summary

Granular cell tumor of the breast is a rare benign neoplasm that may mimic breast carcinoma both clinically and radiologically. Routine histopathology with immunohistochemical studies confirms the diagnosis. Appropriate treatment involves wide local excision. Complete surgical excision is curative.

Phyllodes Tumor

The phyllodes tumor is a rare entity. There are reports of it existence since 1774. In 1827 Chelius described them and in 1838 Johannes Müller coined the "cystosarcoma phyllodes" due to their macro- and microscopic aspect. However, in 1981, the World Health Organization (WHO) proposed eliminating the term cystosarcoma due to the fact that the majority of the lesions are benign, and proposed the name phyllodes tumor [92]. This tumor forms part of a group of tumors known as fibroepithelial lesions, where fibroadenoma is also found, and that possess, as a special characteristic, being composed of epithelial as well as stromal elements.

It is an infrequent entity that represents 0.3–0.9% of breast tumors and 2–3% of all fibroepithelial tumors of the breast [93, 94]. Average age at diagnosis of this group of lesions is 45 years and ranges from 35–55 years. In average, phyllodes tumors present 20 later than the fibroadenoma, which constitutes the most important differential diagnosis [95, 96]. Some cases have been described in males and it has invariably been associated with gynecomastia [93]. Bilaterality or multiple lesions are infrequent.

Etiology

The exact cause of this type of lesion is unknown; however, in 1993, Noguchi et al. [97] analyzed the clonality of fibroadenomas as well as phyllodes tumors by means of PCR of the DNA of the epithelial as well as the stromal component; these authors found that fibroadenomas were polyclonal, more similar to a hyperplastic- than to a neoplastic-type lesion, and that phyllodes tumors showed monoclonal mutations in the cells of the stromal component, more similar to a neoplastic lesion. There are reports of the transformation of fibroadenomas into phyllodes tumors, apparently exhibiting less aggressive behavior [18]. Some factors have been described that behave as stimulants of their growth, including breast trauma, pregnancy, and the increase of estrogen levels; however, their association remains inconclusive due to the rarity of the lesion [93].

Classification

The WHO in 1982 classified this group as benign, borderline, and malignant, taking into account various histological parameters that include grade of cellular atypia in the stroma, mitotic activity in 10 high-power fields, and degree of stromal growth. This classification is depicted in Table 1 [98].

Azzopardi and collaborators [99] proposed another classification that is presented in Table 2, in which the authors considered the same criteria as the WHO, with the addition of degree of pleomorphism. Based on these histologic criteria, the phyllodes tumor is benign in 40–80%, borderline in 10–20%, and malignant in 5–30% of cases [100, 101].

Table 1. World Health Organization (WHO) classification

Criterion	Benign	Borderline	Malignant
Stromal and atypical cellularity	Minimal	Moderate	Marked
Stromal overgrowth	Minimal	Moderate	Market
Mitoses/10high-power fields	0–4	5–9	10 or more
Tumor margins	Well circumscribed with pressing borders	Focal infiltration zone at margins	Infiltrating margins

Table 2. Azzopardi classification

Criterion	Benign	Borderline	Malignant
Tumor margin	Pressing		Infiltrating
Stromal cellularities	Low	Moderate	High
Mitoses/10 power fields	<5	5–9	10 or more
Pleomorphism	Slight	Moderate	Severe

One distinctive characteristic of this tumor group is that the histological aspect or tumor subtype has no direct correlation with the evolution of the disease and its capacity to recur and cause distal metastasis. Thus, cases of metastatic disease have been reported in patients with histologically benign phyllodes tumors [102–104].

Diagnosis

As in all breast lesions, the diagnostic approach to phyllodes tumor should be based on the diagnostic triad formed by clinical exploration, imaging studies, and histopathological confirmation of the lesion [102–105].

Clinical Condition

The characteristic clinical manifestation of the phyllodes tumor comprises the self-detection of a tumor of solid consistency, generally not painful and, as a very characteristic fact in malignant phyllodes tumors, a very rapid increase in volume. Therefore, when faced with rapid growth, this diagnosis should be suspected [96, 106–108].

Average size at diagnosis is approximately 4 cm; In 20% of cases, the lesion can reach >10 cm. Tumors of >40 cm have been described [106].

On palpation, phyllodes tumor is typically a lesion of solid consistency, generally not adhered to the skin or to deep planes, with well delimited borders. In tumors of great dimensions, a prominent collateral venous network and thinning of the skin are frequently observed. Ulceration of the skin associated with local pressure and necrosis rarely presents, and frank cutaneous infiltration by the tumor rarely presents. In recurrent tumors, there is the risk of local infiltration of the thoracic wall [93, 95, 101, 109]. There can be palpable adenopathies in 10 to 15% of cases; however, tumor lymph node infiltration has been described in fewer than 1% cases [93]. In males, clinical presentation is practically the same as in females.

Diagnosis by Imaging

Mastography (MG) and Ultrasound (US) are the main imaging studies utilized for the assessment of phyllodes tumor and at present, Magnetic resonance (MRI) has acquired a preponderant role in the evaluation of these lesions [110].

Mastography

Because phyllodes tumors present as nodules, the mastographic data should be described according to the BI-RADS system. Thus, in the primary mastographic evaluation, the finding corresponds to BI-RADS category 0 (incomplete evaluation), which is indicative of the performance of a complementary study, which is generally an US. The form, contour, and density of the module should be evaluated.

The most frequent form of mastographic presentation is that of a non speculated solid mass with lobulated borders, an oval form or a round form (Figure 4).

With respect to contour, phyllodes tumors are most commonly well circumscribed, sometimes indistinct and, less frequently, obscured. In the benign phyllodes tumor, one frequently observes circumscribed margins, while in the malignant variant, it is possible to observe an infiltrating edge. Generally, lesions are high density, similar to fibroadenomas and, on very few occasions, one can observe calcifications [111, 112] (Figures 5–7).

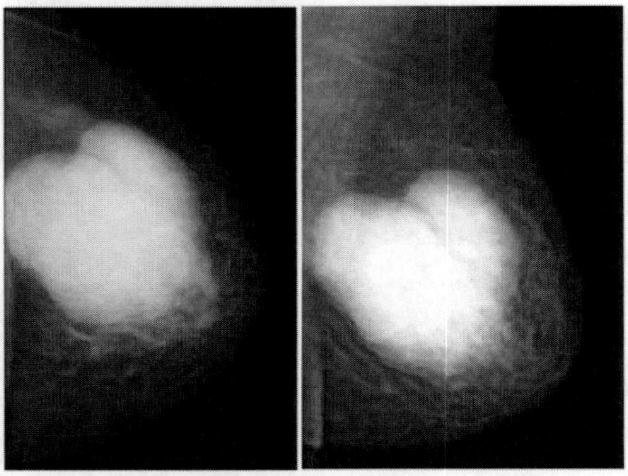

Figure 4A. 75 year old female. Left Mediolateral-oblique (MLO) and Cranial-caudal (CC) projections show a large lobulated lesion, with high density and obscured margins.

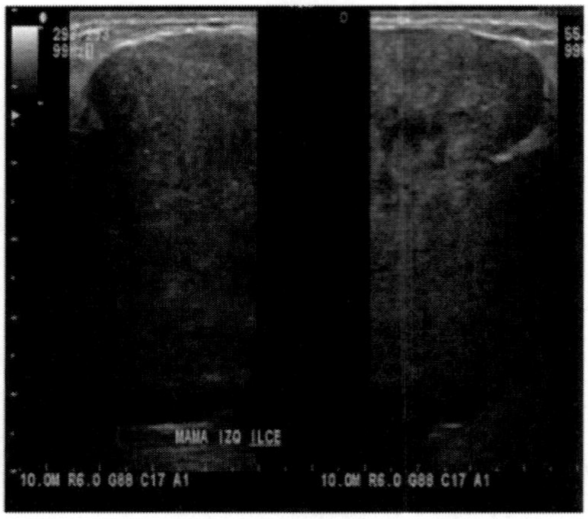

Figure 4B. Ultrasound (US). (C) shows a lobulated mass, of circumscribed margins, heterogeneous, of hypoechoic predominance, with cystic zones in its interior.

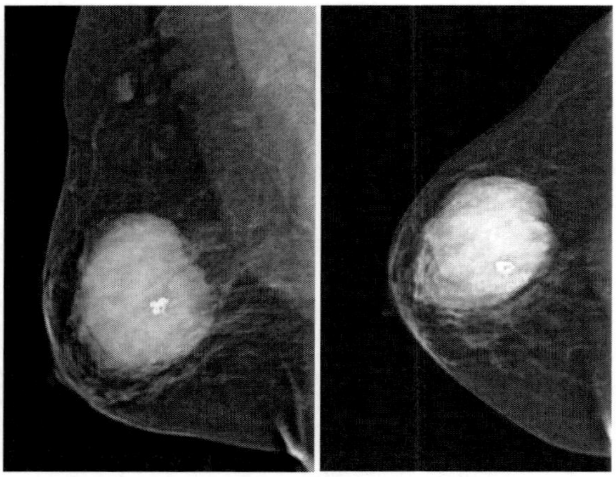

Figure 5A. 51 year old female. Right MLO and CC projections show a mass with lobulated edges and mixed density associated with dystrophic calcifications that occupies the external quadrants.

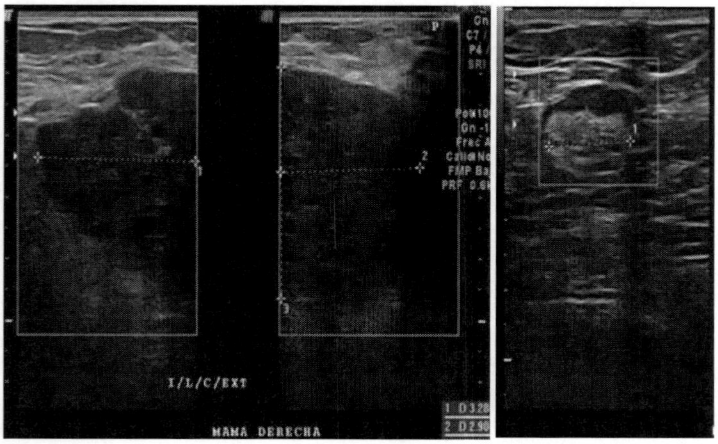

Figure 5B. Ultrasound (US) shows a mass of great size, lobulated with circumscribed margins, of hypoechoic predominance and zones in its interior.

The differential diagnosis should be carried out with benign as well as with malignant lesions. Among the benign lesions with which differential diagnosis should be conducted, the fibroadenoma is the most frequent and probably the most difficult to differentiate. Differential diagnosis should also be established with simple cysts, complicated and complex cysts, solitary papilloma, and multiple papillomas.

Among malignant lesions with which a differential diagnosis must be made are lymphomas, mucinous carcinomas, bone marrow carcinomas, papillary carcinomas, and metastatic breast lesions.

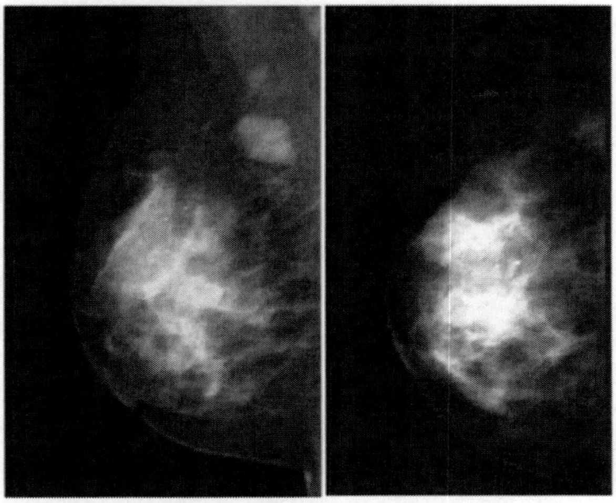

Figure 6A. 41 year old female. Mastography (MG) shows nodule of obscured margins and high density in the Upper outer quadrant (UOQ) of the right breast, as well as dense axillary lymph nodes.

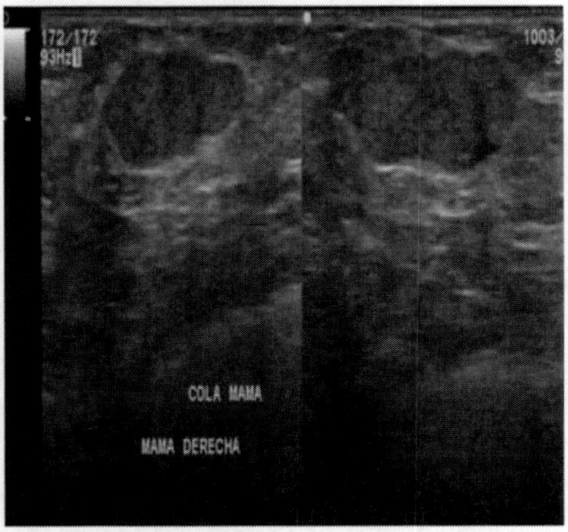

Figure 6B. Ultrasound (US) reveals the presence of a solid nodule, microlobulated, heterogeneous, localized in tail of Spence.

Ultrasound

Similarly to the mastographic findings, the ultrasonographic findings should be described according to the BI-RADS lexicon. These are evaluated, as with all breast nodules, according to form, contour, echogenic halo, and internal echoes. The nodules present as lobulated; in some cases, these can be round or oval. The contours are circumscribed and well defined (Figures 8 and 9), with echogenic halo and low-level, heterogeneous internal echoes. In addition, microcalcifications and posterior acoustic transmission can be observed.

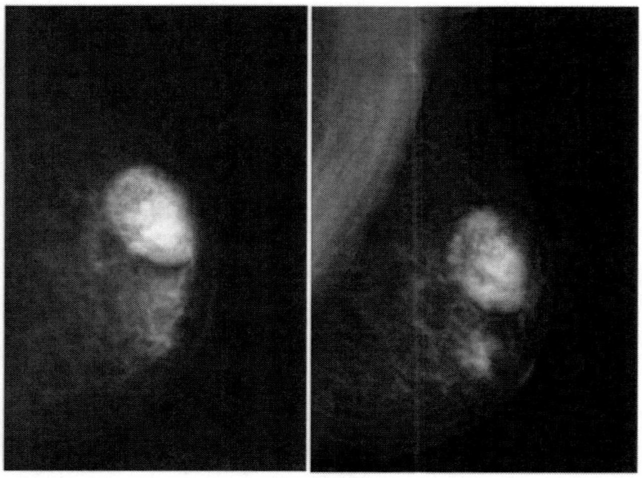

Figure 7A. 27 year old female. Mastography (MG) demonstrated a heterogeneous nodule of partially defined margins, which presents internal radiolucent areas.

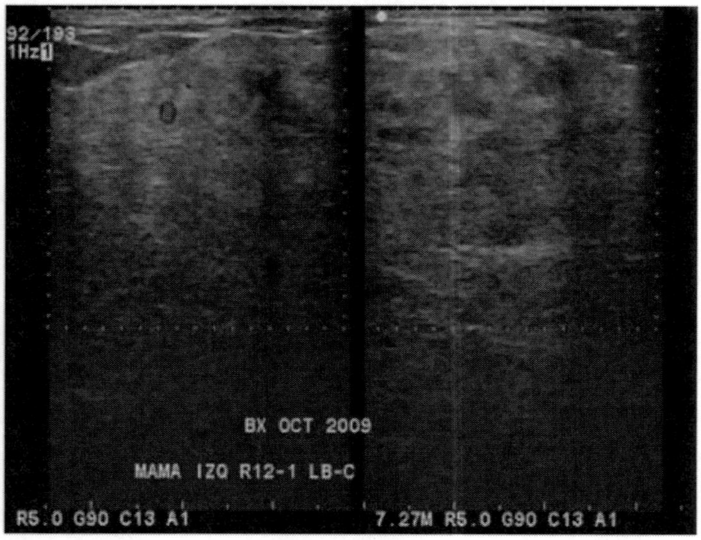

Figure 7B. Ultrasound (US) demonstrates a solid nodule, isoechoic, of partially defined margins.

There is an important superimposition of the ultrasonographic characteristics between phyllodes tumors and fibroadenomas. The diagnosis of phyllodes tumor should be considered if lobulations or internal echoes are observed in the nodule; however, ultrasonographically, a distinction cannot be made among benign, borderline, or malignant phyllodes tumors [113, 114].

Magnetic Resonance

MR is a highly sensitive technique for the detection of breast cancer. Among the most utilized protocols employed for the evaluation of the breast, a 1.5T resonator is used. For the bilateral morphological study, the spatial, high-resolution T2 sequence is utilized, without highlighting or fat saturation on the axial plane. The three-dimensional (3D) dynamic sequences utilize T1 with or without fat saturation according to the criteria of the radiologist, with cuts between 2 and3mm according to the size of the breast. The dose of gadolinium is standard at 0.1mmol/kg with an injection speed of 2ml/second. For the dynamic studies, the sequences are utilized with or without fat saturation and time subtraction.

Similar to the previously described methods, the findings should be described according to BI-RADS terminology. Form, contour, internal structure, septa, signal intensity in T1 and T2, and highlighted patterns should be assessed. The form generally is round or lobulated, the contour is well defined, the internal structure is heterogeneous, and the septa are not highlighted, hypointense in T1 and hypo- or isointense in T2. With regard to the highlighting patterns, the benign lesions present slow initial highlighting with a persistent late phase [115].

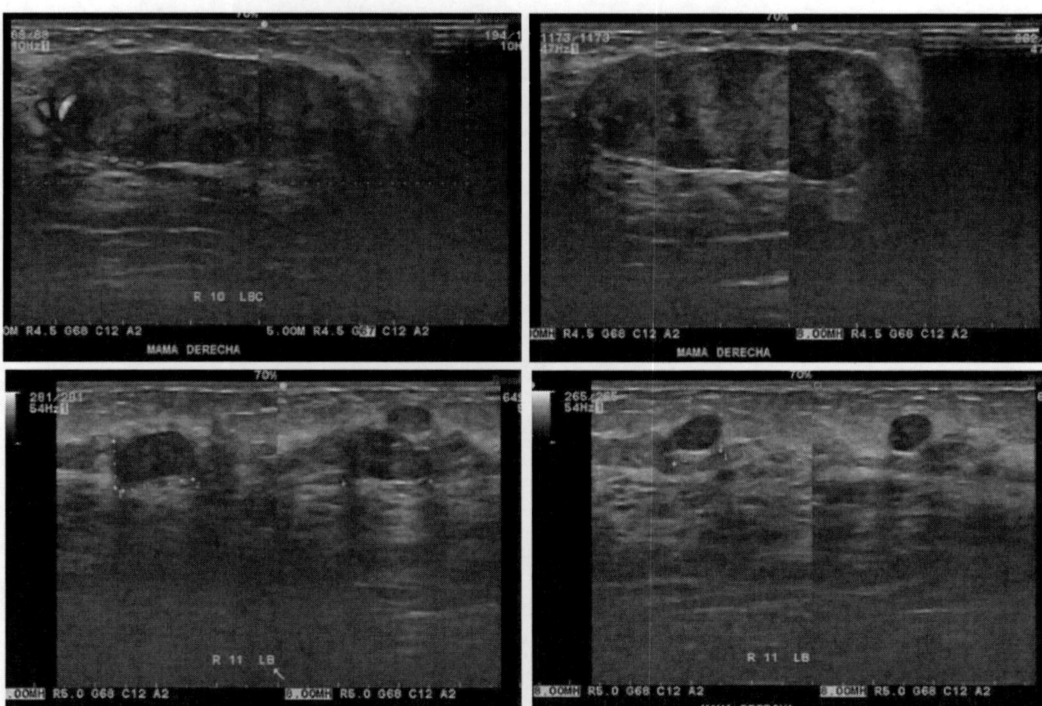

Figure 8. 31 year old female with a 12 week pregnancy Ultrasound (US) demonstrates an oval nodule, circumscribed, heterogeneous, predominantly hypoechoic, with intrinsic vascularity that has increased in size, adjacent to which there are at least three small nodules with similar characteristics.

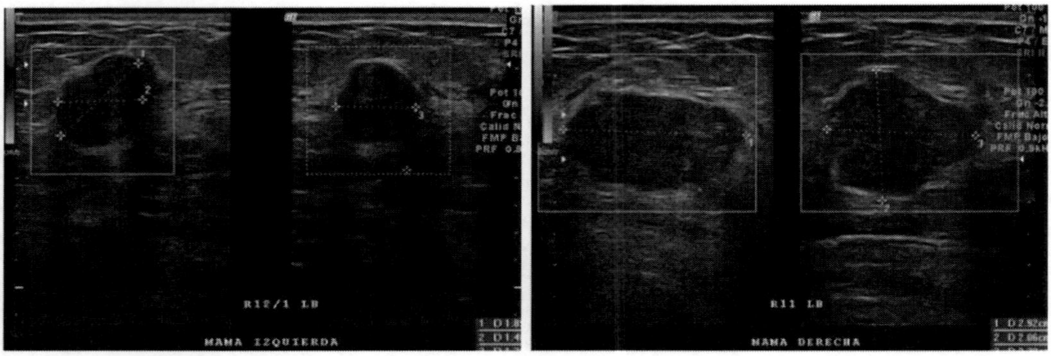

Figure 9. 40 year old female. Ultrasound (US) shows solid, heterogeneous nodules of microlobulated margins in both breasts.

The malignant lesion presents rapid initial highlighting with a persistent plateau or a rapid initial phase with a washout phenomenon. MR can also be useful for differentiation between the benign phyllodes tumor from the malignant variety in some cases [116].

Differential Diagnosis

Lesion	T1	T2	KINETICS
Phyllodes tumor	Intense contrast uptake	Hyperintense	Ascending curve and in plateau
Fibroadenoma	Isointense. Intense impregnation and homogenenous with contrast	Depending on content, iso, hypo, or hyperintense	Ascending curve or in plateau
Papilloma	Hypointense. Intense contrast uptake cap	Intermediate signal	Ascending curve or in plateau
Cysts	Hypointense. Without contrast uptake	Hyperintense	X
Fat necrosis	Hyperintense. Behavior with contrast depends on stage	Hyperintense	Stage-dependent
Lymph nodes	Hyperintense fatty hilium. Intense contrast uptake	Hyperintense.	Washout-type curve
Hematoma and seroma	Hypointense	Hyperintense.	X
IDC (Invasive ductal carcinoma)	Isointense. Reinforce-ment or no mass with contrast	Variable behavior, frequently isointense	Washout-type curve
ILC (Invasive lobular carcinoma)	Isointense. Reinforcement or no mass with contrast	Variable behavior, frequently isointense	Washout-type curve

Histological Diagnosis

The use of fine needle aspiration biopsy (FNA) in the diagnosis of phyllodes tumor is controversial because the diagnostic accuracy reported is variable. Some studies have reported high sensitivity [6, 115], and on some occasions, this has been reported to be around 63% [114]. Therefore, the initial diagnostic procedure that is proposed is the short-needle biopsy (the Trucut biopsy), which has demonstrated 99% sensitivity, a positive predictive value (PPV) of 93%, and a negative predictive value (NPV) of 83%, this in addition to the fact that it is a procedure that can be easily performed in the physician's office with a low index of complications and that is less invasive than open biopsy[117–120].

Phyllodes tumors generally are histologically differentiated from fibroadenomas by their greater stromal cellularity and their mitotic activity [121–123]; however, because stromal cellularity can be heterogeneous, surgical excision of the lesion is suggested for its complete evaluation. Likewise, short-needle biopsy specimens that show marked stromal cellularity, (>2 mitoses/10 high-power fields, and high proliferation indexes, Ki 67 and topoisomerase II) should suggest the possibility of being phyllodes tumors [124, 125].

Although infrequent, these can be found in malignant phyllodes tumors and in sarcomatoid elements such as angiosarcoma, chondrosarcoma, osteosarcoma, leiomyosarcoma, liposarcoma, and rabdomyosarcoma.

The expression of certain biological markers has been studied in phyllodes tumors, such as the proliferation index by Ki67 and the expression index of topoisomerase II, which correlate well between each other, as well as the p53 mutation. These have been used as tools to help to improve diagnostic accuracy and to carry out differential diagnosis between a benign phyllodes tumor and malignant variants, as well as for differentiation with fibroadenomas. It has been reported that the expression of these biological markers is greater in phyllodes tumors than in fibroadenomas. It has been suggested that these markers could be useful in cases of difficult histological diagnosis by hematoxylin and eosin staining (H&E) [104, 124, 126, 127]. Similarly, it has been found that there is an overexpression of the epidermal growth factor receptor (EGFR), reported by Tse and coworkers, with expression rates of 16.2% (48/296) for benign phyllodes tumors, 30.6% (30/98) for borderline, and 56% (33/59) for malignant phyllodes tumors [128]. Recent studies have found certain genetic alterations that are characteristic of benign tumors; gains have been described, mainly in chromosomes 1q, 5q, and 18q, as well as chromosome losses of 13q, 6q, 10q, and 12q. These chromosome imbalances were identified in 83% (25 of 30) of phyllodes tumors, which were present in 55% of morphologically benign tumors compared with 91% of borderline tumors and 100% of benign tumors. It has been suggested that the search for these chromosomal aterations could be useful for differentiating among benign (0–3 mutations), borderline (0–13 mutations), and malignant phyllodes tumors (0–21 mutations) [129, 130]. Chromosome gains1q and 13q are chromosomal alterations are those most frequently found and they are significantly associated for borderline and malignant phyllodes tumors [130].

Differential Diagnosis

Breast lesions with which a differential diagnosis should be established are the following: Fibroadenoma, adenoma, hamartom, lipoma, infantile papillomatosis, carcinoma, sarcoma, and metastatic tumors.

Treatment

Surgery is the cornerstone of treatment for phyllodes tumors. The recommendation is resection of the lesion with a three-dimensional (3D) macroscopic margin of at least 1 cm. This can be performed by means of conservative breast surgery, however, in voluminous lesions; the performance of mastectomy will be required. Formerly, the convetional surgical option consisted of mastectomy; however, multiple studies have reported similar local recurrence rates in comparison with wide, local excision of the tumor whenever the surgical margin is found to be free. This applies to histologically benign as well as to malignant lesions [131–134]. There is no contraindication from the oncologic point of view for performing immediate reconstructive procedures in cases in which mastectomy is necessary. The surgical procedures recommended are abdominal rectal musculocutaneous flaps (ARMF) or wide dorsal flaps for coverage of large resections or as part of reconstructive procedures; similarly, there is evidence of the use of implant-expanders in some cases [135].

Surgical management of the axilla is not routinely indicated because the reported incidence of metastasis to axillary lymph nodes is <1%; resection of the lymph nodes should only be carried out with cytologically confirmed infiltration. The overall survival rate and disease free survival is similar, independently of the type of surgery conducted whenever the surgical margin is the recommended one, despite there being a greater risk of local recurrences with conservative management of the breast [136]. A report exists of the preoperatory embolism of a giant tumor with the purpose of optimizing the surgical treatment and diminishing transoperatory bleeding [137]. The use of short-needle vacuum aspiration in histologically benign phyllodes tumors as a nonsurgical alternative in small lesions has also been reported, permitting complete excision of the lesion and without increasing the risk of recurrences, which are reported in 3.2% [138].

The usefulness of adjuvant radiotherapy in the management of phyllodes tumors is controversial; there are reports of its usefulness in diminishing the risk of local recurrences in malignant tumors whenever margins are unsatisfactory [139, 140]. The combination of some of the following factors can be considered for the indication of adjuvant radiotherapy: voluminous tumor; close margins or positive margins with the impossibility of a new surgical resection, and recurrent and/or malignant tumor [141, 142]. Despite the reporting of the expression of hormone receptors for estrogen and progesterone in up to 50% of phyllodes tumors, the role of hormonal management has not been established [143, 144].

Recurrence and Global Survival

In general, the local recurrence rate has been reported to be between 8 and 40%, with an average of 15%. Distant metastasis has been reported in 1–21%. In benign phyllodes tumors, the local recurrence rate is 4% and the overall survival rate is 96%; however, in borderline and malignant phyllodes tumors, local recurrence rates are higher, posing a 20% risk of distant metastasis for borderline and 22% for maglignant variants. [131, 145, 146].

Local recurrence generally is associated with surgical management, where the main risk factor comprises an inadequate surgical margin (close or positive margin); however, it has also been associated with some histological characteristics, such as histological grade, mitotic activity, and degree of cellular atypia of the stroma [93, 100, 147]. Local metastases are not necessarily associated with distant metastases. Treatment for local recurrences is based on surgical excision and on some occasions, may require resection of the thoracic wall [148–152].

The prognosis of metastatic disease is ominous and generally entertains highly aggressive behavior, with an expected survival period of 6 months [153].

The most frequent site of distant metastasis is the lung, followed by bone and abdomen; these can occur even in the absence of lymph node metastases, and in general, the stromal element is the only histological element identified. The treatment of distal metastatic disease has yet to be defined; the use of chemotherapy is controversial in palliative as well as in adjuvant terrain, due to existing literature in which no benefit is shown in overall survial, expected to be 6.5 months after recurrence [154]. Some authors have reported good palliation of symptoms with single agent chemotherapy and with polychemotherapy; however, the prognosis of these patients is somber with mean survival of 6–36 months [122].

Adenomas of the Breast

Adenomas of the breast are pure benign epithelial lesions, they are divided into tubular adenoma, adenoma of lactancy, apocrine adenoma, ductal adenoma, and pleomorphic adenoma (benign mixed tumor) [155, 156].

Adenoma of the Nipple

This is a rare, benign condition of the nipple that can mimic malignant lesions of the mammary gland, such as carcinoma and Paget's disease [157–160]. Approximately 200 cases have been reported in the world literature [161]. The most frequent form of presentation is as an ulcerative lesion of the nipple, which can be accompanied by pain or pruritus. Average age at presentation is between 45 and 50 years; however, some cases have been reported in infancy [161,162]and exceptional cases have been described in males [163]. Histologically, the tumor is formed of an adenomatous and papillomatous proliferation of the epithelium of lactating breasts with strongly stacked cells with lack of uniform morphology and polarity with intact myoepithelial cells around the ducts [164]. By immunohistochemistry, the glandular epithelium is diffusely positive for 34betaE12, partially positive for CK5/6, and negative for p53 and c-erbB-2, with the myoepithelium positive for p63, smooth muscle actin and calponin. Although this concerns benign tumors, there are reports of cases of malignant transformation; however, this is exceptional [165].

It is highly important to establish the differential diagnosis preoperatively with lesions such as Paget's disease, papillary adenocarcinoma, and intraductal papillary carcinoma, with the purpose of avoiding the performance of excessive treatment [166, 167].

Treatment is based on surgical resection of the lesion with free surgical margins; thus, it is frequently necessary to conduct complete resection of the nipple.

Tubular Adenoma

Tubular adenoma is a benign epithelial breast tumor that represents from 0.12–1.7% of benign breast lesions. It was described for the first time in 1968 by Persaud. Few cases have been reported in the literature, especially in young women at reproductive age; >90% of cases are diagnosed in women under the age of 40. They are considered to be variants of pericannalicular fibroadenomas with the exceptional prominence of an epithelial proliferation similar to that of florid adenosis [168].

Clinically, it presents as a well defined solid lesion that is not associated with alterations of the nipple or of the skin, similar to fibroadenomas, with a generally softer consistency that these. Size varies from 1–7 cm and they are generally present between 2 and 12 months prior to diagnosis.

Macroscopically, tubular adenomas are well circumscribed solid lesions with a fine capsule, on being cut, solid heterogeneous, of slightly yellow coloration [169].

Histologically, the tumor is characterized by the presence of compacted, homogeneous tubular structures associated with an epithelial acinar component with scarce stroma, which can aid in differentiating it from fibroadenomas, in which the stromal component is considerable. The tubular structures generally exhibit small lumina and are generally empty, although sometimes scarce proteinaceous eosinophilic material can be shown [169].

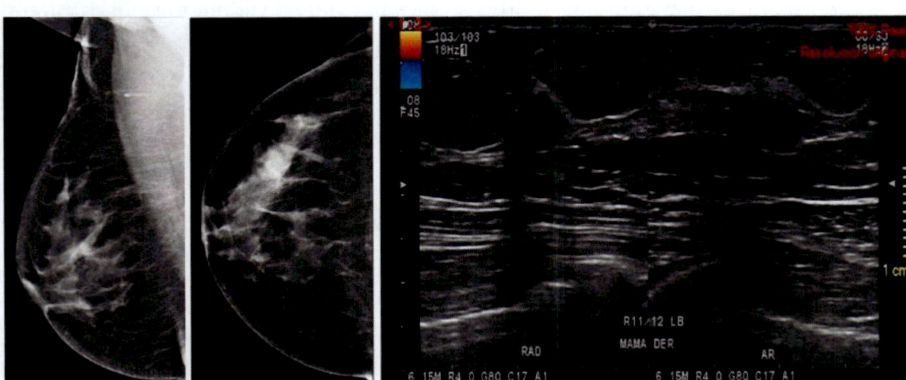

Figure 10. 39 year old female. Cranio-caudal (CC) (a) and Mediolateral-oblique (MLO) (b) projection of the right breast. Focal asymmetry in external quadrants that is partially modified in the MLO projection may be seen. On Ultrasound (US), a nodule is observed of obscured borders in the anterior third of the same quadrant (arrows).

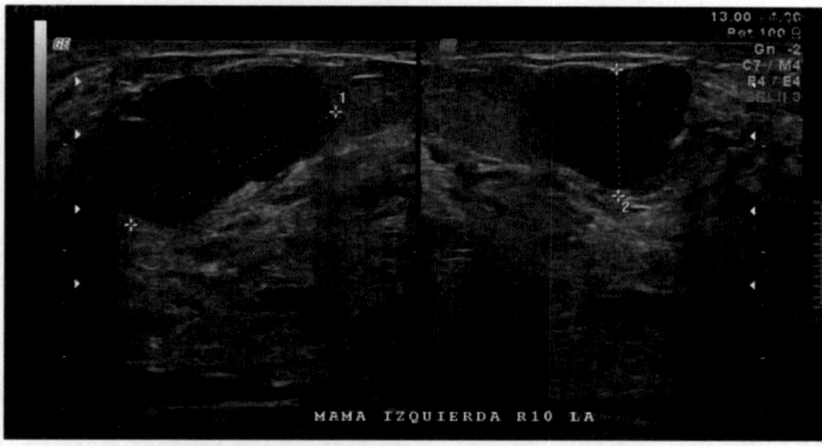

Figure 11. 34 year old female Mammary Ultrasound (US): identified a hypoechoic oval nodule, with macrolobular borders. Histopathological report: tubular adenoma.

It has been found that the morphological characteristics of adenomas clearly mimic some zones present in fibroadenomas; thus, it is suggested that both tumors are histogenetically related, with the stromal component predominating in fibroadenomas and the ductal component predominating in tubular adenomas [170]. Histologically, the differential diagnosis can be established with fibroadenoma, adenoma of the nipple, sclerosing adenosis, eccrine spiradenoma, and tubularcarcinoma. There are reports in the literature of exceptional associations with ductal carcinoma [171].

The clinical and imaging characteristics are similar to those of the fibroadenomas (Figures 10 and 11); therefore, preoperatory diagnosis can on occasion be difficult. In the majority of cases, surgical excision of the lesion is required to establish the definitive diagnosis, this being the definitive treatment of the lesion.

Lactating Adenoma

A lactating adenoma is a benign tumor caused by physiological changes of the breast tissue that take place during pregnancy and lactancy [172]. Sometimes it is interpreted as a variant of the fibroadenoma, tubular adenoma, or lobular hyperplasia [173]. Histologically, adenomas of lactancy are tumors that only contain epithelial elements; macroscopically, it consists of a well defined mass of elastic consistency. At microscopic study, it is composed of acini and densely compacted tubules in lobules separated by scarce connective tissue [174]. The imaging study of choice for evaluation is the US, due to the high density of the breast during the gestational period [175]. By imaging, it is difficult to distinguish the lactating adenoma from a fibroadenoma, because the typical aspect is that of a well circumscribed radiolucent nodule. Sometimes lactating adenomas exhibit fine lobulations and a pseudocapsule and they may occasionally show poorly defined angular borders and posterior acoustic shadowing (Figure 12), which could make it difficult to differentiate from a malignant lesion [176, 177]. The use of MRI is exceptional and its use could be justified in cases of difficult diagnoses [178].

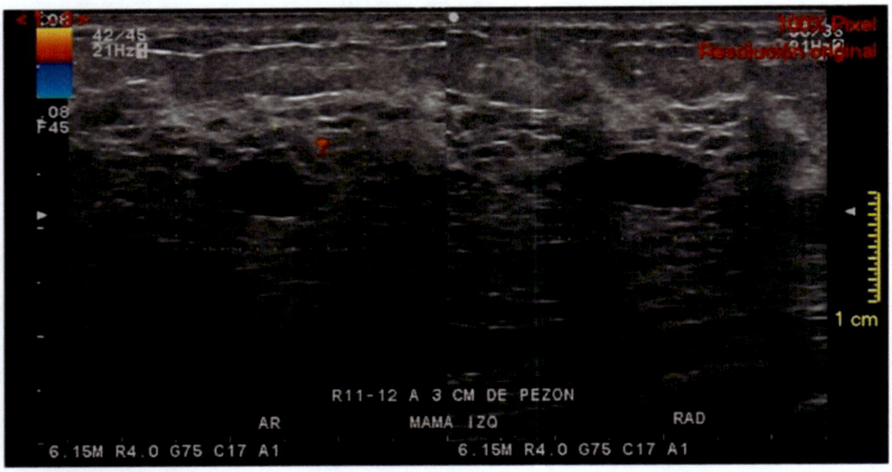

Figure 12. 24 year old female. Breast Ultrasound (US) shows an oval nodule, hypoechoic, with circumscribed borders, without vascularity on application of color Doppler. Histopathological report: Secretory/lactating adenoma (3rd trimester of pregnancy).

Histological diagnosis is achieved through the performance of trucut biopsy; however, a potential complication of this procedure comprises the formation of lactating fistulas, which may contribute to the development of mastitis and the need to interrupt lactancy; thus, this potential complication should be discussed with the patient. The spontaneous resolution of these lesions has been reported; therefore, in some cases, surveillance of the tumor is possible once the pregnancy and lactancy have concluded. Treatment consists of surgical excision of the lesion. No recurrences have been reported following excision. There are reports of the use of bromocriptine as a nonsurgical alternative; however, its results have not been established with certainty.

Rare cases that have developed in ectopic localizations of breast tissue have been reported, such as in the axillary region, thoracic wall, and vulva.

Pleomorphic Adenoma

This is a very rare benign breast tumor. There have been approximately 70 cases reported in the literature [179]. The plemorphic adenoma corresponds to an exceptional localization of its equivalent in the salivary glands.

Histologically, this is composed of epithelial ductal cells, myoepithelial cells, and a mitochondrial matrix.

Immunohistochemically, the ductal cells can be positive for the expression of the estrogen and/or progesterone receptors, and the nucleus of the myoepithelial cells can have reactivity for proteins HMGI-C and HMGI (Y), which indicates a similar histogenesis to that of salivary gland tumors [180]. By means of imaging, it is difficult to distinguish this lesion from other benign breast tumors and the diagnosis is usually arrived at through trucut biopsy. It is important to perform the preoperative histological diagnosis to avoid the employment of excessive treatment.

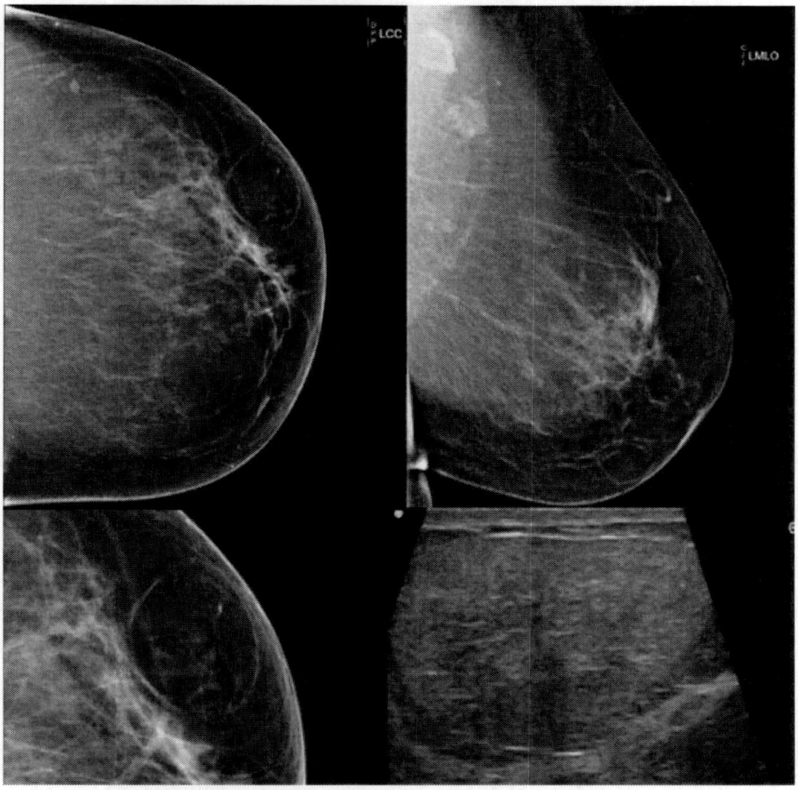

Figure 13. 50 year old female. In the mastography in Cranial-caudal (CC) projection, a circumscribed, oval nodule can be observed, hypodense with fat in its interior (A). In the Mediolateral-oblique (MLO) projection in lower quadrants, a nodule was identified of similar characteristics (B) observed with greater definition in the magnification projection (C). Ultrasound (US) shows an oval nodule in the left breast, circumscribed, isoechoic, localized in R2-3, with vascularity on color Doppler (D).

Lipoma

Lipomas of the breast are rare benign tumors whose incidence is not known with certainty. Clinically, its characteristics are indistinguishable from those originating in other locations. Lipomas are in general well defined and soft. Histologically they are composed of adipose cells with benign characteristics surrounded by a well-defined capsule [181].

Precisely due to their soft consistency, which is very similar to that of normal breast tissue and because of their slow growth, it is possible that lipomas may go unnoticed until reach great dimensions, at which point they may manifest as breast asymmetry because of an increase in the volume of the affected breast [182]. Lipomas are defined as a giant when they reach dimensions of >5cm and a weight of >500gr [183]. Cases have been reported of lipomas with intramuscular origin in the pectoral muscles that can mimic a tumor originating from the gland itself [184]. Fine needle aspiration biopsy (FNA) has not been shown to be useful because the adipose cells that lipomas are comprimed of are similar to those observed within the normal mammary parenchyma. Lipoma is generally an exclusion diagnosis and its importance lies precisely in the differentiation of other lesions, benign as well as malignant. It can be difficult to clinically distinguish a lipoma from its malignant variant, liposarcoma.

On occasion it may be impossible to distinguish between a lipoma and normal fibroadipose tissue, even when evaluating the lesion mastographically and by US. Usually, lipomas are oval hypodense circumscribed nodules with fat in their interior. Uppon US evaluation, an oval isoechoic well circumscribed, nodule without vascularity on color Doppler, with well defined borders and without posterior acoustic shadowing may be observed (Figure 13). Due to its treatment, prognosis, and long-term follow-up, it is important to attempt to make a differential diagnosis preoperatively; thus, magnetic resonance imaging (MRI) has been utilized for this purpose because it possesses high sensitivity for the detection of breast lesions [185].

Definitive treatment consists of surgical excision; however, because giant breast lymphomas may develop, it is sometimes necessary to perform oncoplastic procedures in order to avoid important breast deformities and to achieve a favorable cosmetic result after large breast resections [186–188].

References

[1] Goehring C, Morabia A. Epidemiology of breast disease, with special attention to histologic types. *Epidemiol. Rev*. 1997;19:310–27.

[2] Ferrara A. Benign breast disease. *Radiol. Technol*. 2011;82(5):447M–462M.

[3] Jayasinghe Y, Simmons PS. Fibroadenomas in adolescence. *Curr. Opin. Obstet. Gynecol.* 2009 Oct;21(5):402–6.

[4] Rosen P. Rosen's Breast Pathology. Third ed. Pine J, McGough J, Editors. New York: Wolters Kluwer, Lippincott Williams & Wilkins; 2009.

[5] Sklair-Levy M, Sella T, Alweiss T, Craciun I, Libson E, Mally B. Incidence and management of complex fibroadenomas. *AJR Am. J. Roentgenol*. 2008;190(1): 214–8.

[6] Kollur SM, El Hag IA. FNA of breast fibroadenoma: observer variability and review of cytomorphology with cytohistological correlation. *Cytopathology*. 2006;17(5): 239–44.

[7] Courtillot C, Plu-Bureau G, Binart N, Balleyguier C, Sigal-Zafrani B, Goffin V, et al. Benign breast diseases. *J. Mammary Gland Biol. Neoplasia*. 2005;10(4):325–35.

[8] Gompel A, Levy D, Chaouat M, Forgez P, Rostene W. Apoptosis and aging: breast cells and apoptosis. *Maturitas*. 2001;38(1):39–44.

[9] Branchini G, Schneider L, Cericatto R, Capp E, Brum IS. Progesterone receptors A and B and estrogen receptor alpha expression in normal breast tissue and fibroadenomas. *Endocrine*. 2009 Jun;35(3):459–66.

[10] Schneider L, Branchini G, Cericatto R, Capp E, Brum IS. Gene and protein expression of p53 and p21 in fibroadenomas and adjacent normal mammary tissue. *Endocrine*. 2009;35(1):118–22.

[11] Franco N, Arnould L, Mege F, Picard S-F, Arveux P, Lizard-Nacol S. Comparative analysis of molecular alterations in fibroadenomas associated or not with breast cancer. *Arch. Surg*. 2003;138(3):291–5.

[12] Cavalli LR, Cornélio DA, Wuicik L, Bras AT, Ribeiro EM, Lima RS, et al. Clonal chromosomal alterations in fibroadenomas of the breast. *Cancer Genet Cytogenet.* 2001;131(2):120–4.

[13] Amiel A, Kaufman Z, Goldstein E, Bruchim RB-S, Kidron D, Gaber E, et al. Application of comparative genomic hybridization in search for genetic aberrations in fibroadenomas of the breast. *Cancer Genet Cytogenet.* 2003;142(2):145–8.

[14] Bidgoli SA, Eftekhari T. Role of exogenous and endogenous sources of estrogen on the incidence of breast fibroadenoma: case-control study in Iran. *Asian Pac. J. Cancer Prev.* 2011;12(5):1289–93.

[15] Jayasinghe Y, Simmons P. The occurrrence of two rare neoplasms (breast and ovarian) in adolescent female. *J. Pediatr. Adolesc. Gynecol.* 2009;22(5):99–103.

[16] Estevão RAF, Nazário ACP, Baracat EC. Effect of oral contraceptive with and without associated estriol on ultrasound measurements of breast fibroadenoma: randomized clinical trial. *Sao Paulo Med. J.* 2007;125(5):275–80.

[17] Valdes E, Boolbol S, Cohen J, Flelman S. Malignant transformation of a breast fibroadenoma to cystosarcoma phyllodes: case report and review of the literature. *Am. Surg.* 2005;71:348–54.

[18] Abe M, Miyata S, Nishimura S, Iijima K, Makita M, Akiyama F, et al. Malignant transformation of breast fibroadenoma to malignant phyllodes tumor: long-term outcome of 36 malignant phyllodes tumors. *Breast Cancer.* 2011;18(4):268–72.

[19] Hodges KB, Abdul-Karim FW, Wang M, López-Beltrán A, Montironi R, Easley S, et al. Evidence for transformation of fibroadenoma of the breast to malignant phyllodes tumor. *Appl. Immunohistochem. Mol. Morphol.* 2009;17(4):345–50.

[20] Martínez-Ramos D, Alcalde-Sánchez M, Peñas-Pardo L, Salvador-Sanchís J. Breast fibroadenomas may also contain premalignant and malignant lesions. *CirugEspan* 2009;86(1):51–3.

[21] Morgan JM, Douglas-Jones AG, Gupta SK. Analysis of histological features in needle core biopsy of breast useful in preoperative distinction between fibroadenoma and phyllodes tumour. *Histopathology.* 2010;56(4):489–500.

[22] Skenderi F, Krakonja F, Vranic S. Infarcted fibroadenoma of the breast: report of two new cases with review of the literature. *Diagn. Pathol.* 2013;8(1):38.

[23] Földi M, Klar M, Orlowska-Volk M, Hanjalic-Beck A, Osterloh B, Stickeler E, et al. Ultrasound characteristics of breast fibroadenomas are related to clinical and histological parameters. *Ultraschall Med.* 2010;31(5):475–83.

[24] Zimmermann N, Ohlinger R. Diagnostic value of palpation, mammography, and ultrasonography in the diagnosis of fibroadenoma: impact of breast density, patient age, ultrasonographic size, and palpability. *Ultraschall Med.* 2012;33(7):E151–E157.

[25] Ezer SS, Oguzkurt P, Ince E, Temiz A, Bolat FA, Hicsonmez A. Surgical treatment of the solid breast masses in female adolescents. *J. Pediatr. Adolesc. Gynecol.* 2013;26(1):31–5.

[26] Smith GEC, Burrows P. Ultrasound diagnosis of fibroadenoma - is biopsy always necessary? *Clin. Radiol.* 2008;63(5):511–5; discussion 516–7.

[27] Rosa M. The value of fine needle aspiration Biopsy in the diagnosis and prognostic assessment of palpable breast lesions. *Diagn. Cytopathol.* 2010;40(1):26-34.

[28] D'Orsic C, Bassett L, Feing S, Al E. Illustrated Breast Imaging Reporting and Data System: Illustrated BIRADS. 3rd Resto. American College of Radiology, Editor. 1998.

[29] Stavros A, In. Donnellan K, Martin S, Rothschild R. Benign solid nodules: specific pathologic diagnoses. 1st ed. Philadelphia, PA, USA: Lippincott, Williams and Wilkins; 2004.

[30] Graf O, Helbich TH, Hopf G, Graf C, Sickles EA. Probable benign breast masses at US: is follow-up an acceptable alternative to biopsy? *Radiology*. 2007;244(1):87–93.

[31] Harvey JA, Nicholson BT, Lorusso AP, Cohen MA, Bovbjerg VE. Short-term follow-up of palpable breast lesions with benign imaging features: evaluation of 375 lesions in 320 women. *AJR Am. J. Roentgenol*. 2009;193(6):1723–30.

[32] Leconte I, Abraham C, Galant C, Sy M, Berlière M, Fellah L. Fibroadenoma: can fine needle aspiration biopsy avoid short term follow-up? *Diagn. Interv. Imaging*. 2012;93(10):750–6.

[33] Tea M-KM, Asseryanis E, Kroiss R, Kubista E, Wagner T. Surgical breast lesions in adolescent females. *Pediatr. Surg. Int*. 2009;25(1):73–5.

[34] Amin AL, Purdy AC, Mattingly JD, Kong AL, Termuhlen PM. Benign breast disease. *Surg. Clin. North Am*. 2013;93(2):299–308.

[35] Kaufman C, Littrup P, Freeman-Gibb L. Office -based cryoablation of breast fibroadenomas with long-term follow-up. *Breast J*. 2005;11(5):344–50.

[36] Littrup PJ, Freeman-Gibb L, Andea A, White M, Amerikia KC, Bouwman D, et al. Radiology cryotherapy for breast. *Radiology*. 2005;234(1):63–72.

[37] Hahn M, Pavlista D, Danes J, Klein R, Golatta M, Harcos A, et al. Ultrasound guided cryoablation of fibroadenomas. *Ultraschall Med*. 2013;34(1):64–8.

[38] Fine RE, Staren ED. Percutaneous radiofrequency-assisted excision of fibroadenomas. *Am. J. Surg*. 2006;192(4):545–7.

[39] Fisher C, Hanby A, Robinson L, Mills R. Mammary hamartoma - a review of 35 cases. *Histopathology*. 1992;20(2):99–106.

[40] Charpin C, Mathoulin M, Andrac L. Reappraisal of breast hamartomas. A morphological study of 41 cases. *Pathol. Res. Pract*. 1994;190:362–72.

[41] Herbert M, Sandbank J, Liokumovich P, Yanai O, Pappo I, Karni T, et al. Breast hamartomas: clinicopathological and immunohistochemical studies of 24 cases. *Histopathology*. 2002;41(1):30–4.

[42] Lee W, Sheen-Chen S, Chi S, Huang H. Hamartoma of the breast: an underrecognized disease? *Tumori*. 2008;94:114–5.

[43] Weinzweig N, Botts J, Marcus E. Giant hamartoma of the breast. *Plast. Reconstr. Surg*. 2000;107(5):1216–20.

[44] Chang HL, Lerwill MF, Goldstein AM. Breast hamartomas in adolescent females. *Breast J*. 2009;15(5):515–20.

[45] Venkatesh M, Harish K. Giant breast hamartoma. *Indian J. Surg*. 2009 Feb;71(1):50–1.

[46] Sanal HT, Ersoz N, Altinel O, Unal E, Can C. Giant hamartoma of the breast. *Breast J*. 2006;12(1):84–5.

[47] Birrell AL, Warren LR, Birrell SN. Misdiagnosis of massive breast asymmetry: giant hamartoma. *ANZ J. Surg*. 2012;82(12):941–2.

[48] Murat A, Ozdemir H, Yildirim H, Poyraz AK, Ozercan R. Hamartoma of the breast. *Australas Radiol.* 2007;51 Spec No:B37–B39.

[49] Erdem G, Karakaş HM, Işık B, Fırat AK. Advanced MRI findings in patients with breast hamartomas. *Diagn. Interv. Radiol.* 2011;17(1):33–7.

[50] Farrokh D, Hashemi J, Ansaripour E. Breast hamartoma: mammographic findings. *Iran J. Radiol.* 2011;8(4):258–60.

[51] Tse G, Law B, Ma T, Chan A, Pang L-M, Chu WCW, et al. Hamartoma of the breast: a clinicopathological review. *J. Clin. Pathol.* 2002;55(12):951–4.

[52] Harman M, Ünal Ö, Uðraþ S, Etlik Ö, Kotan Ç. Breast hamartoma: radiologic appearances. *East J. Med.* 2003;8(2):43–5.

[53] Chao T, Chao H, Chen M. Sonographic Features of breast hamartomas. *J. Ultrasound Med.* 2007;26:447–52.

[54] Park S, Oh K, Kim E-K, Son E. Sonographic findings of breast hamartomas emphasis on compressibility 2003. *Yonsei Med. J.* 2003;44(5):847–54.

[55] Georgian-Smith D, Kricun B, McKee G, Yeh E. The mammary hamartoma. Appreciation of additional imaging characteristics. *J. Ultrasound Med.* 2004;8(4):290–3.

[56] Kai M, Tada ÆK, Tamura ÆM. Breast cancer associated with mammary hamartoma. *Breast Cancer.* 2012;19:183–6.

[57] Choi N, Ko ES. Invasive ductal carcinoma in a mammary hamartoma: case report and review of the literature. *Korean J. Radiol.* 2010;11(6):687–91.

[58] Scally N, Campbell W, Hall S, McCusker G, Stirling WJI. Invasive ductal carcinoma arising within a breast hamartoma. *Ir. J. Med. Sci.* 2011;180(3):767–8.

[59] Uliaque CF, Berdun FJP. Carcinoma *in situ* e invasivo dentro de un hamartoma mamario. *Radiologia.* 2010;52(5):487–8.

[60] Baron M, Ladonne J-M, Gravier A, Picquenot J-M, Berry M. Invasive lobular carcinoma in a breast hamartoma. *Breast J.* 2003;9(3):246–8.

[61] Breucq C, Verfaillie G, Perdaens C, Vermeiren B, Stadnik T. Lobular carcinoma located in a breast hamartoma. *Breast J.* 2005;11(6):508–9.

[62] O'Malley F, Pinder S, Mulligan A. Breast Pathology. 2 ed. Philadelphia, PA, USA: Elsevier Saunders; 2011.

[63] Ruiz-Tovar J, Reguero-Callejas ME, Arano-Bermejo JI, González-Palacios F, Cabañas-Navarro L. Notas clínicas Hamartoma mamario. *CirugEspan* 2006;79(3):186–8.

[64] Oikonomou A, Fotiadou V, Panagis A, Prassopoulos P. Case 3177. A case of breast hamartoma. *Euro Radiol.* 2005;(Case 3177):1–6.

[65] Barbaros U, Deveci U, Erbil Y, Budak D. Breast hamartoma: a case report. *Acta Chir Belg.* 2005;105(6):658–9.

[66] Aoyama K, Kamio T, Hirano A, Seshimo A, Kameoka S. Granular cell tumors: a report of six cases. *World J. Surg. Oncol.* 2012;10(1):204.

[67] Adeniran A, Al-Ahmadie H, Mhoney M, Robinson-Smith T. Granular cell tumor of the breast: a series of 17 cases and review of the literature. *Breast J.* 2004;10:528–31.

[68] Filipovski V, Banev S, Janevska V, Dukova B. Granular cell tumor of the breast: a case report and review of literature. *Cases J.* 2009 Jan;2:Case 8551.

[69] Yang WT, Edeiken-Monroe B, Sneige N, Fornage BD. Sonographic and mamographic appearances of granular cell tumors of the breast with pathological correlation. *J. Clin. Ultrasound.* 2006;34(4):153–60.

[70] Gogas J, Markopoulos C, Kouskos E, Gogas H, Mantas D, Antonopoulou Z, et al. Granular cell tumor of the breast: a rare lesion resembling breast cancer. *Eur. J. Gynaecol. Oncol.* 2002;23:333–4.

[71] Patel HB, Leibman AJ. Granular cell tumor in a male breast: mammographic, sonographic, and pathologic features. *J. Clin. Ultrasound*. 2013;41(2):119–21.

[72] Gibbons D, Leitch M, Coscia J, Lindberg G, Molberg K. Fine needle apiration cytology and histologic findings of granular cell tumor of the breast: review of 19 cases with clinical/radiologic correlation. *Breast J.* 2000;6:27–30.

[73] Patel A, Lefemine V, Yousuf SM, Abou-Samra W. Granular cell tumour of the pectoral muscle mimicking breast cancer. *Cases J.* 2008;1(1):142.

[74] Leo C, Briest S, Schütz S, Leinung S. Granular cell tumor of the breast mimicking breast cancer. *Eur. J. Obstet Gynecol. Reprod. Biol*. 2006;27(2):268–70.

[75] IIvan S, Ustundag N, Calay Z, Bukey Y. Benign granular cell tumour of the breast. *Can. J. Surg*. 2005;48:155–6.

[76] Ayub MF, Radhakrishna S, Chakravarthy R. Images: granular cell tumour of the breast mimics a malignancy. *Indian J. Surg. Oncol.* 2012;3(1):47–9.

[77] Gavriilidis P, Michalopoulou I, Baliaka A, Nikolaidou A. Granular cell breast tumour mimicking infiltrating carcinoma. *BMJ Case Rep*. 2013;2012–4.

[78] Akatsu T, Kobayashi H, Uematsu S, Tamagawa E. Granular cell tumor of the breast preoperatively diagnosed by fine needle aspiration cytology. *Surg. Today.* 2004;34:760–3.

[79] El-Aouni N, Laurent I, Terrier P, Mansouri D, Suciu V, Delaloge S, et al. Granular cell tumor of the breast. *Diagn. Pathol*. 2007;35(11):725–7.

[80] Brown AC, Audisio RA, Regitnig P. Granular cell tumour of the breast. *Surg. Oncol.* 2011;20(2):97–105.

[81] Akahane K, Kato K, Ogiso S, Sakaguchi K, Hashimoto M, Ishikawa A, et al. Malignant granular cell tumor of the breast: case report and literature review. *Breast Cancer*. 2012 Mar.

[82] Scaranelo A, Burkhanov K, Crystal P, Mulligaan A. Granular cell tumour of the breast : MRI findings and review of the literature. *Br. J. Radiol*. 2007;80:970–4.

[83] Irshad A, Pope T, Ackerman S, Panzegrau B. Characterization of sonographic and mammographic features of granular cell tumors of the breast. *J. Ultrasound Med.* 2008;27(3):467–75.

[84] Abbas E, Omeroglu A, Kao E, Altinel G, Fleiszer D, Mesurolle B. Granular cell tumor of the breast detected on MRI screening. *Breast J*. 2013;19(5):545–7.

[85] Fanburg-Smith J, Meis-Kindblom L, Fante R, Kindblom L. Malignant granular cell tumor of soft tissue: diagnostic criteria and clinicopathologic correlation. *Am. J. Surg. Pathol.* 1998;22(7):779–94.

[86] Nasser H, Ahmed Y, Szpunar S, Kowalski P. Malignant granular tumor cell: a look into the diagnostic criteria. *Pathol. Res. Pract*. 2011;207(3):164–8.

[87] Sirgi KE, Sneige N, Fanning TV, Fornage BD. Fine-needle aspirates of granular lesions of the breast: report of three cases, with emphasis on differential diagnosis and utility of immunostaining for CD68. *Diagn. Cytopathol.* 1996;15(5):403–8.

[88] Pergel A, Yucel AF, Karaca AS, Aydin I, Sahin DA, Demirbag N. A therapeutic and diagnostic dilemma: granular cell tumor of the breast. *Case Rep. Med.* 2011;2011: 972168.

[89] Celebi AS, Toksoy G, Ozel A, Caliskan KC, Kabukcuoglu F. Granular cell tumor of the breast. *JBR-BTR*. 2012;95(4):235–6.

[90] Qureshi N, Tahir M, Carmichael A. Granular cell tumor of the soft tissues: case report and literature review. *Int. Sem. Surg. Oncol.* 2006;3:21.

[91] Quiroz-Rodríguez G, Robles-Vidal C, Guzmán-Navarro L, Ortiz-Hidalgo C. Granular cell (Abrikossoff) tumor of the breast. *Breast J.* 2006;12(5):494.

[92] World Health Organization. Histologic Typing of Breast Tumors. Histologic Typing of Breast Tumors. 2nd ed. Geneva, Switzterland: World Health Organization (WHO); 1981.

[93] Mishra SP, Tiwary SK, Mishra M, Khanna AK. Phyllodes tumor of breast: a review article. *ISRN Surg*. 2013;2013:361469.

[94] Rosen P. Rosen's Breast Pathology. 2nd ed. New York: Lippincott Williams&Wilkins; 2001.

[95] Flores CA, José E, Guzmán O, Valenzuela AC, Miguel PS. Tumor phyllodes: experiencia institucional. *Ginecol. Obstet. Mex*. 2009;77(12):567–72.

[96] Martín Medrano E, González Blanco I, Sánchez de Río M. Tumor filodes de mama. *Ginecol. Obset. Clin*. 2006;7(1):16–23.

[97] Noguchi S, Motomura K, Inaji H, Imaoka S, Koyama H. Clonal analysis of fibroadenoma and phyllodes tumor of the breast. *Cancer Res*. 1993;53(17):4071–4.

[98] World Health Organization. Histological Typing of Breast Tumor. *Tumori*. 1982;68:181–98.

[99] Azzopardi JG. Sarcoma in the breast. Problems in Breast Pathology, Vol. II. Philadelphia, PA, USA: WB Saunders; 1979. pp. 355–9.

[100] Belkacémi Y, Bousquet G, Marsiglia H, Ray-Coquard I, Magné N, Malard Y, et al. Phyllodes tumor of the breast. *Int. J. Radiat. Oncol. Biol. Phys*. 2008;70:492–500.

[101] Ben Hassouna J, Damak T, Gamoudi A, Chargui R, Khomsi F, Mahjoub S, et al. Phyllodes tumors of the breast: a case series of 106 patients. *Am. J. Surg*. 2006; 192(2):141–7.

[102] Parker S, Harries S. Phyllodes tumours. *Postgr. Med. J*. 2001;77:428–35.

[103] Singer A, Tresley J, Velázquez J, Yepes M. Unusual aggressive breast cancer: metastatic malignant phyllodes tumor. *Radiol. Case*.2013;7(2):24–37.

[104] Tse G, Niu Y, Shi H-J. Phyllodes tumor of the breast: an update. *Breast Cancer*. 2010;17(1):29–34.

[105] Wiratkapun C, Piyapan P, Lertsithichai P, Larbcharoensub N. Fibroadenoma versus phyllodes tumor: distinguishing factors in patients diagnosed with fibroepithelial lesions after a core needle biopsy. *Diagn. Interv. Radiol*. 2013;20(1):27–33.

[106] Liang MI, Ramaswamy B, Patterson CC, McKelvey MT, Gordillo G, Nuovo GJ, et al. Giant breast tumors: surgical management of phyllodes tumors, potential for reconstructive surgery and a review of literature. *World J. Surg. Oncol.* 2008;6:117–25.

[107] Feder J, de Paredes E, Hogge J, Wilken J. Unusual breast lesions: radiologic-pathologic correlation. *Breast Imaging.* 1999;19(S):11–26.

[108] Majeski J, Stroud J. Malignant phyllodes tumors of the breast: a study in clinical practice. *Int. Surg.* 2012;97(2):95–8.

[109] Gonzalo I, Fernández-Carro A, Meneses M. Tumor phyllodes de mama. *Clin. Invest. Gin. Obst.* 2010;37(2):82–4.

[110] Aguilar V, Bauab S, Maranhao N. (2010). Evaluación de los nódulos mamarios - Mamografía y ultrasonido. En: AMOLCA (Ed.). *Mama: Diagnostico por Imagen. Mamografia, Ultrasonografia y Resonancia Magnética.* (1ª ed., tomo 1, pp. 262–64).

[111] Cosmacini P, Veronesi P, Zurrida S, Bartoli C. Mammography in the diagnosis of phyllodes tumors of the breast. Analysis of 99 cases. *Radiol. Med.* 1991;82(1-2):52–5.

[112] Czum J, Sanders L, Titus J, Kalisher L. Breast imaging case of the day. *Radiographics.* 1997;17(2):548–51.

[113] Chao T-C, Lo Y-F, Chen S-C, Chen M-F. Sonographic features of phyllodes tumors of the breast. *Ultrasound Obstet. Gynecol.* 2002;20(1):64–71.

[114] Youn I, Choi SH, Moon HJ, Kim MJ, Kim EK. Phyllodes tumors of the breast: Ultrasonographic findings and diagnostic performance of ultrasound-guided core needle biopsy. *Ultrasound Med. Biol.* 2013;39:987–92.

[115] Orel SG. Differentiation of phyllodes breast tumors from fibroadenomas on MRI. *Breast Dis.* 2006;17(3):231.

[116] Yabuuchi H, Soeda H, Matsuo Y, Okafuji, T et al. Phyllodes tumor of the breast: correlation between MR findings and histologic grade. *Radiology.* 2006;241(3):702–9.

[117] Jacklin RK, Ridgway PF, Ziprin P, Healy V, Hadjiminas D, Darzi A. Optimising preoperative diagnosis in phyllodes tumour of the breast. *J. Clin. Pathol.* 2006; 59(5):454–9.

[118] Houssami N, Ciatto S, Bilous M, Vezzosi V, Bianchi S. Borderline breast core needle histology: predictive values for malignancy in lesions of uncertain malignant potential (B3). *Br. J. Cancer.* 2007;96(8):1253–7.

[119] Komenaka IK, El-Tamer M, Pile-Spellman E, Hibshoosh H. Core needle biopsy as a diagnostic tool to differentiate tumor from fibroadenoma. *Arch. Surg.* 2003;138: 987–90.

[120] Komenaka IK, El-Tamer M, Pile-Spellman E, Hibshoosh H. Core needle biopsy as a diagnostic tool to differentiate phyllodes tumor om fibroadenoma. *Arch. Surg.* 2003;138(9):987–90.

[121] Jacobs TW, Chen Y-Y, Guinee, Jr DG, Holden JA, Cha I, Bauermeister DE, et al. Fibroepithelial lesions with cellular stroma on breast core needle biopsy: are there predictors of outcome on surgical excision? *Am. J. Clin. Pathol.* 2005;124(3):342–54.

[122] Guerrero MA, Ballard BR, Grau AM. Malignant phyllodes tumor of the breast: review of the literature and case report of stromal overgrowth. *Surg. Oncol.* 2003;12(1):27–37.

[123] Pătraşcu A, Popescu CF, Pleşea IE, Bădulescu A, Tănase F, Mateescu G. Clinical and cytopathological aspects in phyllodes tumors of the breast. *Rom. J. Morphol. Embryol.* 2009;50(4):605–11.

[124] Kleer CG, Giordano TJ, Ph D, Braun T, Oberman HA. Features of benign and malignant phyllodes tumors of the breast. *Mod. Pathol.* 2001;14(3):185–90.

[125] Thor AD. Phyllodes tumors of the breast: the role of pathologic parameters. (Abstract). *Breast Dis.* 2006;16(4):357.

[126] Kaya R, Pesterel H, Erdogan G. Proliferating activity in differential diagnosis of benign phyllodes tumor and cellular fibroadenomas: is it helpful? *Pathol. Oncol. Res.* 2001;7(3):213–6.

[127] Yonemori K, Hasegawa T, Shimizu C, Shibata T, Matsumoto K, Kouno T, et al. Correlation of p53 and MIB-1 expression with both the systemic recurrence and survival in cases of phyllodes tumors of the breast. *Pathol. Res. Pract.* 2006;202(10):705–12.

[128] Tse GMK, Lui PCW, Vong JSL, Lau K-M, Putti TC, Karim R, et al. Increased epidermal growth factor receptor (EGFR) expression in malignant mammary phyllodes tumors. *Breast Cancer Res. Treat.* 2009;114(3):441–8.

[129] Jara-Lázaro AR, Tan PH. Molecular pathogenesis of progression and recurrence in breast phyllodes tumors. *Am. J. Transl. Res.* 2009;1(1):23–34.

[130] Lv S, Niu Y, Wei L, Liu Q, Wang X, Chen Y. Chromosomal aberrations and genetic relations in benign, borderline and malignant phyllodes tumors of the breast: a comparative genomic hybridization study. *Breast Cancer Res. Treat.* 2008;112(3): 411–8.

[131] Khosravi-Shahi P. Management of non metastatic phyllodes tumors of the breast: review of the literature. *Surg. Oncol.* 2011;20(4):143–8.

[132] Taira N, Takabatake D, Aogi K. Phyllodes tumor of the breast: stromal overgrowth and histological classification are aseful prognosis-predictive factors for local recurrence in patients with a positive surgical margin. *Jpn. J. Clin. Oncol.* 2007;37(10):730–6.

[133] Sotheran W, Domjan J, Jeffrey M, Wise M, Perry P. Phyllodes tumours of the breast- a retrospective study from 1982–2000 of 50 cases in Portsmouth. *Ann. R. Coll. Surg. Engl.* 2005;87:339–44.

[134] Haberer S, Laé M, Seegers V, Pierga J-Y, Salmon R, Kirova YM, et al. Management of malignant phyllodes tumors of the breast: the experience of the Institut Curie. *Cancer Radiother.* 2009;13(4):305–12.

[135] Crenshaw SA, Roller MD, Chapman JK. Immediate breast reconstruction with a saline implant and AlloDerm, following removal of a phyllodes tumor. (Abstract). *World J. Surg. Oncol.* 2011;9:34.

[136] Macdonald OK, Lee CM, Tward JD, Chappel CD, Gaffney DK. Malignant phyllodes tumor of the female breast: association of primary therapy with cause-specific survival from the Surveillance, Epidemiology, and End Results (SEER) program. *Cancer.* 2006;107(9):2127–33.

[137] Leung JWT, Gotway MB, Sickles EA. Case report: Preoperative embolization of vascular phyllodes tumor of the breast. *AJR.* 2005;94115(March):2004–6.

[138] Park H-L, Kwon S-H, Chang SY, Huh JY, Kim J-Y, Shim JY, et al. Long-term follow-up result of benign phyllodes tumor of the breast diagnosed and excised by ultrasound-guided vacuum-assisted breast biopsy. *J. Breast Cancer*. 2012 Jun;15(2):224–9.

[139] Pezner RD, Schultheiss TE, Paz IB. Malignant phyllodes tumor of the breast: local control rates with surgery alone. *Int. J. Radiat. Oncol. Biol. Phys*. 2008;71(3):710–3.

[140] Barth RJ, Wells WA, Mitchell SE, Cole BF. A prospective, multi-institutional study of adjuvant radiotherapy after resection of malignant phyllodes tumors. *Ann. Surg. Oncol.* 2009;16(8):2288–94.

[141] Chaney AW, Pollack A, McNeese MD, Zagars GK. Adjuvant radiotherapy for phyllodes tumor of breast. *Radiat. Oncol. Investig*. 1998;6(6):264–7.

[142] Belkacémi Y, Bousquet G, Marsiglia H, Ray-Coquard I, Magné N, Malard Y, et al. Phyllodes tumor of the breast. *Int. J. Radiat. Oncol. Biol. Phys*. 2008;70:492–500.

[143] Munawer NH, Md Zin R, Md Ali S-A, Muhammad R, Ali J, Das S. ER, p53 and MIB-1 are significantly associated with malignant phyllodes tumor. *Biomed. J.* 2012; 35(6):486–92.

[144] Sapino A, Bosco M, Cassoni P, Castellano I, Arisio R, Cserni G, et al. Estrogen receptor-beta is expressed in stromal cells of fibroadenoma and phyllodes tumors of the breast. *Mod. Pathol*. 2006;19(4):599–606.

[145] Hawkins R, Schofield J. The clinical and histologic criteria than predict metastases from cystosarcoma phyllodes. *Cancer*. 1992;69:141–7.

[146] Grabowski J, Salzstein SL, Sadler GR, Blair SL. Malignant phyllodes tumors: a review of 752 cases. *Am. Surg*. 2007;73(10):967–9.

[147] Abdalla H, Sakr M. Predictive Factors of Local recurrence and survival following primary surgical treatment of phyllodes tumors of the breast. *J. Egypt Natl. Cancer Inst.* 2006;18(2):125–33.

[148] Kapiris I, Nasiri N, A'Hern R, Healy V, Gui GPH. Outcome and predictive factors of local recurrence and distant metastases following primary surgical treatment of high-grade malignant phyllodes tumours of the breast. *Eur. J. Surg. Oncol.* 2001;27(8):723–30.

[149] Guillot E, Couturaud B, Reyal F, Curnier A, Ravinet J, Laé M, et al. Management of phyllodes breast tumors. *Breast J.* 2011;17(2):129–37.

[150] Ito T, Ito K, Okada T, Murayama K, Hanamura T, Kanai T, et al. Full-thickness chest-wall resection followed by thorax reconstruction for recurrent malignant phyllodes tumor. *Int. J. Clin. Oncol.* 2011;16(2):156–60.

[151] Andrade Neto JD, Terra RM, Fernández A, Rawet V, Jatene FB. Full-thickness chest wall resection for recurrent breast phyllodes tumor. *Ann. Thorac. Surg.* 2007;83(6): 2196–7.

[152] Friedel G, Kuipers T, Engel C, Schopf C, Veit S, Zoller J, et al. Full-thickness chest wall resection for locally recurrent breast cancer. *Thorac. Surg. Sci.* 2005;2:Doc01.

[153] Suzuki-Uematsu S, Shiraishi K, Ito T, Adachi N, Inage Y, Taeda Y, et al. Malignant phyllodes tumor composed almost exclusively of a fibrosarcomatous component: a case report and review of malignant phyllodes tumors with metastases. *Breast Cancer.* 2010;17(3):218–24.

[154] Morales-Vásquez F, González-Angulo A, Broglio K, López-Basave H, Gallardo D, Hortobagyi G, et al. Adjuvant chemotherapy with doxorubicin and dacarbazine has no effect in recurrence-free survival of malignant phyllodes tumors of the breast. *Breast J.* 2007;13(6):551–6.

[155] Guray M. Benign breast diseases: classification, diagnosis, and management. *Oncologist*. 2006;60:435–49.

[156] Onstad M, Stuckey A. Benign breast disorders. *Obstet. Gynecol. Clin. North Am.* 2013;40(3):459–73.

[157] Barsi T, Høyer S, Mortensen J. Adenoma of the nipples. A rare, but essential differential diagnosis. *Ugeskr Laeger*. 1999;161(42):5807–8.

[158] Bianchini GP, De Villa F, Vergine M, Pasta V, Monti M. Rare pathology of the breast: adenoma of the nipple. *G Chir*. 2002;23(5):213–5.

[159] Asagoe T, Hanatani Y, Horie F, Nemoto A, Kidooka K, Shikata J, et al. A case of adenoma of the nipple with breast cancer. *Nippon Geka Gakkai Zasshi*. 1991;92(1): 97–9.

[160] Aftab K, Idrees R. Nipple adenoma of breast: a masquerader of malignancy. *J. Coll. Physicians Surg. Pak.* 2010;20(7):472–4.

[161] Sugai M, Murata K, Kimura N, Munakata H, Hada R, Kamata Y. Adenoma of the nipple in an adolescent. *Breast Cancer*. 2002;9(3):254–6.

[162] Clune JE, Kozakewich HP, VanBeek CA, Labow BI, Greene AK. Nipple adenoma in infancy. *J. Pediatr. Surg*. 2009;44(11):2219–22.

[163] Fernández-Flores A, Suárez-Peñaranda J-M. Immunophenotype of nipple adenoma in a male patient. *Appl. Immunohistochem. Mol. Morphol*. 2011;19(2):190–4.

[164] Marsch WC, Nürnberger F. Adenoma of the nipples. *Z. Hautkr*. 1979;54(24):1067–72.

[165] Ermilova VD, Seredin VP. Adenoma of the nipple with malignant degeneration. *Arkh. Patol.* 1987;49(12):59–61.

[166] Interlandi A, Busacca G. Adenomas of the nipple. *Minerva Chir*. 2002;57(5):699–702.

[167] Sánchez Pedreño P, Rivera F, Ortega I, González Campora R, Galera Davidson H, Camacho F. Adenoma of the nipple. Clinico-pathologic review of 16 cases. *Med. Cutan Ibero Lat Am.* 1984;12(2):123–7.

[168] Salemis N, Gemenetzis G, Karagkiouzis G. Tubular adenoma of the breast: arare presentation and review of the literature. *J. Clin. Med. Res*. 2011;4(1):64–7.

[169] Ravindra S, Suguna BV. Cytomorphology of tubular adenoma breast-a case report. *Indian J. Pathol. Microbiol.*2006;49(2):267–8.

[170] Hertel BF, Zaloudek C KR. Breast adenomas. *Pathol. Res. Pract.* 1995;191(12):1222–30.

[171] Domoto H, Tsuda H, Miyakawa K, Shinoda A, Nanasawa T. Invasive ductal carcinoma associated with tubular adenoma of the breast. *Pathol. Int.* 2002;52(3):244–8.

[172] Yu JH, Kim MJ, Cho H, Liu HJ, Han S-J, Ahn T-G. Breast diseases during pregnancy and lactation. *Obstet. Gynecol. Sci*. 2013;56(3):143–59.

[173] Choudhury M, Singal MK. Lactating adenoma-cytomorphologic study with review of literature. *Indian J. PatholMicrobiol*. 2001. p. 445–8.

[174] James K, Bridger J, Anthony PP. Breast tumour of pregnancy ('lactating adenoma'). *J. Pathol.* 1988;156:37–44.

[175] Bock K, Duda VF, Hadji P, Iwinska-Zelder J, Ramaswamy A, Schmidt S, et al. Sonographic variability of lactating adenoma demonstrated by a longitudinal evaluation of 4 cases. *Ultraschall Med.* 2001;22(4):176–81.

[176] Darling ML, Smith DN, Rhei E, Denison CM, Lester SC, Meyer JE. Lactating adenoma: a diagnosis of exclusion. *Breast J.* 2000;6(4):252–6.

[177] Eid S, Dos Santos E, Boisserie-Lacroix M, Grelet P, Rivel J. Lactating adenoma: radiologic aspects. A case report. *J. Radiol.* 2001;82(3 Pt 1):264–7.

[178] Magno S, Terribile D, Franceschini G, Fabbri C, Chiesa F, Di Leone A, et al. Early onset lactating adenoma and the role of breast MRI: a case report. *J. Med. Case Rep.* 2009;3:43.

[179] Mizukami Y, Takayama T, Takemura A, Ichikawa K, Onoguchi M, Miyati T, et al. Pleomorphic adenoma of the breast. *Radiat. Med.* 2008;26(7):442–5.

[180] Sato K, Ueda Y, Shimasaki M, Ozaki M, Nitta N, Chada K, et al. Pleomorphic adenoma (benign mixed tumor) of the breast: a case report and review of the literature. *Pathol. Res. Pract.* 2005;201(4):333–9.

[181] Lanng C, Eriksen BØ, Hoffmann J. Lipoma of the breast: a diagnostic dilemma. *Breast.* 2004;13(5):408–11.

[182] Rodríguez LF, Shuster BA, Milliken RG. Giant lipoma of the breast. *Br. J. Plast. Surg.* 1997;50(4):263–5.

[183] HawaryHB. Breast lipoma. *Ann. Saudi Med.* 1999;19(2):174–6.

[184] Pant R, Poh ACC, Hwang SG. An unusual case of an intramuscular lipoma of the pectoralis major muscle simulating a malignant breast mass. *Ann. Acad. Med. Singapore.* 2005;34(3):275–6.

[185] Gaskin CM, Helms CA. Lipomas, lipoma variants, and well-differentiated liposarcomas (atypical lipomas): results of MRI evaluations of 126 consecutive fatty masses. *AJR Am. J. Roentgenol.* 2004;182(3):733–9.

[186] Bonomi S, Salval A, Settembrini F, Musumarra G, Rapisarda V. Breast reshaping with dermaglandular flaps after giant lipoma removal: versatility of oncoplastic techniques. *Aesthet. Plast. Surg.* 2012;36(2):355–8.

[187] Grossman J, Menes T, Lahat G, Gur E, Weiss J, Barnea Y. Use of the oncoplastic reduction pattern technique following removal of a giant breast lipoma. *Ann. Plast. Surg.* 2011;67(2):106–8.

[188] Ribeiro RC, Saltz R, España Quintera LF. Breast reconstruction with parenchymal cross after giant lipoma removal. *Aesthet. Plast. Surg.* 2008;32(4):695–7.

In: Benign Disease of the Breast
Editors: J. de la Garza Salazar, C. Arce Salinas et al.
ISBN: 978-1-63321-624-2

Chapter 11

Mastalgia

Claudia Arce-Salinas, Rebeca Ramirez-Morales, Alberto Alvarado-Miranda and Fernando Lara-Medina
Medical Oncology Department
Instituto Nacional Cancerologia-Mexico, Mexico City, DF, Mexico

Abstract

Mastalgia is a common entity in women and may also occasionally be present in men. Pain usually presents with slight intensity; however, up to 11% of persons affected can experience moderate or intense pain that limits their Activities of daily living (ADL).

Mastalgia is classified as cyclic and non-cyclic, the former often associated with hormonal changes of the menstrual cycle. Clinically; the pain usually is bilateral and affect the upper external quadrants.

Non cyclic mastalgia is not related with the menstrual cycle; it is generally unilateral with variable localization. Multiple causes have been described, among which the following are highlighted: large and pendulous breasts that may develop stretching-related Cooper's ligament pain; this pain can also be accompanied by neck, back, shoulder, and head pain, as well as a rash underneath the pendulous breast. Other causes could be related with infectious diseases, ductal ectasia, and breast cancer; however, these are uncommon.

Diagnosis is based on the clinical manifestations and sometimes, breast ultrasound or mammography is required.

Treatment is administered according to the cause of the breast pain, and for cyclic mastalgia, Nonsteroidal anti-inflammatory drugs (NSAID) could be useful.

Introduction

Breast pain or mastalgia is a common entity in women and can occasionally also be present in men. The clinical evolution is important in determining the cause of the pain. The pain usually presents with slight intensity; however, up to 11% of the persons affected can experience moderate or intense pain that limits their Activities of daily living (ADL).

Incidence and Risk for Cancer

It has been reported that up to 70% of women experience mastalgia during their lifetime [1].

To date, there is no evidence that mastalgia is associated with an increased risk for cancer [2,3]. Rogulskiand colleagues [4] carried out a study to evaluate the risk for cancer of mastalgia; the authors evaluated 112 premenopausal women with noncyclic mastalgia and compared these with 182 control women who presented for a clinical screening examination. All were submitted to mastography and breast Ultrasound (US). The risk of breast cancer was evaluated with the assessment models of Gail and of Tyrer-Cuzick. The analysis reported that women with mastalgia had a lesser risk for cancer compared with the controls: the 5-year Gail model showed a risk of 0.66 ± 0.4% vs. 0.77 ± 0.4% (p =0.000) and the Tyrer-Cuzick model reported a 5-year risk of 0.85 ± 0.4% vs. 0.95 ± 0.3% (p = 0.002), while the Gail model showed a lifetime risk of 8.98 ± 3.6% vs. 9.6 ± 3.9% (p = 0.015) and the Tyrer-Cuzick model reported a lifetime risk of 8.3 ± 3.1% vs. 8.9 ± 2.7% (p = 0.045).

On the other hand, in the Edinburgh study [1], which consisted of a survey of 8,504 patients who presented with mastalgia as their main symptom, 220 of these (2.7%) subsequently developed cancer.

Etiology

The Aberrations of Normal Development and Involution (ANDI) classification describes mastalgia as a benign disorder deriving from hormonal activity [5].

Preece [6] initially classified mastalgia in six categories, which included cyclic mastalgia, ductal ectasia, Tietze syndrome, trauma, sclerosingadenosis, and cancer. Later, this classification was simplified to cyclic and noncyclic mastalgia [7].

Cyclic mastalgia is usually associated with the hormonal changes of the menstrual cycle; it begins with luteal phase and cedes with the initiation of menstruation. The most frequent clinical manifestation is bilateral pain, diffuse, which affects the external quadrants; on occasion, the pain can extend to the thoracic wall; on the other hand, the pain can be constant or intermittent [8].

As previously mentioned, cyclic pain is caused by hormonal changes associated with ovulation. The estrogens stimulate the ductal elements, progesterone stimulates the stroma, and ductal secretion is stimulated by Prolactin (PRL); all of these changes are those mainly responsible for cyclic menstrual pain. To a lesser extent, the pain can be the consequence of pharmaceutical agents, principally hormonal, such as contraceptive drugs and Hormone replacement therapy (HRT).

Cyclic mastalgia can have important clinical repercussions; a study that evaluated 1,171 premenopausal women reported that 11% of these had moderate pain, with affectation in their sexual activity in 48%, in physical activity in 37%, in social activity in 12%, and in academic activities in 8% [9,10].

Noncyclic mastalgia is not related with the menstrual cycle, is generally unilateral, and is of variable localization. Multiple causes have been described, among which the following are highlighted: large and pendulous breasts can develop stretching-related Cooper's ligament pain; this pain can also be accompanied by neck, back, shoulder, and head pain, as well as a rash underneath the pendulous breast.

It has been suggested that diet and lifestyle can influence the development of noncyclic pain; however, noncontrolled studies have not demonstrated a harmful effect of caffeine on breast pain [11,12], although some patients have referred improvement with suspension of the ingestion of caffeine, possibly due to the placebo effect. A case-control study was published by Lubin et al. [13], in which the authors analyzed 854 cases histologically diagnosed as benign breast disease were matched with 755 surgical controls and with 723 controls from the neighborhood. The study did not demonstrate an association with the consumption of coffee and the development of benign breast pathology. Ingestion of methylxanthines was similar in the cases as well as in controls at 302, 312, and 313 mg, respectively.

Nicotine may increase breast pain by incrementing epinephrine levels that, which induce a stimulatory effect of the Adenosine monophosphate (AMP) cycle. Smoking cessation improves mastalgia [14,15], although it also has been suggested that this fact is due to the placebo effect.

Up to one third of patients who were administered HRT can experience noncyclic pain, which can cede spontaneously over time [16,17]. Other causes of noncyclic mastalgia are described as follows:

Ductal ectasias characterized by distention of the subareolar ducts due to inflammation and subsequent infection, with the penetration of lipid material into the ducts; all of these facts favor acute pain, localized, and fever. The acute process is usually resolved and can leave a subareolar nodule as a sequela. A study demonstrated that the degree of ductal dilatation is correlated with the intensity of noncyclic pain [18].

Mastitis or breast abscesses are other causes of pain that, although more common during the first postpartum month and during lactancy, can also occur in women who are not breast-feeding; the cause generally is due to an obstruction in the duct. At the beginning of lactancy, the nipple and the areolar region are submitted to inflammation and edema. This edema results in a relative obstruction of the milk flow, which can become a favorable environment for the bacterial growth of cutaneous flora, such as *Staphylococcus aureus* and *Streptococcus* spp., which leads to bacterial mastitis. The clinical manifestations of mastitis and of the breast abscess are diffuse breast pain; on exploration, the breast is found with edema and erythema with or without areas of fluctuation.

Inflammatory breast cancer can be another cause of pain; the clinical characteristic is rapidly progressive pain accompanied by an increase in breast volume and skin changes (orange peel), without evidence of fever or leukocytosis.

Hidradenitis suppurativa can involve the breast; its clinical manifestation is that of a painful nodule. Other causes of breast pain include pregnancy, thrombophlebitis, trauma, macrocytosis prior to surgical interventions, and drugs (antidepressives, cardiovascular agents, antibiotics, and hormones) [19].

On occasion, mastalgia can possess an extramammary origin, with the most common origin in the thoracic wall; other causes include antecedents of trauma and the presence of scarring. In other cases, pain can be referred from the dorsal region (vertebral or extravertebral), as well as by pulmonary, esophageal, cardiac, or biliary diseases. Referred pain usually presents in the lateral part of the breast, can have a burning sensation, and can be localized or diffuse. Thoracic wall-associated pain frequently originates in the pectoralis major muscle and is related with physical activities; in these cases, the pain can be reproduced when the patient is requested to place their hand on the iliac crest and to push forward. When thoracic pain presents bilaterally, accompanied by parasternal pain that mainly affects the fifth costosternal joint, it can be the consequence of osteochondritis, or if it affects the second to the fifth costosternal joint, it can be the consequence of Tietze syndrome, which is commonly bilateral. Other causes of thoracic-wall pain can be arthritis, as well as radicular pain. Spinal and paraspinal alterations occur more frequently in women with problems with the neck and thoracic column associated with osteoarthritis.

Post-thoracotomy syndrome is an uncommon clinical manifestation. In the scarring process, it simulates the effect of a baby sucking; it can be accompanied by an increase in serum concentration of PRL, lacteal production, and breast pain [20].

Clinical History

It is recommended to always question the patient about the frequency and severity of the pain, as well as about factors that can trigger or improve the latter. Additionally, it is always necessary to question the patient concerning whether the pain is bilateral, its association with menstrual cycles or with pregnancy, the patient's physical activity, as well as the presence of systemic symptoms such as fever and local symptoms such as erythema, antecedents of recent trauma and, above all, to investigate whether the pain limits the patient's ADL.

Physical Examination

It is suggested to intentionally seek out the signs suggestive of malignancy; in addition, the four quadrants of the breast should be examined systematically, these including the subareolar area, the axilla, and the supra- and infraclavicular regions, with the patient in a seated position as well as in the ventral decubitus position. It is also necessary to investigate changes in the skin, the symmetry and contours of the breasts, and the position of the nipples, scars, skin retraction, edema or erythema of the skin, delimiting the presence of tumors or nipple discharge and identifying localized areas of pain.

Imaging Studies

If the pain is diffuse and the symptoms are those of classic mastalgia, complementary imaging studies such as US or masmmography are not required. However, some patients may not agree with this approach; in this case, it is recommended to carry out a breast US if the women is aged <30 years or if she has no risk factors for developing breast cancer [21]. For women >30 years of age, a masmmography with complementary US are recommended.

Within the scenario of suspicious findings of malignancy, mastography should be performed regardless of the patient's age.

For patients with focal pain without associated tumor, guided breast US or masmmography are indicated. In a retrospective study of 257 patients with localized pain without palpable mass, US detected breast cancer in three patients (1.2%) at the site of the pain, and cancer was detected in no patient with Breast Imaging Reporting and Data System

(BI-RADS) classification categories 1, 2, or 3 [22]. Of 36 patients with localized pain without palpable mass and with BI-RADS category 1 masmmography, 25 of these had a mass diagnosed by US, 26 of these lesions corresponded to cysts, and six were benign tumors; cancer was not diagnosed in this subgroup. Mammographic alterations require follow-up.

Treatment

After making the diagnosis of cyclic mastalgia evident, it is necessary to reassure to patients that they do not have cancer; the fact produces adequate relief in the majority of women [19]. Local heat and analgesics can relieve the pain. In severe cases, analgesics or steroids can be applied directly.

For patients requiring treatment, multiple therapies have been evaluated; however, those most recommended are based on observational or case-control studies. To date, evidence of randomized studies is scarce. We list here the most utilized therapeutic measures:

- *Diet and lifestyle*: The role of the diet and lifestyle changes in cyclic pain improvement is not clear. Observational studies have demonstrated that a diet low in fats (15% of calories) and high in complex carbohydrates can be effective [19,23,24]. The elimination of caffeine has not been effective in controlled assays; however, elimination of caffeine appears to produce improvement in some women [25,26]. There is non conclusive evidence on the role of vitamin E [27] and on that of evening primrose oil in the reduction of pain[28]. Pruthi and colleagues [29] conducted a randomized, double-blind, placebo-compared study in which the authors evaluated the usefulness of vitamin E in comparison with evening primrose oil for the treatment of mastalgia. Patients were randomized into the following four treatment arms; the first was administered vitamin E 1,200 IU/day; the second comprised evening primrose oil 3 gr/day; the third consisted of the combination of both, and the fourth, placebo; in total, 41 patients were included. The results demonstrated improvement in pain in the groups that received active treatment, but this was not so in the placebo group. Dhar and colleagues [30] reported 100% improvement in mastalgia as well as in nodule control with Ormeloxifene (centchroman); this drug is a nonselective antiestrogen and has the advantage of not producing the side effects common to contraceptives, such as nausea, vomiting, weight gain, and dizziness. A randomized study [31] included 135 patients assigned to two groups: Group 1 included 67 women who were given Ormeloxifene 30 mg on alternate days, and Group 2, which included 68 women treated with evening primrose oil 3 gr/day. In a 6-month follow-up, improvement was demonstrated in 86% of Group 1 women, compared with 23% of Group 2 women, with statistical significance ($p<0.05$); the sole side effect was delay in menstruation of 7–10 days.
- *Support brassiere*: The use has been widely recommended of a support brassiere without metal under wiring in the reduction of mastalgia, especially in women with pendulous breasts [32]. The use of these brassieres during exercise has shown to reduce pain related with breast movement [33,34].

- *Compresses:* Some women obtain pain relief on applying hot compresses or ice or gentle massage. Cold compresses are recommended during the obstructive phase of mastitis to diminish milk production regionally; this decreased intraductal pressure, resulting in better pain control.
- *Medical treatment:* Acetaminophen or Nonsteroidal anti-inflammatory drugs (NSAID) can be employed to diminish pain [6]. Topical NSAID can be employed with clinical benefit [35–37].
- In women who employ HRT or who utilize hormonal contraceptives, pain can be reduced on diminishing the dose of estrogen or on suspending the therapy [38]. Oral contraceptives can reduce the severity and duration of breast pain in women with cyclic pain [39,40]. Progesterone can also improve the pain in some women [41,42]. Danazol is the only drug approved by the Food and Drug Administration (FDA) in the U.S. for the treatment of mastalgia. Danazol is effective in improving breast pain and sensitivity; however, it produces an androgenic effect, which has limited its use [43–45]. In a randomized study conducted by Lakhmich and Tejwani et al.[46], the authors evaluated the effectiveness of Ormeloxifene compared with Danazol in 81 patients with mastalgia; they reported that after 12 weeks of treatment, pain control, evaluated by the Visual Analog Scale (VAS) was 89.7% for patients treated with Ormeloxifene in comparison with 69.4% of women treated with Danazol (p = 0.0001); 3 months after suspending treatment, pain control was maintained in favor of Ormeloxifene (p =0.019). Another drug evaluated for the treatment of severe mastalgia was Tamoxifen 10 mg/day [47]; however, this drug is associated with side effects that include hot flashes, joint pain, cramps in pelvic limbs, in addition to the development of venous thrombosis, vascular events, endometrial cancer, and cataracts.

Other drugs that affect the production of estrogens or Prolactin (PRL), such as bromocriptine and Gonadotropin-releasing hormone (GnRH) agonists, have been evaluated [47,48]; however, they are not recommended for the severe adverse events than can present.

Prognosis

Prognosis is variable and depends on the age of the patient at the onset of pain [49]. In some series, it has been reported that cyclic pain resolves spontaneously in 20–30% of cases within the first 3 months; however, there can be transitory recurrences [50]. In another series of cases of noncyclic mastalgia, breast pain resolved spontaneously in 50% of patients [51]. Pain relief can be spontaneous or even related with hormone-measured events, such as pregnancy or menopause [49].

Summing up and Recommendations

1. The majority of cases with mastalgia are associated with benign conditions, such as cyclic pain, fibrocystic changes, or cysts.

2. Breast pain is common in the premenstrual stage. A detailed clinical history aids in establishing the cyclic character.
3. Evaluation of breast pain is conducted by means of a complete clinical history and physical examination. Clinical judgment should be employed in deciding on the performance of imaging studies, such as masmmography or guided US.
4. For women <30 years of age, US is the optimal study; however, imaging studies are not necessary in the majority of cases.
5. In cases of focalized findings, such as pain and masses, masmmography or guided US is indicated.
6. Treatment with analgesics and a support brassiere can be useful for many women. Other useful drugs can be NSAIDs, Tamoxifen and Danazol; however, it is necessary to consider the side effects of these drugs prior to arriving at a decision concerning their use.

Approach for the diagnosis and treatment of mastalgia

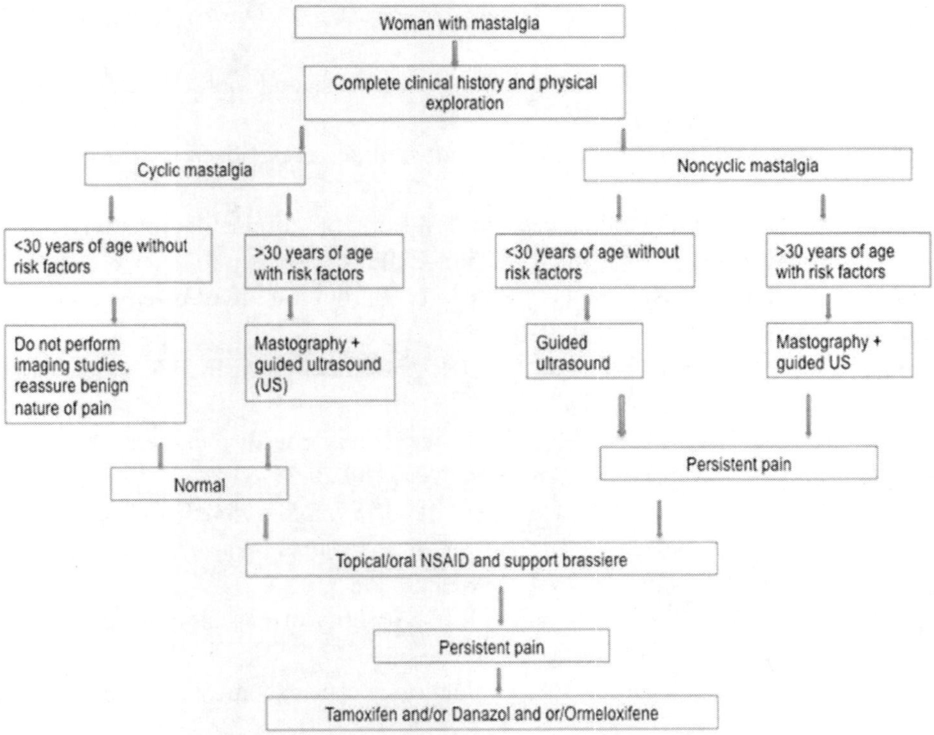

References

[1] Iddon J, Dixon JM. Mastalgia. *BMJ* 2013;347:f3288. doi: 10.1136/bmj.f3288.

[2] Aiello EJ, Buist DS, White E, Seger D, Taplin SH. Rate of breast cancer diagnoses among postmenopausal women with self-reported breast symptoms. *J. Am. Board Fam. Pract.* 2004;17(6):408–415.

[3] Smith RL, Pruthi S, Fitzpatrick LA. Evaluation and management of breast pain. *Mayo. Clin.* Proc. 2004;79(3):353–372.

[4] Rogulski L, Bińczyk J. Estimated breast cancer risk and screening outcomes among premenopausal women with non-cyclic mastalgia. *Ginekol. Pol.* 2013;84:754–757.

[5] Hughes LE, Mansel RE, Webster DJT. Aberrations of normal development and involution (ANDI): a new perspective on pathogenesis and nomenclature of benign breast disorders. *Lancet* 1987;2:1316–9.

[6] Preece PE, Hughes LE, Mansel RE, et al. Clinical syndromes of mastalgia. *Lancet* 1976;2:670–3.

[7] Maddox PR, Harrison BJ, Mansel RE, et al. Non-cyclical mastalgia: an improved classification and treatment. *Br. J. Surg.* 1989;76:901–4.

[8] Davies EL, Gateley CA, Miers M, Mansel RE. The long-term course of mastalgia. *J. R. Soc. Med.* 1998;91:462–4.

[9] Ader DN, Browne MW. Prevalence and impact of cyclic mastalgia in a United States clinic-based sample. *Am. J. Obstet. Gynecol.* 1997;177:126–32.

[10] Ader DN, South-Paul J, Adera T, Deuster PA. Cyclical mastalgia: prevalence and associated health and behavioral factors. *J. Psychosom. Obstet. Gynaecol.* 2001;22: 71–6.

[11] Levinson W, Dunn PM. Non-association of caffeine and fibrocystic breast disease. *Arch. Intern. Med.* 1986;146:1773–5.

[12] Jacobson MF, Liebman BF. Caffeine and benign breast disease. *JAMA* 1986;255: 1438–9.

[13] Lubin F, Ron E, Wax Y, et al. A case-control study of caffeine and methylxanthines in benign breast disease. *JAMA* 1985;253:2388–2392.

[14] Heyden S, Muhlbaier LH. Prospective study of"fibrocystic breast disease" and caffeine consumption. *Surgery* 1984;96:479–84.

[15] Abraham GE. Nutritional factors in the etiology of the premenstrual tension syndromes. *J. Reprod. Med.* 1983;28:446–64.

[16] Archer DR, Fischer LA, Rich D, et al. EstracevsPremarin for treatment of menopausal symptoms: dosage comparison study. *Adv. Ther.* 1992;9:21–31.

[17] Greendale GA, Reboussin BA, Hogan P, et al. Symptom relief and side effects of postmenopausal hormones: results from the Postmenopausal Estrogen/Progestin Interventions *Trial. Obstet. Gynecol.* 1998;92:982–8.

[18] Peters F, Diemer P, Mecks O, Behnken L LJ. Severity of mastalgia in relation to milk duct dilatation. *Obstet. Gynecol.* 2003;101:54–60.

[19] Smith RL, Pruthi S, Fitzpatrick LA. Evaluation and management of breastpain. *Mayo. Clinic. Proc.* 2004;79:353-372

[20] Morley JE, Dawson M, Hodgkinson H, Kalk WJ. Galactorrhea and hyperprolactinemia associated with chest wall injury. *J. Clin. Endocrinol. Meta.*b 1977;45:931–5.

[21] Morrow M. The evaluation of common breast problems. *Am. Fam. Physician* 2000;61:2371–8.

[22] Leddy R, Irshad A, Zerwas E, et al. Role of breast ultrasound and mammography in evaluating patients presenting with focal breast pain in the absence of a palpable lump. *Breast J.* 2013;19:582-589.

[23] Boyd NF, McGuire V, Shannon P, et al. Effect of a low-fat high-carbohydrate diet on symptoms of cyclical mastopathy. *Lancet* 1988;2:128–32.

[24] Goodwin PJ, Miller A, Del Giudice ME, et al. Elevated high-density lipoprotein cholesterol and dietary fat intake in women with cyclic mastopathy. *Am. J. Obstet. Gynecol.* 1998;179:430–7.

[25] Levinson W, Dunn PM. Nonassociation of caffeine and fibrocystic disease. *Arch. Intern. Med.* 1986;146:1773-1775.

[26] Heyden S, Fodor JG. Coffee consumption and fibrocystic breasts: an unlikely association. *Can. J. Surg.* 1986;29:208-211.

[27] Parsay S Olfati F, Nahidi S. Therapeutic effects of vitamin E on cyclic mastalgia. *Breast J.* 2009;15:510-514. doi: 10.1111/j.1524-4741.2009.00768.x. Epub 2009 Jul 14.

[28] Blommers J, de Lange-De Klerk ES, Kuik DJ, et al. Evening primrose oil and fish oil for severe chronic mastalgia: a randomized, double-blind, controlled trial. *Am. J. Obstet. Gynecol.* 2002;187:1389–4.

[29] Pruthi S, Wahner-Roedler DL, Torkelson CJ, et al. Vitamin E and evening primrose oil for management of cyclical mastalgia: a randomized pilot study. *Altern. Med. Rev.* 2010:1:59–65.

[30] Dhar A, Srivastava A. Role of centchroman in regression of mastalgia and fibroadenoma. *World. J. Surg.* 2007;31:1178–1184.

[31] Sharma N, Gupta A, Jha PK, Rajput P. Mastalgia cured! Randomized trial comparing centchroman to evening primrose oil. *Breast J.* 2012;18:509–510.

[32] Wilson MC, Sellwood RA. Therapeutic value of a supporting brassière in mastodynia. *Br. Med. J.* 1976;2:90.

[33] Hadi MS. Sports brassiere: is it a solution for mastalgia? *Breast J.* 2000;6:407–9.

[34] Mason BR, Page KA, Fallon K. An analysis of movement and discomfort of the female breast during exercise and the effects of breast support in three cases. *J. Sci. Med. Sport* 1999;2:134–44.

[35] Colak T, Ipek T, Kanik A, et al. Efficacy of topical nonsteroidalantiinflammatory drugs in mastalgia treatment. *J. Am. Coll. Surg.* 2003;196:525–30.

[36] No Authors listed. Diclofenac gel for osteoarthritis. *Med Lett Drugs* Ther 2008;50:31.

[37] No Authors listed.A diclofenac patch (Flector) for pain. *Med. Lett. Drugs Ther.* 2008;50:1.

[38] Dixon JM. Hormone replacement therapy and the breast. *BMJ* 2001;323:1381–2.

[39] Graham CA, Sherwin BB. A prospective treatment study of premenstrual symptoms using a triphasic oral contraceptive. *J. Psychosom. Res.* 1992;36:257–66.

[40] Bancroft J, Rennie D. The impact of oral contraceptives on the experience of perimenstrual mood, clumsiness, food craving and other symptoms. *J. Psychosom. Res.* 1993;37:195–202.

[41] Euhus DM, Uyehara C. Influence of parenteral progesterones on the prevalence and severity of mastalgia in premenopausal women: a multi-institutional cross-sectional study. *J. Am. Coll. Surg.* 1997;184:596–604.

[42] Uzan S, Denis C, Pomi V, Varin C. Double-blind trial of promegestone (R 5020) and lynestrenol in the treatment of benign breast disease. *Eur. J. Obstet. Gynecol. Reprod. Biol.* 1992;43:219–27.

[43] O'Brien PM, Abukhalil IE. Randomized controlled trial of the management of premenstrual syndrome and premenstrual mastalgia using luteal phase-only danazol. *Am. J. Obstet. Gynecol.* 1999;180:18–23.

[44] Srivastava A, Mansel RE, Arvind N, et al. Evidence-based management of mastalgia: a meta-analysis of randomised trials. *Breast* 2007;16:503–12.

[45] Fentiman IS, Caleffi M, Hamed H, Chaudary MA. Dosage and duration of tamoxifen treatment for mastalgia: a controlled trial. Br. J. Surg. 1988;75:845–6.

[46] LakhmichandTejwani P, Srivastava A, Nerkar H, et al. Centchroman regresses mastalgia: a randomized comparison with danazol. *Indian J Surg* 2010;73(3):199–205. doi: 10.1007/s12262-010-0216-z.

[47] Parlati E, Polinari U, Salvi G, et al. Bromocriptine for treatment of benign breast disease. A double-blind clinical trial versus placebo. *Acta. Obstet. Gynecol. Scand.* 1987;66:483–8.

[48] Sismondi P, Biglia N, Giai M, Defabiani E. GnRH analogs in benign breast disease and breast cancer chemoprevention. A challenge for the year 2000. *Eur. J. Gynaecol. Oncol.* 1994;15:108–14.

[49] Wisbey JR, Kumar S, Mansel RE, et al. Natural history of breast pain. *Lancet* 1983;2:672–4.

[50] Kumar S, Mansel RE, Scanlon MF, et al. Altered responses of prolactin, luteinizing hormone and follicle stimulating hormone secretion to thyrotropin releasing hormone/gonadotropin releasing hormone stimulation in cyclical mastalgia. *Br. J. Surg* 1984;71:870–3.

[51] Gateley CA, Mansel RE. Management of the painful and nodular breast. *Br. Med. Bull* 1991;47:284–94.

In: Benign Disease of the Breast
Editors: J. de la Garza Salazar, C. Arce Salinas et al.
ISBN: 978-1-63321-624-2

Chapter 12

Gynecomastia

Osvaldo Armando Quiroz-Sandoval, Carlos Robles-Vidal, Alberto Mitsuo Leon-Takahashi and Angel Herrera-Gomez
Instituto Nacional Cancerologia-Mexico, Mexico City, DF, Mexico

Abstract

Gynecomastia is a benign enlargement of the breast attributable to proliferation of the ductal elements and that is usually self-limited. Its prevalence ranges from 24–65% when asymptomatic, but when it is symptomatic, this is markedly lower. It occurs as a result of metabolic, endocrine, congenital, or acquired hypogonadal disorders, producing increased estrogenic secretion, decreased testosterone synthesis, and less androgen sensitivity.

The treatment of gynecomastia depends upon its etiology, duration, severity, and the presence of pain, and it is a multidisciplinary problem that requires endocrinological, surgical, oncological, and psychological management. Observation is the best approach, with reevaluation in men with drug-induced gynecomastia or with an underlying, treatable disorder such as hypogonadism or hyperthyroidism. If the gynecomastia persists for >3 but <6 months, administration of Tamoxifen is justified. Finally, if gynecomastia persists for >1 or 2 years, surgery is the best option because the breast tissue has probably become fibrotic and unresponsive to drug therapy.

Introduction

Gynecomastia is a benign enlargement of the breast attributable to proliferation of the ductal elements and is a common clinical condition in men. It often presents as a diffuse or a discrete retroareolar lump, while merely excessive breast adipose tissue is termed lipomastia or pseudogynecomastia; both can generally be differentiated by careful palpation, in which subareolar tissue is compared with adjacent subcutaneous fat [1]. The term is derived from the Greek *gyne* (woman) and *mastos* (breast). In some cases, it may be due to an imbalance between circulating estrogens and androgens in the blood, but its etiology is broad and varied [2].

Prevalence

The prevalence of asymptomatic gynecomastia in male population ranges from 24–65% and symptomatic gynecomastia is markedly lower [3, 4]. Three distinct peaks are recognized in the age distribution of patients with physiological gynecomastia. The first peak occurs in the neonatal period, in which 60–90% of all newborns develop brief transient enlargement of a palpable breast tissue due to transplacental passage of estrogen stimulation. This stimulus disappears as estrogens are removed from neonatal circulation; the resulting breast tissue usually disappears in 2–3 weeks. The second peak originates in puberty during the early teenage years. About 50–70% of all adolescent boys develop breast enlargement during puberty, which usually begins between the ages of 10 and 12 years, with highest prevalence between 13 and 14 years of age. This breast enlargement during puberty is followed by a complete involution, which usually occurs between the ages of 16 and 17 years. A relative excess of plasma estradiol compared with testosterone has been implicated in the pathogenesis of peripubertal gynecomastia [1, 2, 5]. The last peak is found in the mature population (senile gynecomastia); 30–65% of men have palpable breast tissue enlargement, with highest prevalence at 50–80 years of age); another high prevalence takes place in men with a Body mass index (BMI) of >25 kg/m^2, which relates to declining levels of testosterone and aromatization and with an increase in the estrogen: androgen ratio. [6, 7]. Another interesting group is hospitalized men who develop gynecomastia at a high ratio (70%); finally, in autopsy studies, evidence of gynecomastia is found in 40–50%, and the frequency of bilateral engagement is about 25–72%. In hospitalized men, the proportion with gynecomastia is even higher (70%). In autopsy studies, histologic evidence of gynecomastia is found in 40–55% of all men, and the frequency of bilateral engagement is about 25–75% [8, 9]. It is likely that many cases of gynecomastia are not reported in men with mammary volume increase.

Etiology

Gynecomastia occurs as a result of metabolic, endocrine, congenital, or acquired hypogonadal disorders and as increased estrogenic states, the result of estrogen-secreting neoplasms. Increased aromatization is found to occur in Sertoli cell tumors of the testes, in trophoblastic and non-trophoblastic germ cell tumors, hyperthyroidism, Klinefelter's syndrome, and in those patients receiving Spironolactone [10]. The androgen resistance syndrome due to impaired activity of the enzymes involved in the biosynthesis of testosterone can also be associated with gynecomastia [11].

Pharmacological gynecomastia may occur due to increased estrogen activity, estrogen secretion, decreased testosterone synthesis, and less androgen sensitivity. It can also occur from increased estrogenic effects from the metabolic conversion of exogenous androgens into estrogenic compounds. Many pharmaceutical preparations, prescription medicines, and recreational drugs have been implicated with this group [2].

Idiopathic gynecomastia is, however, the most common cause of breast enlargement, accounting for up to 25%. Additional cases can also be attributed to physiological causes (persistent pubertal gynecomastia), while drug-induced gynecomastia accounts for around 10–25% of the cases. Other causes of gynecomastia can be attributed to uncommon pathological conditions such as congenital anorchia, Klinefelter's syndrome, testicular feminization, hermaphroditism, primary adrenal carcinoma, hyperprolactinemia (9%), chronic liver disease (8%), primary hypogonadism (8%), secondary hypogonadism (2%), testicular tumors (3%), hyperthyroidism (2%), chronic renal insufficiency (1%), and malnutrition [12, 13]. Carcinoma of the male breast is a rare cause of breast enlargement that is not classified as a cause of gynecomastia, but that needs to be differentiated from it. It is extremely uncommon at 50 years of age. Male breast cancer accounts for <1% of all breast cancers and for about 0.2% of all cancers in male patients.

Classification

Webster in 1934 classified gynecomastia into three subtypes according to the nature of the proliferated tissues (glandular, fatty glandular, simple primarily fatty). In 1973, Simon classified patients with gynecomastia into three categories according to the physical aspects of the disease. Currently, this is applicable in surgical practice and is based on the amount of breast enlargement with or without skin redundancy [14, 15] (Table 1).

Table 1. Simon's classification

I	Minor breast enlargement without skin redundancy
IIa	Moderate breast enlargement without skin redundancy
IIb	Moderate breast enlargement with skin redundancy
III	Gross breast enlargement with skin redundancy that simulates a pendulous female breast

Simon BE, Hoffman S, Kahn S. Classification and surgical correction of gynaecomastia. Plast Reconstr Surg 1973;51:48

Histology

Breast tissue cells express estrogen receptors, which have a stimulating effect, and androgen receptors, which have an inhibitory effect. There are also receptors for prolactin and various growth factors such as Insulin-like growth factor 1 (IGF1), Insulin-like growth factor 2 (IGF2), Platelet-derived growth factor (PDGF), and Epidermal growth factor (EGF); there is a positive imbalance in the action of these stimuli and the proliferation of ductal epithelium occurs with hyperplasia and edema of the connective tissue and increased vascularization in periductal stroma. Patients with early symptomatic gynecomastia present common pathological findings of the early or florid stage, such as hyperplasia of the ductal epithelium, extensive proliferation and infiltration of the edematous periductal tissue with inflammatory cells, loss of stroma, and increased subareolar fat growth. This proliferation is susceptible to regression if the determining factors disappear [6, 16].

In the quiescent or fibrous stage, the glandular elements become less prominent and stromal fibrosis is the predominant histologic finding. Examination of breast tissue in asymptomatic patients who develop chronic breast enlargement (>1 year) usually shows dilated ducts with periductal stroma fibrosis and hyalinization with increased subareolar fat [9, 17] (Figure 1).

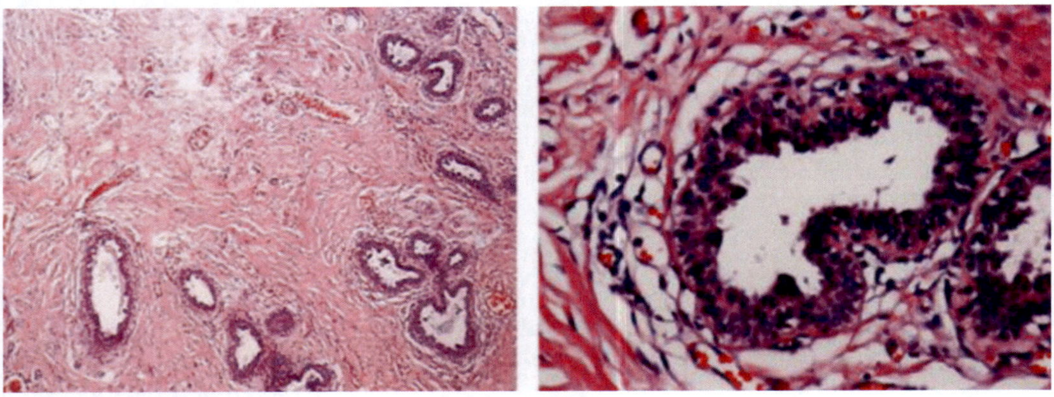

Figure 1. Proliferation of glandular epithelium surrounded by hypocellular fibrous stroma Delineated duct by cubic to cylindrical epithellium with scarce luminal secrerion.

There is no relation between the cause of the gynecomastia and histologic appearance [16].

Pathophysiology

Gynecomastia in adults is often multifactorial. The basic mechanisms of true physiological gynecomastia are thought to comprise either relative decrease in androgen production, absolute increase in estrogen production and increased availability of estrogen precursors for peripheral conversion into estradiol, or increased end-organ sensitivity to estrogen metabolites [15]. Exposure of breast tissue to estrogen causes duct growth, mammary stroma, and fat deposit. Breast lobules develop and proliferate under the influence of prolactin and progesterone. The testes secrete several sex steroid hormones with masculinizing effects denominated androgens, testosterone, dihydrotestosterone, and androstenedione. Induced stimulation of Gonadotropin-releasing hormone (GnRH) stimulated Luteinizing hormone (LH); testosterone is formed on interstitial Leydig cells located between the interstices between the seminiferous tubules, constituting up to 20% of testicular mass from puberty until age 50 years, which shows a rapid decrease, reaching, by the age of 80 years, 20–50% of the maximum (500–700 ng/dl). These are nearly nonexistent during childhood (<50 ng/dl), but usually are abundant throughout fetal development (250 ng/dl) from the genital ridge. This is due to their formation from coelomic epithelial proliferation and condensation of the underlying mesenchyme by the fetus from week 7 of embryonic development and for 10 weeks or more after birth by placental chorionic gonadotropin-stimulated testicles. Similarly, the adrenal glands secrete at least five different androgens, although the masculinizing activity of these hormones constitute <5% of those of the adult male, and they do not induce significant male characters except for hair growth in armpits and pubis. In both testes and adrenal glands, androgens may be synthesized from cholesterol or directly from acetyl coenzyme A. After discharge from the testes, 97% of testosterone is bound loosely to plasma albumin or with higher affinity to the Sex hormone binding globulin pathway (SHBG), at about 40%, where it is maintained in circulation to be fixed in the target tissues or degraded into inactive compounds, androsterone, and dehydroepiandrosterone, which are conjugated into glucuronides or sulfates excreted in bile or urine. The imbalance between free testosterone and estrogen affected by serum levels of SHBG is the proposed mechanism of gynecomastia under certain conditions, such as hyperthyroidism, chronic liver disease, and the use of some medications such as spironolactones [16]. Local production of estrogens enhanced aromatase activity in the breast, decreased local estrogen inactivation, and decreased local production of testosterone from androstenedione and changes androgen or estrogen receptors. The prevalence of these conditions increases with advanced age and nearly 50% of men aged >70 years have a low free testosterone concentration [14, 18].

Estrogen production takes place in the liver, where up to 80% of estradiol and production of estradiol and a lesser proportion in aromatase-mediated adipose tissue can be observed. The remainder of the conversion of noncirculating testosterone and androstenediol into estradiol is produced in the Sertoli cells (15% of circulating estradiol) [19].

Endogenous Estrogen Overproduction

Excessive Testicular Secretion of Estrogens

Although the increased incidence of testicular tumors occurs once pubertal development is completed, this type of tumor can cause gynecomastia in adolescents. According to reported studies, the incidence of testicular tumors in men with gynecomastia is 3%, and in 7–11% of cases it comprises the only clinical finding at the time of diagnosis [20]. Endocrine manifestations of testicular tumors can be produced by direct synthesis of androgens or estrogens by the tumors; synthesis of the gonadotropins stimulates secondary secretion of androgens or estrogens or an alteration of the peripheral metabolism of androgens. The hypothalamic-pituitary-testicular axis finely regulates levels of circulating sex steroids. Testosterone directly regulates LH secretion at both hypothalamic and pituitary levels; Leydig cells under the control of LH produce testosterone and Sertoli cells under the control of FSH and sensitive to intratesticular levels of testosterone produce the estradiol necessary for the maturation of germ cells. An abnormality in this sensitive control system that leads to progressive elevations in gonadotropin concentrations may be etiologically important in both germ-cell and non-germ-cell tumors. Estrogen dominance with an elevated estrogen/testosterone ratio can be observed in any testicular neoplasm and may result in gynecomastia [21].

Leydig Cell Tumors

Gynecomastia is found in 20–30% of patients with Leydig cell tumors of the testis, which is present in only 2% of all testicular tumors and which in the majority of cases represents a benign neoplasm (85–90%). Although they can occur at any age, Leydig cell tumors are generally observed in young and middle-aged men, principally in boys aged from 6–10 years who present with precocious puberty and in men aged 26–35 years who present with a testicular mass, gynecomastia, impotence, and loss of libido. Leydig cell tumors aromatize more androgen precursors into estrogens and directly secrete increased quantities of estradiol, which raises the serum levels of estrogen and suppresses LH release from the pituitary gland, leading to decreased production of testosterone [22]. Estrogens also stimulate the production and glycosylation of SHBG, raising serum SHBG levels. Because testosterone is more tightly bound to SHBG than to estradiol, a rise in the SHBG level leads to a decrease in the free testosterone concentration, further increasing the free estrogen-to-free androgen ratio, which leads to secondary hypogonadism due to inhibited gonadotropin secretion caused by increasing estradiol levels [23, 24]. Leydig cell tumors are small and in some cases tend to be nonpalpable; testicular Ultrasound (US) may be helpful and surgery is the treatment-of-choice.

Sertoli Cell Tumors

The Sertoli cell tumors that originate comprise a subset of sex-cord tumors that constitute <1% of all testicular tumors; the majority is benign, multifocal, and bilateral, and occurs in boys and young men. When these are malignant (20%), they are unilateral, usually extend to other organs, and frequently occur at older ages (between 38–74 years of age, with an average age of 39 years). Sertoli cells tumors can occur spontaneously (60%) without any endocrine effect or can be associated with hormonal and genetic disorders, such as Peutz-Jeghers syndrome (PJS), Carney complex syndrome (CNC), and tuberous sclerosis [25]. PJS is a rare autosomal dominant disease with variable and incomplete penetrance characterized by hamartomatous gastrointestinal polyposis and mucocutaneous hyperpigmentation, with an elevated risk for cancer at many sites and is associated with testicular sex-cord and Sertoli cell tumors; it is caused by a mutation in the serine-threonine kinase gene *STK11* on chromosome 19p13.3 and presents an estimated incidence of 1 in 8,300–29,000 births. Sertoli cell tumors in PJS overexpress aromatase, leading to significant production of estrogens and markedly elevated serum estrogen levels. These tumors often present with rapid growth, gynecomastia, and advancing bone age [26, 27].

CNC is an autosomal dominantly inherited syndrome with variable expressivity and complete penetrance (70–80% at age 40 years) and is characterized by spotty skin pigmentation, cardiac and cutaneous myxoma, and endocrine overactivity produced by an inactivating mutation of the 1-alpha regulatory subunit of Protein kinase A (PRKAR1A) located on chromosome 17q22-24, a key component of the c-AMP (cyclic-Adenosine monophosphate) signaling pathway implicated in endocrine tumorigenesis. The presence of testicular tumors appears in 33% of patients affected by CNC when diagnosed. In the majority of cases, these are Large-cell calcifying Sertoli cell tumors (LCCSCT) and, in exceptional cases, Leydig cell tumors. They are usually nonpalpable, bilateral, and multifocal (50%) tumors with poor potential for malignancy, are easily diagnosed by the presence of bilateral testicular microcalcifications observed on testicular US, and may be hormonally active, resulting in pre- and peripubertal gynecomastia due to an increase in peripheral aromatization [28]. High frequency of tumor-associated syndrome presentation in CNC is always necessary in order to perform an additional echocardiogram to rule out the possibility of myxoma, which in turn can be a cause of sudden death [29].

Around 10% of testicular tumors arise from an undescended testis and the Relative risk (RR) of testicular cancer in cryptorchidism is 5–7%. Germ-cell tumors of the testes that contain chorionic elements secrete human Chorionic gonadotropin (hCG), which in addition to aromatizing circulating Dehydroepiandrosterone (DHEA) in estrogen, may stimulate Leydig cells to produce estradiol, leading to a relative or absolute systemic excess of estrogens [29]. Feminizing tumors of the adrenal gland are undifferentiated and produce estrogen or DHEA, which is aromatized in peripheral tissues. Congenital adrenal hyperplasia, caused by a deficit of 3β hydroxysteroid-dehydrogenase, 11 β-hydroxylase, or 21-hydroxylase, also gives rise to an increase in the aromatization of androgens into estrogens [30].

With an estimated prevalence in autopsy studies ranging from 7% in patients >70 years of age to 1% in patients <30 years of age, gynecomastia usually appears to be the first symptom in men with adrenal tumors, which are often associated with Cushing's syndrome. Patients with feminizing adrenal adenomas present with gynecomastia (98%), breast tenderness (42%), and testicular atrophy (52%). Its pathogenesis is related with estrogen secretion by tumoral overproduction of corticosteroids (which are normally produced in the adrenal cortex), although the dominant action is maintained by weak estrogens such as estrone and estriol. A work-up for excess pheochromocytoma and cortisol should be performed and the evaluation of feminization should include estradiol and estrone levels [31, 32]. It is not unusual for these in principle to be considered benign, but they often metastasize, manifesting with the same functionality as the primary tumor. Thus, it is advisable to monitor their evolution. Up to 76% of adrenal carcinomas are functional, among which 2–10% of patients have some degree of feminization. However, it is attributed to the conversion of androstenedione into estrogen, and not to direct secretion of estrogen by the cortex. A review of adrenal incidentalomas recommended that all adrenal masses >4 cm, functioning adenomas, and adrenal carcinomas should be resected. Even after complete resection, 43% of patients with adrenal carcinoma develop metastatic disease, with a 73% mortality rate and an average 8.7 months after diagnosis. No significant data on treatment exist with chemotherapies other than Mitotane. Feminization associated with adrenal carcinoma may be achieved with Tamoxifen; gynecomastia usually corrects after adrenalectomy [33–35].

Exogenous Estrogen Administration

Prostate Cancer

The prevalence of gynecomastia in patients with prostate cancer treated with hormonal therapy based on systemic estrogen is around 71% in the first 6–9 months of hormonal therapy, up to 49% in those treated with nonsteroidal antiandrogens and up to 25% in those treated with LHRH analogues. In patients with bilateral orchiectomy, an incidence has been reported of gynecomastia of up to 10% [36].

Radiation therapy with prophylactic purposes at a low dose of 10–12 Gy to the breast tissue has reported good results for the prevention or treatment of Bicalutamide-induced gynecomastia; however, the long-term risk for developing a radiation-induced tumor in these patients has not been clarified. The use of Tamoxifen appears to have better results by reducing the risk of gynecomastia in patients with treatments based on antiandrogenic or estrogenic agonist drugs [37, 38]. In a comparative study by Perdona, the efficacy of Tamoxifen 10 mg/day vs. radiotherapy with a low dose in the management of Bicalutamide (150 mg) monotherapy induced gynecomastia.

These findings were in agreement with those published by Boccardo and Saltzstein [39, 40]. Fradet in 2007 conducted a double-blind, multicenter trial to define the optimal Tamoxifen dose for treating Bicalutamide-induced gynecomastia without compromising disease control. Two hundred eighty two patients with prostate cancer were randomized to receive Bicalutamide 150 mg/daily plus Tamoxifen 1, 2.5, 5, 10, or 20 mg/daily vs. placebo for 12 months. At 6 and 12 months, Tamoxifen exhibited a decrease in the incidence of breast symptoms with better results at the 20-mg/day dose [41].

Absolute Deficiency of Androgens

Primary Hypogonadism

The causes of primary hypogonadism are congenital or acquired for testicular failure with low or absent secretion of testosterone and consequent increase in LH levels and which can increase estradiol secretion by Leydig cell; in Klinefelter's syndrome, bilateral testicular anorchia or defects in enzymes (17-reductase cetosteroid) converts androstenedione into testosterone. Testosterone replacement therapy in men with primary hypogonadism often reduces in gynecomastia.

Klinefelter's Syndrome

This is a group of chromosomal disorders in which there is at least one extra X chromosome to a normal male karyotype. Many boys with 47XXY appear to enter puberty normally, with a tendency for declining testosterone concentrations at late adolescence and early adulthood. With a decrease in androgen production, secondary sexual characteristics do not completely develop, and features of eunuchoidism and gynecomastia can develop. Over 56–88% of patients with Klinefelter's syndrome have gynecomastia; in these cases, in addition to poor secretion of androgens by testis dysfunction due to testicular atrophy, an increase in aromatase activity, decreased androgen levels, and elevated gonadotropin levels are shown [42]. Patients with Klinefelter's syndrome have been found to have plasma estradiol levels that are, on average, up to twice those of normal men. This modest difference renders the magnitude of the risk of developing breast cancer approximately 60 times greater, with an incidence of 1:400 per 1:1,000 patients. Possible reasons for this large RR are that men with Klinefelter's syndrome have an estradiol-to-testosterone ratio that is several-fold higher than that of karyotypically normal men, or that there is increased peripheral conversion of testosterone into estradiol in men with Klinefelter's syndrome compared with karyotypically normal men [43]. Another possibility is that the presence of two X chromosomes per se might increase the genetic risk of breast cancer in men with Klinefelter's syndrome [44]. Due to this increased incidence of breast cancer, excisional techniques are preferred for the treatment of gynecomastia, as they allow a full histopathological study of the surgical specimen [45, 46].

Disordered Enzymes of Testosterone Biosynthesis

Ketoconazole, Metronidazole, and Spironolactone can inhibit various enzymes in the testosterone biosynthesis pathway and lead to decreased testosterone production resulting in gynecomastia.

Secondary Hypogonadism

In secondary hypogonadism (due to failure in the pituitary-hypothalamic axis, secondary to hypothalamic tumors, radiation, surgery, or drugs), an overall decrease in gonadal steroids, androgens, and estrogens occurs; thus, gynecomastia is not as common, although it may appear to be due to an altered androgen-to-estrogen ratio by persistent peripheral aromatization of androgenic precursors of the adrenal gland into estrogens [47].

Pituitary adenomas are epithelial neoplasms that correspond to 15% of intracranial tumors, with an incidence of 1–7.6 per 100,000 persons and in up to 25% of autopsies. Incidence increases with age and these are more common between the ages of 30 and 60 years. Up to 70% of pituitary adenomas are hormonally active, while the remainder is considered nonfunctional.

Pituitary gland tumors produce hypogonadism by means of two mechanisms: destruction of secreting GnRH cells, or by inhibition of GnRH secretion when there is prolactinemia. Pharmacological gynecomastia also includes increased estrogenic effects from metabolic conversion of exogenous androgens into estrogenic compounds. Spironolactone and Ketoconazole inhibit the biosynthesis of testosterone and can result in significant gynecomastia.

Spironolactone can also increase the aromatization of testosterone into estradiol, decreasing the testosterone production rate by the testes and displacing testosterone from SHBG, thereby increasing its metabolic clearance rate, because estradiol and estrone bind less avidly to SHBG than testosterone does [48]. Spironolactone can act as an antiandrogen by binding to androgen receptors and displacing or preventing binding of testosterone and dihydrotestosterone to their receptors, increasing the bioavailable fraction of estrogen to a greater extent than androgen does [46].

In a placebo-controlled trial, low doses of Spironolactone used in the treatment of heart failure could cause certain endocrine side effects as important as breast pain, impotence, decreased libido, and gynecomastia; gynecomastia will occur in nearly every male who takes a ≥100 mg/day dose of Spironolactone, as observed in patients receiving large doses for liver failure [49, 50].

In patients receiving highly active antiretroviral therapy, there is fat-redistribution lipodystrophy-like syndrome described as pseudogynecomastia. However, true gynecomastia has also been associated in patients receiving Efavirenz, possibly by a co-existing hypogonadism or due to an estrogen-like effect [51].

Hormone Imbalance

The pubertal state is associated with a thirty-fold rise in testosterone concentration, with only a three-fold increase in the estrogen level [52]. This relative imbalance or altered ratio may lead to true gynecomastia, which may be attributable to excessive estrogen action, deficient androgen action, or a combination of these effects on the breast tissue.

Diminished Androgen Concentration

This is commonly encountered in older men as a part of a normal aging process and in patients with primary and secondary hypogonadism. Adipose tissue is a major aromatization site; with increasing age, there is often increasing adiposity. In addition, there is evidence that there may be increased aromatase activity in adipose cells with aging. Although prolactin receptors have been demonstrated in breast tissue, including gynecomastia, hyperprolactinemia probably plays an indirect role in gynecomastia by causing central hypogonadism. The majority of men with gynecomastia do not have elevated serum prolactin levels, and not all men with hyperprolactinemia develop gynecomastia. Acute prolactin treatment produced an increase in progesterone receptor and a decrease in androgen receptor content. The resulting increase in progesterone receptor expression and the decrease in androgen receptor expression could promote breast tissue growth and result in gynecomastia.

Receptor-Mediated Pathogenesis

Androgen receptors could possess a genetic defect or be blocked by certain medications such as Bicalutamide, and the estrogen receptors could be activated by certain medications or environmental exposure [16]. Displacement of androgen from breast androgen receptors can occur with drugs such as Spironolactone, Cyproterone acetate, Flutamide, and Cimetidine. Digoxin has a structural homology to estrogen and could lead to an activation of estrogen receptors in breast tissue. Enhanced estrogen receptor sensitivity has also been implicated in the cause of idiopathic gynecomastia, and the increased aromatization of androgen into estrogen within breast tissue may also be responsible. In addition, expanded CAG trinucleotide repeats in exon 1 of the androgen receptor gene can lead to partial androgen insensitivity of the androgen receptor to circulating androgens and may explain why some men, even with normal circulating androgen levels, develop gynecomastia [14].

Altered Serum Androgen: Estrogen Ratio

Puberty

Prepubertal gynecomastia accounts for 5% of the total and is characterized by increased breast tissue without other secondary sexual characteristics [53.]

Patients with pubertal gynecomastia have normal estradiol, testosterone, dehydroepiandrosterone-sulfate levels, and a normal estrogen-testosterone ratio. However, some reports have shown a transient increase in estradiol concentration and wider fluctuations of estradiol at adult levels prior to those of testosterone at the onset of puberty in boys who develop gynecomastia, with an absolute increase in the 24-h concentration of estradiol, which may reflect increased conversion of adrenal androgens into estrogens and which may occur independently of and prior to the maturation of the hypothalamic-pituitary-gonadal axis; eventually, exposure to hormonal imbalance leads to proliferation of glandular tissues, i.e., ductal hyperplasia [54, 55].

Leptin is also implicated as an etiologic agent. The mammary gland expresses leptin receptors capable of increasing aromatase activity in adipose stromal cells and breast tissue. Some reports show an increase in circulating levels of leptin in obese children with pubertal gynecomastia [56].

Pubertal gynecomastia is usually observed between the ages of 10 and 13 years, is often <4 cm in length, and usually resolves spontaneously within 6 months to 2 years of onset. However, in some instances, it may persist after completion of puberty and into adulthood, resulting in persistent pubertal gynecomastia. The influence of genetic factors is unknown, but Lawrence in 2004 communicates familial history in nearly one half of the patients in their series [57].

Another theory suggests the existence of estrogenic dominance at the onset of puberty, when the nocturnal and pulsatile secretion of LH begins. Because its secretion only occurs nocturnally, the inhibitory effect on the proliferation of breast tissue of testosterone after LH stimulation will be exercised only at night.

At the level of the adrenal gland, this produces a weak androgen secretion that will be aromatized peripherally and converted into estrogens throughout the day, having only the compensatory effect at night, with the stimulating estrogenic effect prevailing during the rest of the day. This situation must be reversed when, at the end of puberty, LH secretion continues maintains throughout the entire day.

Aging

Increased aromatization is found to occur physiologically because of aging, together with a gradual increase in the body fat tissue relative to a lean body mass. Adipose tissue is an active site of extraglandular aromatization of testosterone into estradiol and of androstenedione into estrone.

In addition, there tends to be a gradual decrease in testosterone production by the aging testes and an increase in SHBG levels, resulting in a decreasing free testosterone concentration with a reciprocal increase in the LH level. Also, old men may be likely to take some gynecomastia-associated medications [58]. The high prevalence of asymptomatic gynecomastia in older men raises the question of whether or not this should be considered physiological due to the normal aging process, to the enhanced aromatization of androgens in subareolar fat tissue, as well as to the age-related decrease in testosterone production. Because the excessive aromatization of androgens has been shown to be present in many patients with gynecomastia, it is unclear why aromatase inhibitors have not been more successful in the treatment of these patients [46].

Starvation

Gynecomastia associated with malnutrition usually appears when weight regain occurs and is probably due to liver dysfunction; increased caloric intake determines an increase in the production of both estrogen and androgen, but the liver dysfunction generated during malnutrition renders estrogen degradation difficult, resulting in an increase of the estrogen:androgen ratio [59].

Renal Failure/Dialysis

In the case of renal failure, men are often hypogonadal with defects in testicular steroidogenesis. Increased uremia can lead to damage in the Leydig cells, causing a decrease in testosterone concentrations and associated elevation of gonadotropin levels; serum prolactin levels are elevated because of decreased renal clearance and increased production, which relates to a functional disturbance in the hypothalamic regulation of prolactin secretion. Furthermore, starvation is common in patients with renal failure before dialysis and protein-restricted diets are part of their treatments; after initiation of dialysis, their nutritional status improves and dialysis-associated gynecomastia resolves spontaneously after 1 or 2 years [60].

Hepatic Cirrhosis

Prevalence of gynecomastia in patients with cirrhosis is thought to be around 67%; however, Cavanaugh in 1990 reported that the prevalence is not different from that of patients hospitalized with similar ages [61]. However, chronic liver disease can give rise to several hormonal changes that may, theoretically, increase the risk for developing gynecomastia; a decrease in androstenedione clearance enables the increase in serum concentrations, which in turn allows greater estrone aromatization, resulting in its conversion into estradiol [62]. Furthermore, it has been reported that serum progesterone and SHBG levels are also increased in patients with cirrhosis, decreasing free testosterone levels. Consequently, these same patients also develop secondary hypogonadism due to the testicular atrophy that accompanies these [62, 64].

Hyperthyroidism

Attributable to increased peripheral conversion by aromatization of testosterone to estradiol and androstenedione to estrone in extraglandular tissues and increased serum SHBG levels, 10–40% of men with thyrotoxicosis develop gynecomastia that resolves with correction of the hyperthyroid state [65–67]. LH levels are also elevated and contribute to enhanced estradiol concentrations relative to testosterone production by Leydig cells in the testis. Free testosterone levels are normal or low, while free estradiol levels are high. High serum levels of progesterone have also been reported in men with hyperthyroidism, although its biologic significance and relation to gynecomastia remains unclear [68].

Drugs

Many medications and recreational drugs have been associated with gynecomastia. Although a causal relationship is well established with some drugs, the mechanism is unclear for the majority of the latter. Medications that cause gynecomastia are widely categorized by their hormone-like action. Type 1 drugs act like estrogens, type 2 drugs enhance endogenous estrogen formation, type 3 drugs inhibit testosterone synthesis and its action, and type 4 drugs are represented by several drugs that act by unknown mechanisms [16] (Table 2)

Table 2. Medications cause gynecomastia

Type 1. Act like estrogens	Type 2. Enhance endogenous estrogen formation	Type 3. Inhibit testosterone synthesis and its action	Type 4. Act by unknown mechanisms
• Diethylstilbestrol • Digitalis (Digoxin) • Steroid (Stanozolole) • Oral contraceptive pills • Estrogen-containing cosmetics.	• Gonadotrophin - related GnRH (Triptoreline, Leuprorelin) • Clomiphene	• Chemotherapeutic drugs (Alkylating agents, Vinca alkaloids, Methotrexate, Imatinib) • Aldosterone antagonists (Spironolactone, Splerenone) • Antiandrogens (Flutamide, Gosereline, Bicalutamide, Cyproterone) • Antifungal drugs (Itraconazole, Ketoconazole) • 5-alpha reductase inhibitors (Finasteride, Dutasteride) • Proton pump inhibitors (Omeprazole) • H2 Antihistamines (Cimetidine, Ranitidine) • Benzodiazepines (Diazepam) • Metronidazole • D-Penicillamine	• Tricyclic antidepressants • Antipsychotics (Methylphenidate) • ACE inhibitors (Captopril, Enalapril) • ARBs AT_1-receptor antagonists • Calcium channel blockers • Alpha adrenergic receptor antagonists (Alfulzosina, Tamsulosin, Terazosin, Doxazosin, Prazosin) • NSAIDs (Sulindac) • Antibiotics (Antiretroviral drugs, Isoniazid) • Antiadrenergic of central action (Clonidine, Methyldopa, Reserpine) • Antiemetics (Domperidone, Dimethicone Metoclopramide) • Statins • Allopurinol • Amiodarone • Phenytoin • Teophylline • Methadone • Heroin • Cannabis • Alcohol

Modified form: Rahmani S, Turton P, Shaaban A, et al. Overview of gynecomastia in the modern era and the Leeds gynecomastia investigation algorithm. Breast J 2011;17(3):246-255.

Decreased Androgen Action

Androgen Receptor Defects

Partial or complete X-linked androgen insensitivity is due to defects in the androgen receptor structure as a result of mutations characterized by high serum testosterone levels, which lack inhibitory activity in breast tissue, and high blood levels of gonadotropins leading to an increase in the synthesis of estradiol as in primary hypogonadism [69]. A relationship has been described between the insensitivity of androgen receptors and the number of unstable repetitions of the glutamine codon CAG in tandem exon 1 of the androgen receptor gene *Xq11-12* in patients with Kennedy's disease (X-linked bulbospinal neuropathy characterized by slowly progressive muscle weakness and late-onset atrophy), where >40 repetitions on average have been documented [70]. Such repeats have been described in lower numbers in male patients with prostate cancer, hepatocellular carcinoma, and intellectual disability [71].

Male Breast Cancer

Male breast cancer is a rare cause of breast enlargement that is not classified as a real cause of gynecomastia; it accounts for about 0.2% of all of the cancers diagnosed in male patients and is extremely uncommon >50 years of age. However, it needs to be differentiated from true causes of gynecomastia during clinical evaluation [21]. Men with a familial history of breast cancer in relatives have a 2.5-times increased risk of developing breast cancer, and those with the *BRCA2* mutation have a 100-fold greater risk of developing breast cancer [45]. A higher incidence of breast cancer in patients with gynecomastia has not been detected in relation to the remainder of the male population, except in patients with Klinefelter's syndrome [72, 73].

Evaluation

Gynecomastia is common in infancy, adolescence, and in middle-aged-to-older-adult males. Pseudogynecomastia, which is often observed in obese men, refers to fat deposition without glandular proliferation and does not require evaluation. It may be uni- or bilateral and is diagnosed on examination as a palpable mass of tissue at least 0.5 cm in diameter (usually underlying the nipple). Idiopathic and drug-induced gynecomastia is usually unilateral; however, in pubertal and hormonal cases, the changes are often bilateral [74]. Complete clinical evaluation may be sufficient to establish the cause in patients with gynecomastia (Figure 1).

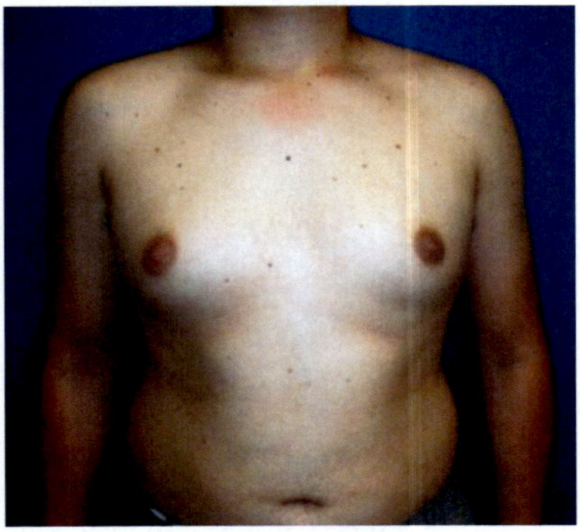

Figure 1. Clinical presentation of gynecomastia (courtesy of Fernado Magallanes M.D. The American British Cowdray Medical Center).

Clinical evaluation should include time of evolution, history of drugs or medication intake and the associated symptoms, patient's age and phenotype, hair distribution, secondary sexual characteristics, and palpation of the testes, determining size, symmetry, and the presence of masses to rule out alcoholism, hypo- or hyperthyroidism, liver diseases, adrenal and renal failure, and testicular tumors. Physical examination of gynecomastia is performed with the patient in a supine position, arms placed behind head, and taking the breast tissue between the forefinger and thumb, sliding and approximating them closer to perceive contact with a consistent structure that corresponds to the underlying breast tissue. In patients with true gynecomastia, a rubbery or firm mound of tissue that is concentric with the nipple-areola complex is palpated, whereas in patients with pseudogynecomastia, no such mound of tissue is found.

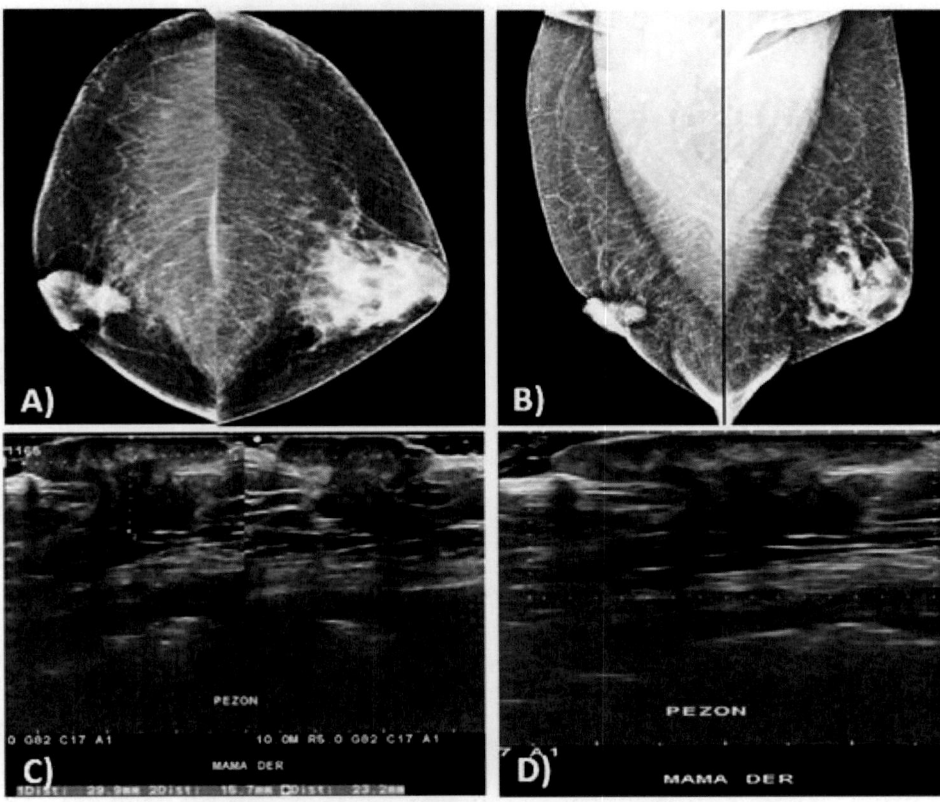

Figure 2. Male 76 years old who started with a 6-month retroareolar mass in the right breast. Clinically with right nipple retracted. A) and B) Mammography in CC and MLO projections where an area of retroareolar high density in left breast is identified that does not retract nipple or adjacent structures; in right subareolar region a radiopaque nodule is seen, not well defined that retracts the nipple. C) Ultrasound showing right retroareolar lobulated tumor, which was biopsied resulting infiltrating dual carcinoma SBR 7. D) Left retroareolar ultrasound where a diffuse hypoechoic area is observed corresponding to a left nodular gynecomastia.

However, in clinical practice, there is a clear mismatch between amount of breast tissue determined by palpation and measurement of glandular tissue provided by US, because manual palpation does not take into account the proportion of measurement corresponding to subcutaneous fat tissue components. Hence, it is necessary to measure the skin fold in the area adjacent to the breast and to correlate it with the full breast. Physical breast physical examination determines the relationship between glandular and adipose tissue, degree of ptosis, cutaneous excess, presence of nodules or palpable masses, altered nipple-areola complex, and the presence of secretions through the nipple [75].

In patients with suspected gynecomastia, a bilateral Mediolateral oblique view (MLO) mammographic projection and bilateral breast US is recommended. Only 1% of mammograms in men reveal breast cancer [75]. Despite the low incidence of breast cancer in men, we are forced to discard it as one of the differential diagnoses (Figure 2).

From the point of view of gynecomastia, three types of mammographic patterns have been identified: nodular; diffuse, and dendritic. Nodular or focal type is characterized by an increased rounded, retroareolar appearance density, it represents an early florid stage of ductal and stromal proliferation, US and mammographic findings are a subareolar hypoechoic mass with fan-shaped density, and ductal prominence may occur; these findings are consistent with an early reversible pathology, with <1 year of evolution.

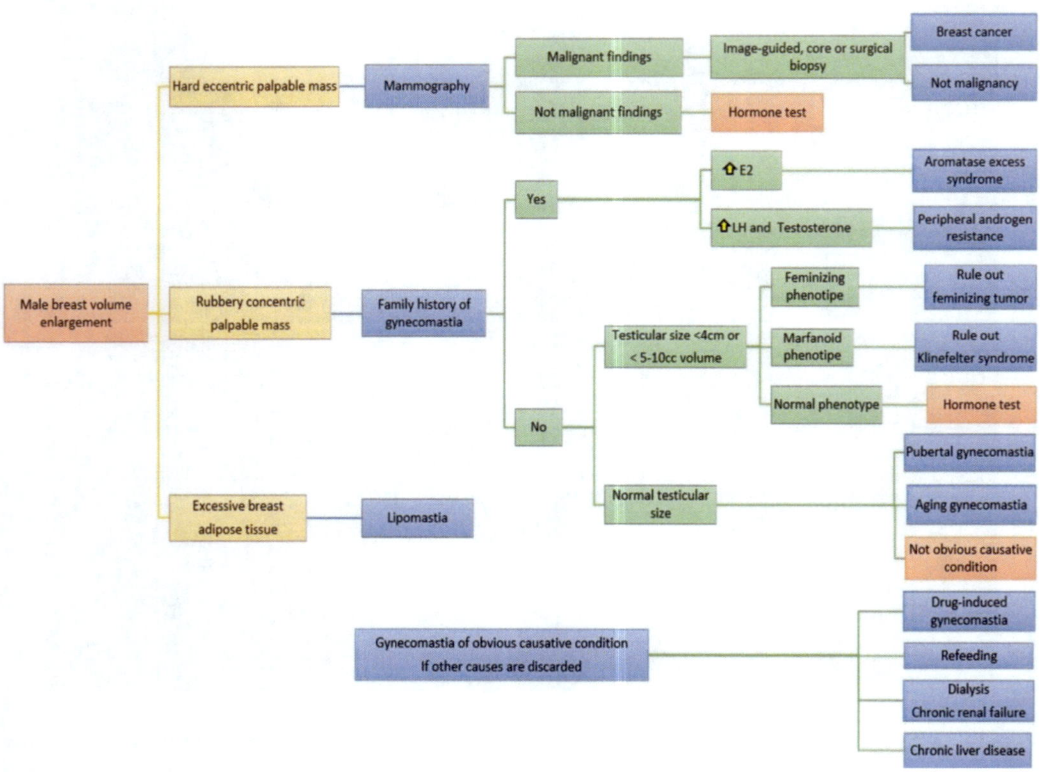

Figure 3. Initial evaluation of gynecomastia.

The dendritic type corresponds to a fibrotic phase and is mammographically identified as a subareolar flame-shaped density, ranging from retroareolar region to the deeper tissues, which are usually irreversible. US can identify a retroareolar, stellate-shaped central mass with finger-like projections into the deeper tissues. The diffuse type is observed in patients with systemic hormonal replacement. It may occur in patients with prostate cancer and mammographically is identified as a heterogeneous, dense breast tissue resembling a female breast. US identifies a female-like breast tissue [76, 77].

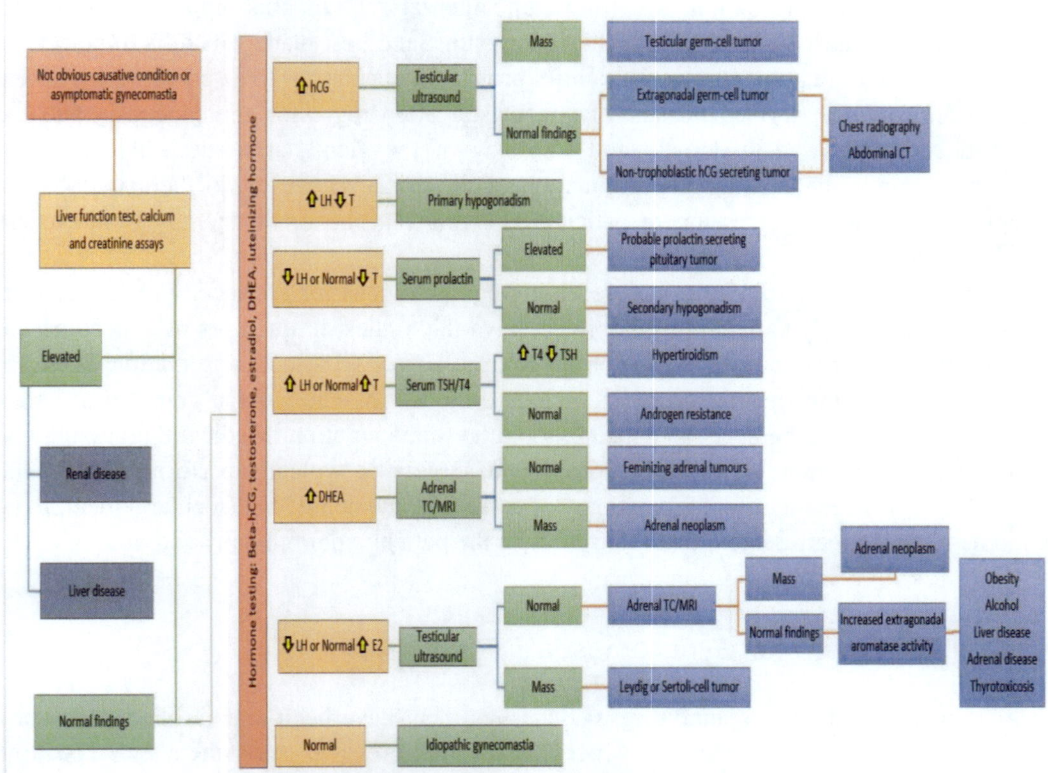

Modified from: Braunstein GD. Gynecomastia. NEJM 1993;328:490-495.

Figure 4. Not obvious causative gynecomatia evaluation.

No supplementary examinations are conducted routinely, requesting a diagnostic profile according to the clinical findings. If the physical examination reveals signs of feminization, such as reduction in testicular size (<4 cm in length or a volume of 5–10 cc), alteration in hairy distribution, and eunuchoid phenotype, the existence of a feminizing tumor should be evaluated. In these cases, determination of a hormonal profile is indicated, measuring serum levels of testosterone, estradiol, LH, and dehydroepiandrosterone. In addition to a marfanoid phenotype, the request for a karyotype is indicated to rule out Klinefelter's syndrome (Figures 3 and 4).

Treatment

Overall, gynecomastia is a benign condition and is usually self-limited. Over time, fibrotic tissue replaces symptomatic proliferation of glandular tissue and the tenderness resolves [78]. The treatment of gynecomastia depends upon its etiology, duration, severity, and the presence of pain, and it is a multidisciplinary problem that requires endocrinological, surgical, oncological, and psychological management, but in many cases gynecomastia resolves without therapy. The major factor that influences the approach is the duration of gynecomastia. The majority of pubertal gynecomastia resolves within 6 months; however, in 8% of cases, gynecomastia continued to be detected at 2 years. Although evidence is lacking to support a recommendation for follow-up intervals, 6 months appears reasonable. Gynecomastia is most symptomatic in the first months, and best management is to detect the specific cause and treat this during the painful proliferative phase or to discontinue drugs that cause it and only observe it, because gynecomastia often regresses spontaneously and the drug-induced, decreased tenderness and softening of the glandular tissue will usually be apparent within 1 month after discontinuation of the drugs. However, in therapeutic trials, complete spontaneous regression in patients receiving placebo or no therapy is much less frequent [79].

Gynecomastia is common in men receiving antiandrogens for advanced prostate cancer; other drugs, such as Verapamil or Nifedipine, have the highest frequencies of gynecomastia, as does the use of aldosterone antagonist (Spironolactone) [80]. If observation does not resolve the symptoms, treatment options include drug therapy and surgical removal of breast glandular tissue, with the decision depending on the time evolution. Medical therapy may be effective early (<6 months) in active phase and surgery is typically performed when the fibrotic stage has been reached. Indications for early therapy include breast enlargement, pain, tenderness, and embarrassment that interfere with the patient's normal daily activities.

Medical Treatment for Gynecomastia

The majority of studies analyzing medical treatment have been uncontrolled; thus, they are difficult to interpret because gynecomastia may resolve spontaneously. The few randomized, double-blind, placebo-controlled trials generally have been limited by small samples [46]. Information on drug therapy is limited; several pharmacological agents have been used to manipulate the hormonal imbalances thought to cause gynecomastia. However, studies that evaluated their efficacy were in general small and uncontrolled, rendering inference challenging. Androgens, selective estrogen receptor modulators, and aromatase inhibitors are used, but none induce complete regression and none have been approved by the U.S. Federal Drug Administration (FDA) for the treatment of gynecomastia. The use of dihydrotestosterone (a nonaromatizable androgen) has been reported as effective for gynecomastia in uncontrolled studies. The use of Tamoxifen or Raloxifene appears to decrease breast volume; however, complete breast regression is not achieved with this treatment and it could be effective for patients with painful gynecomastia. Devoto et al. in 2007 conducted a study with 33 patients between 12 and 62 years of age with gynecomastia, obtaining complete clinical responses in 62% of cases after the application of Tamoxifen for 6 months, 52% in patients with gynecomastia >4 cm, in 90% in those with smaller masses (p <0.05), in 55% of patients with gynecomastia longer that 2 years of evolution, and 70% in those with less [81]. Tamoxifen has also been reported to avoid estrogenic effects deriving from adjuvant hormone therapy used in prostate cancer. Lawrence et al. [82]. in a retrospective review evaluated patients with persistent pubertal gynecomastia who received Raloxifene (60 mg/day) or Tamoxifen (10–20 mg/day) for 3–9 months. Nearly 90% in both groups reported a decrease in gynecomastia, but patients in the Raloxifene group experienced a reduction of >50% in breast glandular tissue; 3 of the 10 patients in the Raloxifene group and 1 of 15 in the Tamoxifen group had complete resolution of gynecomastia in both breasts. Finally, this review is inconclusive concerning the efficacy of the drugs compared to no treatment or to placebo. Similar results were reported in another case series of 37 patients who used Tamoxifen; reductions in pain and nodule size were observed in all patients without long-term adverse effects [83].

Another trial included 16 men with gynecomastia randomly assigned to receive Tamoxifen (10 mg/day) vs. placebo; there was a statistically significant reduction in tenderness and breast size with Tamoxifen, but no patient experienced complete remission [84]. In another study with long-term follow-up, at a 20-mg/day dose for 3 or more months, Tamoxifen resulted in complete regression of gynecomastia in 60% of patients and partial regression in 20% [85].

In relation to aromatase inhibitors, Plourde, in a randomized double-blind controlled trial in patients with pubertal gynecomastia >3 cm in length, included 38 patients treated with Anastrozole 1 mg/day and 35 patients treated with placebo. A reduction of >50% of the initial volume with Anastrozole was observed in 38.5% of patients treated with the latter and in 31.4% of those treated with placebo. Only 1 of the 38 patients treated with Anastrozole had complete remission after 6 months of treatment, and this did not occur in any of the patients treated with placebo.

Also reported was an increase of the testosterone:estradiol ratio in 166% of patients treated with Anastrozole vs 39% in patients treated with placebo [86]. Other important group of patients is men with gynecomastia due to androgen deprivation therapy for prostate cancer; prevalence is approximately 15% in men treated with gonadotropin-releasing hormone agonist combined with an antiandrogen; however, prevalence is as high as 75% when antiandrogen monotherapy is used [87].

The use of prophylactic radiation therapy directed at the breast has been somewhat successful in preventing new-onset gynecomastia in several small studies; however, Tamoxifen has also been used successfully in this situation and appears to be superior to both radiotherapy and Anastrozole. [82, 89, 90].

Surgical Treatment for Gynecomastia

Surgical correction is considered the therapeutic gold standard and should be considered for patients whose gynecomastia does not regress spontaneously or with medical therapy and for patients with considerable discomfort or psychological distress. For adolescents, surgery is not recommended until adult testicular size is attained. According to Córdova and Moschella, the aims of surgical treatment include flattening of the thorax, elimination of the inframammary fold, positioning of the nipple-areola complex, removal of skin redundancy, symmetrization, and scar containment [91]. There are no clear guidelines in the surgical management of gynecomastia because the different interventions were tested only in case series, not in randomized trials. The most widely used techniques for the treatment of grades I-II gynecomastia provide for direct surgical excision of the glandular tissue by means of a peri- or transareolar approach [92] (Figure 5).

The extent of surgery depends upon the severity of the breast enlargement and whether there is also excess adipose tissue present; surgical approaches have been numerous and have included subcutaneous mastectomy, breast reduction, Mammotome device, liposuction, or a combination of these techniques [93]. The classic surgical approach with semicircular periareolar incision described by Webster was the standard procedure for the excision of gynecomastia [94].

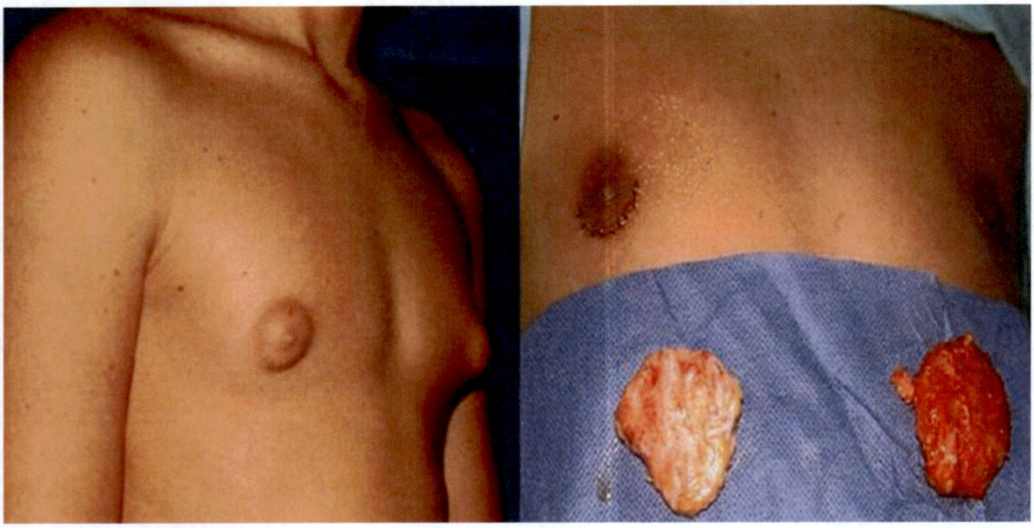

Figure 5. Treatment of gynecomastia with subareolar resection (courtesy of Fernando Magallanes M.D. The American British Cowdray Medical Center).

However, surgical management has undergone significant changes over the past decades, ranging from a predominantly open approach to that involving liposuction alone for removing glandular breast tissue; this procedure was introduced by Teimourian and Pearlman in 1983 in search of a surgical technique that reduces scars [95], but the most important disadvantage of liposuction as an exclusive procedure is the lack of histologic verification. Resection of the glandular tissue using a peri- or transareolar approach with or without liposuction has been successfully employed [95, 97]. In patients with significant associated adipose component, traditional liposuction can optimize the result to improve the contour of the chest region. In grade III gynecomastia, surgical evaluation must additionally include resection of excess skin, utilizing techniques equivalent to reduction mammoplasty (inverted T approach). Other therapeutic alternatives in treatment evaluation include ultrasonic liposuction, transaxillary endoscopic adenectomy, and shaver [98]. In patients with a prominent fatty component, liposuction complements the treatment for improving the contour of the chest region. Although excisional techniques have good results, they are not exempt from complications. Courtiss analyzed the complications of 101 patients who underwent 192 breast surgeries with excisional techniques; in all cases, the author reported a high rate of complications including overcorrection (18.7%), unattractive scar (18.7%), hematoma (16.1%), seroma (9.4%), and undercorrection (21.9%) [99]. Cosmetic surgery is required for patients with marked gynecomastia or for those who develop excessive sagging of the breast tissue, and many different techniques and approaches are in current use and are likely to be influenced by the degree of breast enlargement, as well as by the proportion of glandular and fibrous vs. adipose tissue present [100]. More recent studies advocate the use of liposuction alone, emphasizing its superior esthetic results and decreased complication rates, but an approach using minimal incision with endoscopy or a pull-through technique were presented for a better esthetic result [101–103].

In one study, a semicircular-periareolar inferior incision proved to be a practical approach in mild-to-moderate gynecomastia [104]. Since the description of the pull-through technique in 1996 by Morselli, minimally invasive treatment for gynecomastia has undergone several modifications. The use of liposuction is especially attractive in cases of gynecomastia with fatty dominance, although those with moderate glandular component represent no great difficulty with the use of a Toledo V-dissector cannula, according to the technique described by Lista and Hammand in 2008 [105]. Another option is ultrasonic liposuction, which employs cannulas that vibrate at 20,000 cycles per second, transforming mechanical energy into heat. Proponents of the technique claim that it is possible to adequately remove the glandular tissue further promoting good skin retraction, even allowing the treatment of some patients with grade III gynecomastia [106]. Disadvantages of ultrasonic liposuction comprise expensive equipment, skin burns, and unsuitable tissue for histopathological examination (Figure 6).

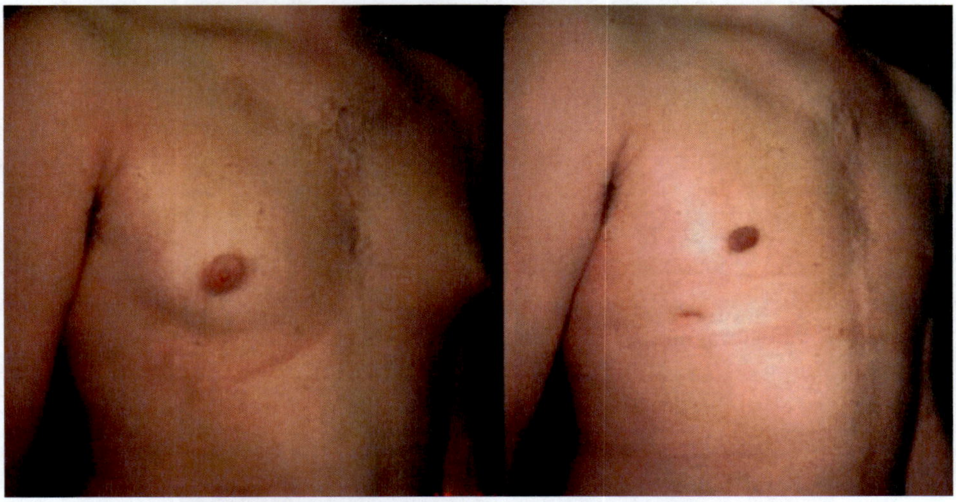

Figure 6. Treatment of gynecomastia with ultrasonic liposuction (courtesy of Fernando Magallanes M.D./The American British Cowdray Medical Center).

The shaver system is an orthopedic device utilized to wear down articular surfaces; it consists of a powered motor that provides rotary motion to a cannula, and a vacuum system that enables collection of the tissue. The shaver system has enabled the effective, controlled, and gradual resection of fibrous glands that, moreover, affords harvesting into small fragments for histopathological examination. It has also led to good postoperative skin retraction, enabling the treatment of patients with grade IIB gynecomastia with no additional skin removal. One disadvantage is the high cost of the equipment. Finally, the main advantage of the endoscopic axillary adenectomy is leaving no visible scars on the anterior chest area. However, it is a time-consuming technique that requires special equipment and videoendoscopic instruments to create an optical cavity in which to work and it can be more difficult to obtain a symmetrical result [107].

In general, in the overall complications rate, which ranges from 15.5–41%, overweight is considered a risk factor for complications. The potential complications of surgical therapy include tissue sloughing, contour irregularity, hematoma or seroma formation, and numbness of the nipple-areolar area.

It is very important for the surgical procedure to be performed by an experienced surgeon, to decrease complication rates and to achieve the best cosmetic result [108]. In another recent study with 733 patients, 402 patients were treated with subcutaneous (s.c.)

mastectomy and 331 patients were operated on using liposuction techniques. In the mastectomy group, periareolar incision was more prevalent (49%), less so inverted T incision (6%), but increased on using inframammary fold incision (10%). But this never exceeded the percentage of complete concentric periareolar incision: 53 (12%) patients using Mammotome (a vacuum-assisted biopsy device) excision. The liposuction group included 145 (38%) patients with liposuction alone and 241 (62%) with US-assisted liposuction.

The patients' overall dissatisfaction in each group was 14% of patients with mastectomy and 12% with liposuction techniques with their related complications including hematomas, seromas, nipple-areola complex necrosis, persisting pain, recurrence, and an ugly scar. There was no difference in the overall incidence of complications between the two groups, but the liposuction group was associated with few complications from an esthetic point of view and there were no nipple/areola necrosis and scars. Reoperation rates in the mastectomy group were 1.4 and 0.5% in the liposuction group. Finally, another important finding was age disparity; the patients who customarily underwent mastectomy were within the 40–60 years-of-age group, whereas liposuction was most commonly performed in patients aged 20–40 years, and patients with a firm or fibrous breast disk continued to require open surgery [109]. Treatment of gynecomastia necessitates an individualized operational approach, mainly depending on symptoms (lump or enlargement) and specific indications to improve the satisfaction rate and reduce complications. Newer, less invasive techniques that require minimal surgical incision have recently emerged and may offer faster recovery and lower rates of local complications [110]. Histologic analysis is recommended in true gynecomastia corrections because unexpected histologic findings, such as papilloma, may occur in 3% of cases [111].

Oncoplastic Techniques in the Management of Gynecomastia

Horizontal Mammoplasty

Horizontal breast mammoplasty produces a reduction in breast volume in the horizontal axis; thus, it is best indicated in those with horizontal dermoglandular axis distribution and conical projection with minimal ptosis. The main limitation of this technique is the presence of marked ptosis, especially when the nipple-areola complex is situated below the submammary groove, because in these cases, vertical mammoplasty will constitute the best alternative [112, 113].

Vertical Mammoplasty

The vertical mammoplasty pattern is the best alternative for a large ptotic component gynecomastia, with a nipple-areola complex located below the submammary groove with resection volumes exceeding 150 g. The main objective of this pattern is cephalic mobilization of the nipple-areola complex and significant excision of breast tissue in and skin on each breast. Like their female counterparts, male patients with low-volume gynecomastia and minimal ptosis are not candidates for this technique [105].

Circular Mammoplasty

The main indication for circular mammoplasty in the male is tuberous breast (congenital disorder of collagen deposition during pubertal breast development) associated or not with gynecomastia.

In these cases, circular mammoplasty is the procedure-of-choice to reduce the tubular projection of the nipple-areola complex and at the same time, the approach allows for removal of glandular tissue when it is associated with gynecomastia. Another indication of this pattern is through conical projection gynecomastia with a volume <150 g. Counterindications of this approach include patients with breast volume >200 g or with a large ptotic component, because this procedure cannot allow significant excision of the glandular tissue and fails to remedy the existing ptosis. Sometimes this can be a slight central defect that corrects after 4–6 months in nearly 100% of cases. In cases in which deformities persist after surgical treatment, lipofilling (autologous fat tissue installation) can be a promising technique [107, 114].

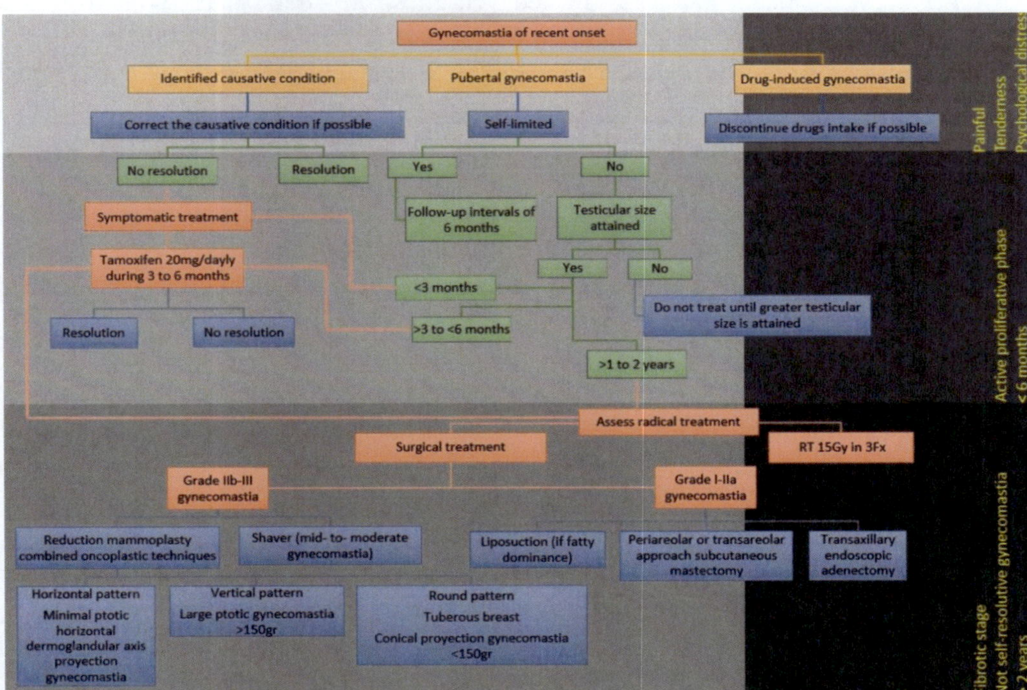

Figure 7. Treatment of gynecomastia.

In conclusion, and initially for the majority of men with gynecomastia, observation is the best approach, and reevaluation in men with drug-induced gynecomastia or with an underlying treatable disorder such as hypogonadism or hyperthyroidism. If the gynecomastia persists for more than 3 but less than 6 months, administration of Tamoxifen is justified.

Finally, if gynecomastia persists for more than 1 or 2 years, surgery is the best option because the breast tissue has probably become fibrotic and unresponsive to drug therapy (Figure 7).

References

[1] Narula HS, Carlson HE. Gynecomastia. *Endocrinol. Metab. Clin. North Am.* 2007;36(2):497-519.

[2] Devalia HL, Layer GT. Current concepts in gynaecomastia. *Surgeon* 2009 Apr;7(2):114-119.

[3] Georgiadis E, Papandreu L, Evangelopoulou C, et al. Incidence of gynaecomastia in 954 young males and its relationship to somatometric parameters. *Ann. Hum. Biol.* 1994;21:579-587.

[4] Nuttall FQ. Gynecomastia as a physical finding in normal men. *J. Clin. Endocrinol. Metab.* 1979;48:338-340.

[5] Nydick M, Bustos J, Dale JH, et al. Gynecomastia in adolescent boys. *JAMA* 1961;178:449-454.

[6] Bannayan GA, Hajdu SI. Gynecomastia: clinicopathologic study of 351 cases. *Am. J. Clin. Pathol.* 1972;57:431-437.

[7] Pirke KM, Doerr P. Age related changes in free plasma testosterone, dihydrotestosterone and oestradiol. *Acta Endocrinol.* 1975;80(1):171-178.

[8] Niewoehner CB, Nuttall FQ. Gynecomastia in a hospitalized male population. *Am. J. Med.* 1984;77:633-638.

[9] Williams MJ. Gynecomastia: its incidence, recognition and host characterization in 447 autopsy cases. *Am. J. Med.* 1963;34:103-112.

[10] Cleland WH, Mendelson CE, Simpson ER. Effects of aging and obesity on aromatase activity of human adipose cells. *J. Clin. Endocrinol. Metab.* 1985;60:174-177.

[11] Ruth EJ, Hassan MM. Gynecomastia: pathophysiology, evaluation and management. *Mayo. Clin. Proc.* 2009;84(11):1010-1015.

[12] Braunstein GD. Gynaecomastia. NEJM 1993;328(7):490-495.

[13] Glass AR. Gynecomastia. *Endocrinol. Metab. Clin. North Am.* 1994;23:825-837.

[14] Simon BE, Hoffman S, Kahn S. Classification and surgical correction of gynaecomastia. (Abstract). *Plast. Reconstr. Aesthet Surg.* 1973;51:48.

[15] Rahmani S, Turton P, Shaaban A, et al. Overview of gynecomastia in the modern era and the Leeds gynaecomastia investigation algorithm. *Breast J.* 2011;17(3):246-255.

[16] Nicolis GL, Modlinger RS, Gabrilove JL. A study of the histopathology of human gynecomastia. *J. Clin. Endocrinol. Metab.* 1971;32:173-178.

[17] Andersen JA, Gram JB. Gynecomasty: histological aspects in a surgical material. *Acta. Pathol. Microbiol. Scand.* (A) 1982;90:185-190.

[18] Harman SM, Metter EJ, Tobin JD, et al. Longitudinal effects of aging on serum total and free testosterone levels in healthy men. *J. Clin. Endocrinol. Metab.* 2001;86:724-731.

[19] Coen P, Kulin H, Ballantine T, et al. An aromatase-producing sex-cord tumour resulting in prepubertal gynaecomastia. *NEJM* 1991;324(5):317-322.

[20] Daniels IR, Layer GT. Testicular tumours presenting as gynecomastia. *Eur. J. Surg.* Oncol 2003;29:437-439.

[21] Walsh PC. The endocrinology of testicular tumors. *Recent Results Cancer Res.* 1997;60:196-201.

[22] Bercovici JP, Nahoul K, Tater D, et al. Hormonal profile of Leydig cell tumors with gynecomastia. *J. Clin. Endocrinol. Metab.* 1984;59:625-630.

[23] Bercovici JP, Tater D, Khoury S, et al. Leydig cell tumor with gynecomastia: hormonal effects of an estrogen-producing tumor. J. Clin. Endocrinol. Metab. 1981;53:1291.

[24] Braunstein GD. Aromatase and gynecomastia. (Abstract). *Endocr. Relat. Cancer* 1999;6:315.

[25] Kratzer SS, Ulbright TM, Talerman A, et al. Large cell calcifying Sertoli cell tumor of the testis, contrasting features of six malignant and six benign tumors and a review of the literature. *Am. J. Surg. Pathol.* 1997;21:1271-1280.

[26] Young S, Gooneratne S, Straus FH, et al. Feminizing Sertoli cell tumors in boys with Peutz-Jeghers syndrome. *Am. J. Surg. Pathol.* 1995;19:50-58.

[27] Amos CI, Keitheri-Cheteri MB, Sabripour M, et al. Genotype-phenotype correlations in Peutz-Jeghers syndrome. *J. Med. Genet.* 2004;41:327-233.

[28] Eladio LG, Daniel KM, Margarita GB. Carney complex. *Endocrinol. Nutr.* 2011;56(6):308-314.

[29] Aboutorabi R, Feiz zadeh B, Rajabian R. Gynecomastia secondary to choriocarcinoma in a man with persistent Mullerian duct. *Int. J. Endocrinol. Metab.* 2005;3:140-142.

[30] Wasniewska M, Raiola G, Galati MC, Salzano G, Rulli I, Zirilli G, et al. Non-classical 21-hydroxylase deficiency in boys with prepubertal or pubertal gynecomastia. *Eur. J. Pediatr.* 2008;167(9):1083-1084.

[31] Zayed A, Stock JL, Liepman MK, et al. Feminization as a result of both peripheral conversion of androgens and direct estrogen production from an adrenocortical carcinoma. *J. Endocrinol. Invest.* 1994;17:275-278.

[32] Phan AT. Adrenal cortical carcinoma- review of current knowledge and treatment practice. *Hematol. Oncol. Clin. North Am.* 2007;21:489-507.

[33] Shen WT, Sturgeon C, Duh QY. From incidentaloma to adrenocortical carcinoma: the surgical management of adrenal tumors. *J. Surg. Oncol.* 2005;89:186-192.

[34] Allolio B, Fassnacht M. Clinical review: Adrenocortical carcinoma- Clinical update. *J Clin. Endocrinol. Metab.* 2006;91:2027-2037.

[35] Michael T, Nina J, Curtiss B. Feminizing adrenal neoplasms: case presentations and review of the literature. *J. Clin. Oncol.* 2011;29(6):127-130.

[36] McLeod DG, Iversen P. Gynecomastia in patients with prostate cancer: a review of treatment options. *Urology* 2000;56:713-720.

[37] Dicker AP. The safety and tolerability of low dose irradiation for the management of gynecomastia caused by antiandrogen monotherapy. *Lancet Oncol.* 2003;4:30-36.

[38] Van Poppel H, Tyrrell CJ, Haustermans K, et al. Efficacy and tolerability of radiotherapy as treatment for bicalutamide-induced gynaecomastia and breast pain in prostate cancer. *Eur. Urol. J.* 2005;47:587-592.

[39] Perdona S, Autorino R, De Placido S, et al. Efficacy of tamoxifen and radiotherapy for prevention and treatment of gynaecomastia and breast pain caused by bicalutamide in prostate cancer: a randomised controlled trial. *Lancet Oncol.* 2005;6(5):295-300.

[40] Di Lorenzo G, Autorino R, Perdona S, et al. Management of gynecomastia in patients with prostate cancer: a systematic review of treatment options. *Lancet Oncol.* 2005;6:972-979.

[41] Fradet Y, Egerdie B, Anderson M, et al. Tamoxifen as prophylaxis for prevention of gynecomastia and breast pain associated with bicalutamide 150 mg monotherapy in patients with prostate cancer: a randomized, placebo-controlled, dose-response study. *Eur. Urol. J.* 2007;52(1):106-115.

[42] Smyth CM, Bremner WJ. Klinefelter syndrome. *Arch. Intern. Med.* 1998,158:1309-1314.

[43] Wang C, Baker HWG, Burger HG, et al. Hormonal studies in Klinefelter's syndrome. *Clin. Endocrinol.* 1975;4:399-411.

[44] Lynch HT, Kaplan AR, Lynch JF. Klinefelter syndrome and cancer. A family study. *JAMA* 1974;229:809-811.

[45] Swerdlow AJ. Cancer incidence and mortality in men with Klinefelter syndrome: a cohort study. *J. Natl. Cancer Inst.* 2005;97(16):1204-1210.

[46] Fentiman IS, Fourquet A, Hortobagyi GN. Male breast cancer. *Lancet* 2006;367:595-604.

[47] Braunstein GD. Gynecomastia. *NEJM* 2007;357:1229-1237.

[48] Rose LI, Underwood RH, Newmark SR, et al. Pathophysiology of spironolactone-induced gynecomastia. (Abstract). *Ann. Intern. Med.* 1977;87:398.

[49] Dobs AS, Meikle AW, Arver S, et al. Pharmacokinetics, efficacy, and safety of a permeation-enhanced testosterone transdermal system in comparison with bi-weekly injections of testosterone enanthate for the treatment of hypogonadal men. (Abstract). *J. Clin. Endocrinol. Metab.* 1999;84:3469.

[50] The Copenhagen Study Group for Liver Diseases. Testosterone treatment of men with alcoholic cirrhosis: a double-blind study. *Hepatology* 1986;6:807.

[51] Jover F, Cuadrado JM, Roig P, et al. Efavirenz-associated gynecomastia: report of five cases and review of the literature. *Breast J.* 2004;10:244.

[52] Bidlingmaier F, Knorr D. Plasma testosterone and estrogens in pubertal gynaecomastia. Z Kinderheilkd 1973;115(1):89-94.

[53] Einav-Bachar, Philip M, Aurbach-Klipper Y, Lazar L. Prepubertal gynecomastia: aetiology, course and outcome. *Clin. Endocrinol.* 2004;61:55-60.

[54] Moore DC, Schlaepfer LV, Paunier L, et al. Hormonal changes during puberty: V. Transient pubertal gynecomastia: abnormal androgen-estrogen ratios. *J. Clin. Endocrinol. Metab.* 1984;58:492-499.

[55] Ruth EJ, Hassan MM. Gynaecomastia: pathophysiology, evaluation and management. *Mayo. Clin. Proc.* 2009;84(11):1010-1015.

[56] Dundar B, Dundar N, Erci T, et al. Leptin levels in boys with pubertal gynecomastia. *J. Pediatr. Endocrinol. Metab.* 2005;18:929-934.

[57] Lawrence SE, Faught KA, Vethamuthu J, et al. Beneficial effects of raloxifene and tamoxifen in the treatment of pubertal gynecomastia. *J. Pediatr.* 2004;145:71-76.

[58] Swerdloff RS, Wang C. Androgen deficiency and aging in men. *West J. Med.* 1993;159:579.

[59] Mahoney CP. Adolescent gynecomastia. Differential diagnosis and management. *Pediatr. Clin. North Am.* 1990;37:1398-1404.

[60] Schmitt GW, Shehadeh I, Sawin CT. Transient gynecomastia in chronic renal failure during chronic intermittent hemodialysis. *Ann. Intern. Med.* 1968;69:73-79.

[61] Cavanaugh J, Niewoehner CB, Nuttall FQ. Gynecomastia and cirrhosis of the liver. *Arch. Intern. Med.* 1990;150(3):563-565.

[62] Farthing MJG, Green JRB, Edwards CRW, et al. Progesterone, prolactin, and gynecomastia in men with liver disease. *Gut.* 1982;23:276-279.

[63] Gordon GG, Olivo J, Rafil F, et al. Conversion of androgens to estrogens in cirrhosis of the liver. *J. Clin. Endocrinol. Metab.* 1975;40:1018-1026.

[64] Van Thiel DH. Ethanol: its adverse effects upon the hypothalamic-pituitary-gonadal axis. *J. Lab. Clin. Med.* 1983;101:21-33.

[65] Olivo J, Gordon GG, Rafii F, Southren AL. Estrogen metabolism in hyperthyroidism and in cirrhosis of the liver. *Steroids* 1975;26:47.

[66] Ford HC, Cooke RR, Keightley EA, et al. Serum levels of free and bound testosterone in hyperthyroidism. *Clin. Endocrinol.* 1992;36:187-192.

[67] Harmeet SN, Harold EC. Gynecomastia. *Endocrinol. Metab. Clin. North Am.* 2007;36:497-519.

[68] Nomura K, Suzuki H, Saji M, et al. High serum progesterone in hyperthyroid men with Graves' disease. *J. Clin. Endocrinol. Metab.* 1988;66(1):230-232.

[69] Melo KF, Mendonca BB, Cillerbeck AC, et al. Clinical hormonal, behavioral, and genetic characteristics of androgen insensibility syndrome in a Brazilian cohort; five novel mutations in the androgen receptor gene. *J. Clin. Endocrinol. Metab.* 2003;88:3241-3250.

[70] Dejager S, Bry-Gauillard H, Brickert E, et al. A comprehensive endocrine description of Kennedy's disease revealing androgen insensitivity linked to CAG repeat length. *J. Clin. Endocrinol. Metab.* 2002;87:3893-3901.

[71] Mahoney CP. Adolescent gynecomastia. Differential diagnosis and management. *Pediatr. Clin. North Am.* 1990;37:1398-1404.

[72] Cohen IK, Pozez AL, McKeown JE. Gynecomastia. In: Courtis EH (Editor). Male Aesthetic Surgery. St. Louis, MO, USA: Mosby; 1991.

[73] Rohrich RJ, Ha RY, Kenkel JM et al. Classification and management of gynecomastia: defining the role of ultrasound-assisted liposuction. *Plast. Reconstr. Aesthet. Surg.* 2003;111:909-923.

[74] Aboutorabi R, Feiz zadeh B, Rajabian R. Gynecomastia secondary to choriocarcinoma in a man with persistent Mullerian duct. *Int. J. Endocrinol. Metab.* 2005;3:140-142.

[75] Hines SL, Tan WW, Yasrebi M, et al. The role of mammography in male patients with breast symptoms. *Mayo. Clin. Proc.* 2007;82(3):297-300.

[76] Cheri N, Mark DK, Michael E, et al. Male breast disease: pictorial review with radiologic-pathologic correlation. R*adioGraphic*s 2013;33:763-779.

[77] Lattin GE Jr, Robert A, et al. Diseases of the male breast: radiologic-pathologic correlation. *RadioGraphics* 2013;33:461-489.

[78] Johnson R, Hassan M. Gynecomastia: pathophysiology, evaluation, and management. *Mayo. Clin. Proc.* 2009;84(11):1010-1015.

[79] Gruntmanis U, Braunstein GD. Treatment of gynecomastia. *Curr. Opin. Investig. Drugs* 2001;2(5):643.

[80] Eckman A, Dobs A. Drug-induced gynecomastia. Expert Opin Drug Saf 2008;7(6):691.

[81] Devoto CE, Madariaga AM, Lioi CX, et al. Influence of size and duration of gynecomastia on its response to treatment with tamoxifen. *Rev. Med. Chil.* 2007;135(12):1558-1565.

[82] Lawrence SE, Faught KA, Vethamuthu J, Lawson ML. Beneficial effects of raloxifene and tamoxifen in the treatment of pubertal gynecomastia. *J. Pediatr.* 2004; 145(1):71-76.

[83] Derman O, Kanbur NO, Kutluk T. Tamoxifen treatment for pubertal gynecomastia. Int *J. Adolesc. Med. Health.* 2003;13(4):339-363.

[84] Parker LN, Gray DR, Lai MK, Levin ER. Treatment of gynecomastia with tamoxifen: a double-blind crossover study. *Metabolism* 1986;35(8):705.

[85] Derman O, Kanbur N, Kilic I, et al. Long term follow-up of tamoxifen treatment in adolescents with gynecomastia. *J. Pediatr. Endocrinol. Metab* 2008;21:449-453.

[86] Plourde PV, Reiter EO, Jou HC, Desrochers PE, Rubin SD, Bercu BB, et al. Safety and efficacy of anastrozole for the treatment of pubertal gynecomastia: a randomized, double-blind, placebo-controlled trial. *J. Clin. Endocrinol. Metab.* 2004;89(9):4428.

[87] Dobs A, Darkes MJ. Incidence and management of gynecomastia in men treated for prostate cancer. *J. Urol.* 2005;174:1737-1742.

[88] Viani GA, Bernardes da Silva LG, Stefano EJ. Prevention of gynecomastia and breast pain caused by androgen deprivation therapy in prostate cancer: tamoxifen or radiotherapy? *Int. J. Radiat. Oncol. Biol. Phys.* 2012 Jul 15;83(4):e519-e524.

[89] Tyrrell CJ, Payne H, Tammela TL, Bakke A, Lodding P, Goedhals L, et al. Prophylactic breast irradiation with a single dose of electron beam radiotherapy (10 Gy) significantly reduces the incidence of bicalutamide-induced gynecomastia. *Int. J. Radiat. Oncol. Biol. Phys.* 2004 60:476-483.

[90] Boccardo F, Rubagotti A, Battaglia M, Di Tonno P, Selvaggi FP, Conti G, et al. Evaluation of tamoxifen and anastrozole in the prevention of gynecomastia and breast pain induced by bicalutamide monotherapy of prostate cancer. *J. Clin. Oncol.* 2005;23:808-815.

[91] Córdova A, Moschella F. Algorithm for clinical evaluation and surgical treatment of gynaecomastia. *Plast. Reconstr. Aesthet. Surg.* 2008;61:41-49.

[92] Calderón W, Arriagada J, Godoy M, et al. Vía transareolomamilar para el tratamiento de la ginecomastia. *Rev. Chil. Cir.* 1985;37:140-144.

[93] Carlson HE. Approach to the patient with gynecomastia. *J. Clin. Endocrinol. Metab.* 2011;96:15-21.

[94] Webster JP. Mastectomy for gynaecomastia through a semicircular intra-areolar incision. *Ann. Surg.* 1946;124:557-575.

[95] Teimourian B, Pearlman R. Surgery for gynecomastia. *Aesthet. Plast. Surg.* 1983;7:155-157.

[96] Handschin AE, Bietry D, Hüsler R, Banic A, Constantinescu M. Surgical management of gynecomastia- a 10-year analysis. *World J. Surg.* 2008;32:38-44.

[97] Harold E. Approach to the patient with gynecomastia. *J. Clin. Endocrinol. Metab.* 2011;96(1):15-21.

[98] Castillo DP. Ginecomastia. *Cuad. Cir.* 2003;17:52-57.

[99] Courtiss EH. Gynecomastia: analysis of 159 patients and current recommendations for treatment. *Plast. Reconstr. Aesthet. Surg.* 1987;79:740-753.

[100] Ridha H, Colville RJ, Vesely MJ. How happy are patients with their gynaecomastia reduction surgery? *Plast. Reconstr. Aesthet. Surg*. 2009;62:1473-1478.

[101] Hodgson EL, Fruhstorfer BH, Malata CM. Ultrasonic liposuction in the treatment of gynecomastia. *Plast. Reconstr. Aesthet. Surg*. 2005;116:646-653.

[102] Rohrich RJ, Ha RY, Kenkel JM, et al. Classification and management of gynecomastia: defining the role of ultrasound-assisted liposuction. *Plast. Reconstr. Aesthet. Surg*. 2003;111:909-923.

[103] Hammond DC, Arnold JF, Simon AM, et al. Combined use of ultrasonic liposuction with the pull through technique for the treatment of gynecomastia. *Plast. Reconstr. Aesthet. Surg*. 2003;112:891-895.

[104] Li CC, Fu JP, Chang SC, Chen TM, Chen SG. Surgical treatment of gynecomastia: complications and outcomes. *Ann. Plast. Aesthet. Surg*. 2012 Nov;69(5):510-515.

[105] Benigno AN. Cirugía oncológica de la mama. Técnicas oncoplásticas y reconstructivas. 3ª ed Barcelona, *España: Elsevier Masson*; 2013. pp. 207-215.

[106] Gingrass MK, Shermak MA. The treatment of gynecomastia with ultrasound-assisted lipoplasty. *Perspect. Plast. Surg*. 1999;12:101-106.

[107] Ohyama T, Takada A, Fujikawa M, et al. Endoscope-assisted transaxillary removal of glandular tissue in gynecomastia. *Ann. Plast. Surg*. 1998;40:62-64.

[108] Hammond DC. Surgical correction of gynecomastia. *Plast. Reconstr. Aesthet. Surg*. 2009;124(1 Suppl):61e-68e.

[109] Song YN, Wang YB, Huang R, He XG, Zhang JF, Zhang GQ, et al. Surgical treatment of gynecomastia: mastectomy compared to liposuction technique. *Ann. Plast. Surg*. 2013 May 2. [Epub ahead of print]

[110] Prado AC, Castillo PF. Minimal surgical access to treat gynecomastia with the use of a power-assisted arthroscopic-endoscopic cartilage shaver. *Plast. Reconstr. Aesthet. Surg*. 2005;115(3):939-942.

[111] Handschin AE, Bietry D, Hüsler R, et al. Surgical management of gynecomastia- a 10 year analysis. *World J. Surg*. 2008;32(1):38-44.

[112] Celebioglu S, Ertas NM, Ozdil K, et al. Gynecomastia treatment with subareolar glandular pedicle. *Aesthet. Plast. Surg*. 2004;28(5):281-286.

[113] Tashkandi M, Al-Qattan MM, Hassanain JM, et al. The surgical management of high grade gynecomastia. *Ann. Plast. Surg*. 2004 Jul;53(1):17-20.

[114] Persichetti P, Berloco M, Casadei RM, et al. Gynecomastia and the complete circumareolar approach in the surgical management of skin redundancy. *Plast. Reconst. Aesthet. Surg*. 2001;107(4):948-954.

In: Benign Disease of the Breast
Editors: J. de la Garza Salazar, C. Arce Salinas et al.
ISBN: 978-1-63321-624-2

Chapter 13

Imaging Studies for Benign Lesions of the Breast

Yolanda Villaseñor-Navarro*, Lesvia Olivia Aguilar-Cortazar, Cecilia Magdalena Pavon-Hernandez, Martha Patricia Perez-Badillo and Irma Perez-Zuñiga

Radiology Department, Instituto Nacional Cancerologia-Mexico, Mexico City, DF, Mexico

Abstract

Among diseases that affect the breast, those that are benign are the most frequent. The majority of lesions are clinically diagnosed or are found as the result of imaging studies in symptomatic women, with breast pain, palpable mass, and the nipple discharge comprising the most frequent symptomatology. These benign diseases of the breast include developmental abnormalities, inflammatory lesions, epithelial and stromal proliferations, and neoplasms.

With the use of imaging studies, such as mammography, ultrasound, magnetic resonance and, more recently molecular studies, it is possible to detect and evaluate breast lesions, recognizing that the gold standard in establishing the diagnosis is carried out by means of a biopsy of the lesions and their histological study.

Screening mammography has demonstrated its usefulness in the reduction of mortality. Most recently this application is the object of debate due to its limited sensitivity in dense breast, as well as to its specificity. The latter increases the number of false positives that give rise to over diagnosis and even overtreatment of women, which then exerts a psychological, social, and economic impact on the population.

With the introduction of digital imaging, more advanced methods have become possible, especially tomosynthesis in digital mammography. Tomosynthesis removes overlaying tissues, which improves detection of a subtle lesion, distortion of the architecture, characterization of masses and of the asymmetry of the density, and precise measurements of the lesion by means of a better delineation of the lesion's borders.

* Corresponding author: Yolanda Villaseñor-Navarro. Radiology Department, Instituto Nacional Cancerologia-Mexico, Mexico City, DF. Mexico.

Among the benefits of tomosynthesis, we find improvement in the sensitivity of detection of breast cancer, in the evaluation of the lesion's dimensions and characterization, as well as in diminution in recall. As for the evaluation of response to treatment, mammography plus tomosynthesis exhibit a precision similar to that of magnetic resonance and superior to that of digital mammography alone and ultrasound.

Breast ultrasound demonstrates different applications: it is especially utilized for differentiating between cystic lesions and solid nodules with high specificity. In combination with mammography, ultrasound contributes to differentiation between solid benign and malignant lesions. Breast ultrasound can be performed in B mode, compound images, images with harmony for better visualization of breast lesions, and the reduction of imaging artifacts. Application of Doppler and contrast agents for measuring tumor blood flow and elastography, given the hardness of a tumor, aid in differentiating between benignancy and malignancy, and also assist as a method-of-choice for guiding breast biopsies and other interventional procedures. Taken together, with the application of BI-RADS for characterization of nodules observed by ultrasound, these techniques have improved diagnosis of the breast ultrasound.

It is important to note that the role of magnetic resonance of the breast has been established as a complement of conventional, diagnostic techniques such as mammography and ultrasound. Magnetic resonance of the breast permits the detection and characterization of benign lesions, primary breast cancers, recurrence, and allows evaluation of response to therapy.

To date, the fundamental objective of imaging studies has been the detection of nonpalpable lesions, which has been complied with for during several decades thanks to mammography. However, today one must search of ever smaller lesions, utilizing one or various imaging methods that additionally permit the characterization of these lesions with adequate specificity in the diagnosis of cancer.

Mammography continues to be the imaging method-of-choice for screening in the breast with sensitivity for detection of breast cancer of 70.8% in patients aged 40–44 years and of 84.5% in patients 75–89 years of age. One limitation of mammography is that it is a biplanar study, even when its target organ is three-dimensional or volumetric, which results in tissue over position. Another limitation is dense breasts, which has given rise to the advent of novel imaging techniques or tools [43], as is the case of digital mammography, tomosynthesis, computed tomography, different ultrasound techniques, nuclear medicine studies (SPECT, PET, PET/CT, PEM) and magnetic resonance, studies that allow to simultaneously obtain different types of information. The former provides anatomical information, while nuclear medicine studies contribute functional information and where magnetic resonance delivers a combination of both.

Once a breast lesion is detected by clinical evaluation and/or by imaging studies, it is not always possible to determine with certainty its benign nature as there can also be a suspicion of breast cancer. This makes it necessary to conduct a cytological or histological biopsy.

Introduction

Among the diseases that affect the breast, the benign diseases are the most frequent. These include a set of conditions that while not mortal, can in some cases increase the risk for breast cancer. The majority of the lesions are diagnosed clinically or are the result of imaging studies in asymptomatic women who have breast pain, palpable mass, and nipple discharge as the most frequent symptomatology [1].

Among benign breast diseases we can include developmental abnormalities, inflammatory lesions, epithelial and stromal proliferations, and neoplasms. These occur with greatest frequency in the second decade of life, with a peak between the fourth and fifth decades. It is of utmost importance to recognize the characteristics of a benign disease and to establish its diagnosis, thus imaging studies show particular indications and contribute to the characterization of breast lesions.

With the use of imaging studies, such as Mammography, Ultrasound (USG), Magnetic resonance (MR) and, more recently, molecular studies, it is possible to detect and evaluate breast lesions. Accurate diagnosis is achieved by means of a biopsy of the lesions. At present this can be carried out via a percutaneous biopsy with a needle, avoiding diagnostic surgical procedures that are reserved for when the diagnosis is one of a lesion of risk or, in the case of the diagnosis of a malignant lesion, for its treatment.

Imaging studies in general demonstrate two basic indications: detection in asymptomatic women and diagnosis in symptomatic women (pain, palpable mass, nipple secretion, etc.), where the presence of a mass, calcifications, or distortions is found. It is noteworthy that there are other indications for imaging studies applied to the evaluation of the breast which are as follows: assessment of local and distal disease extension; status of contralateral breast; appraisal of response to treatment; providing women who received treatment with follow-up; evaluating the presence of residual disease; finalizing treatment; and evaluating recurrences.

Each of these lesions should be categorized according to the BI-RADS system (Breast Imaging- and Reporting Data System) [2], in which BI-RADS 1, 2, and 3 are considered negative and BI-RADS 2 is applied for benign findings.

From its creation to the present, BI-RADS has included different imaging modalities for the evaluation of breast findings by mammography, USG and, more recently, Magnetic resonance (MR) (Figures 1-8).

Figures 8a-f Mammographic image of the different types of benign calcifications.

Mammography

Different controlled randomized assays have demonstrated that reduction of breast cancer-associated mortality can be carried out with screening mammographies [3-8] (Figures 9a-f). Figures 9a-f Woman aged 58 years, first screening mammography.

Mammography shows limited sensitivity and specificity (83.5%, range, 71-96%, and 90.9%, respectively) in direct relation to breast density [9-12].

False negatives occur mainly in dense breast because the lesions are obscured principally due to tissue superimposition. With digital mammography, accurate diagnosis increased in some groups of women with dense breast [13]. With the introduction of digital imaging, advanced imaging methods have been made possible, especially tomosynthesis.

Tomosynthesis avoid tissue super positioning, thus improving the detection of subtle lesions, architectural distortion, characterization of masses and of the asymmetry of the density, and accurate measurement of the lesion by means of better delineation of the lesion's borders [14] (Figures 10a-c).

Digital mammography with tomosynthesis presents the same basic components of a digital mammography.

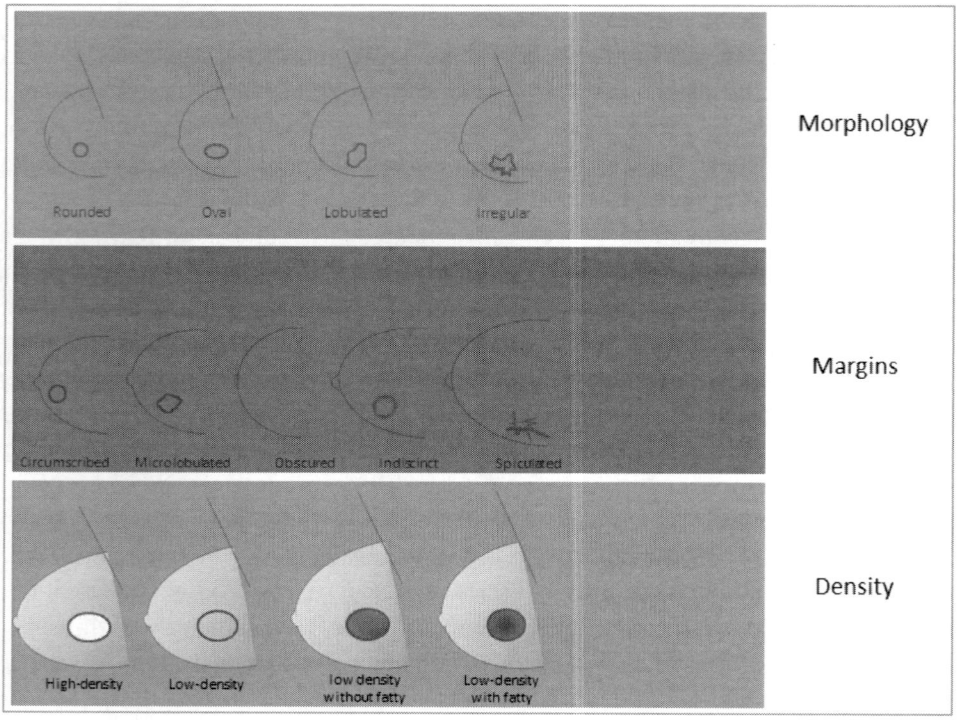

Figure 1. Characterization of nodular images by mammography. The nodules observed on mammography should be evaluated according to their morphology, margins, and density.

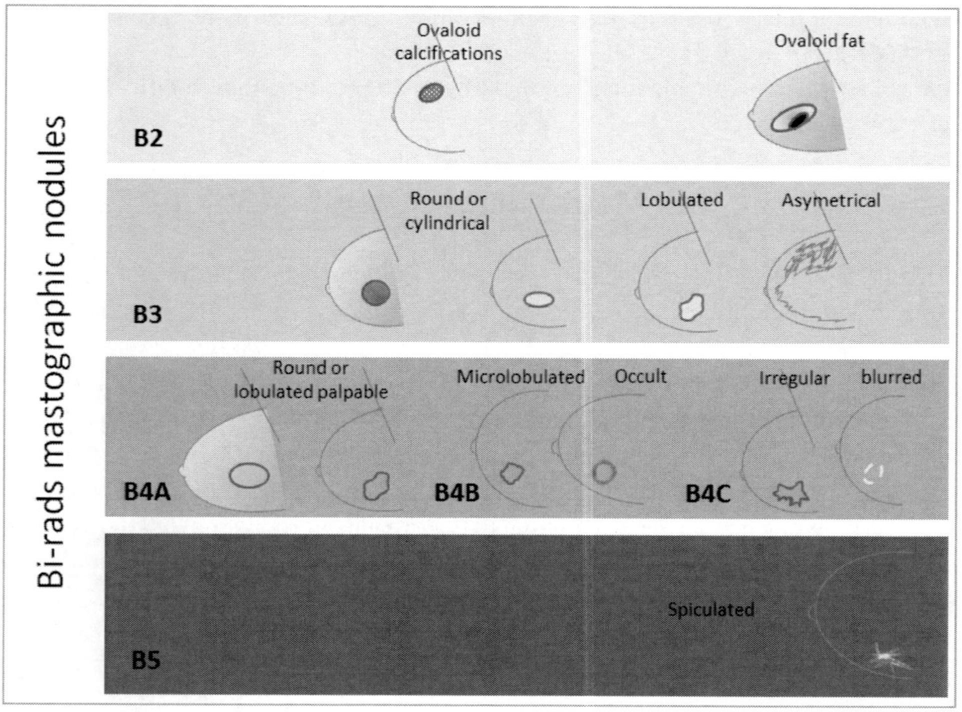

Figure 2. Characterization of the nodules observed on mammography in the BI-RADS system, with BI-RADS 2 conclusive of benign nodule.

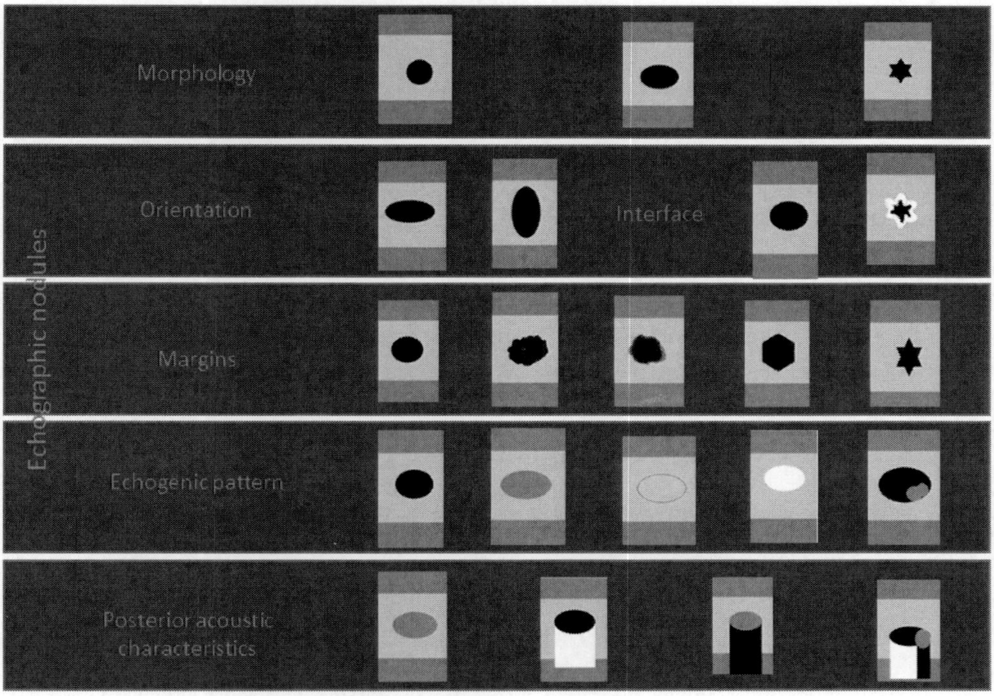

Figure 3. Echographic findings. The nodules should be described in relation to their morphology, orientation, margins, echographic pattern, and posterior acoustic characteristics.

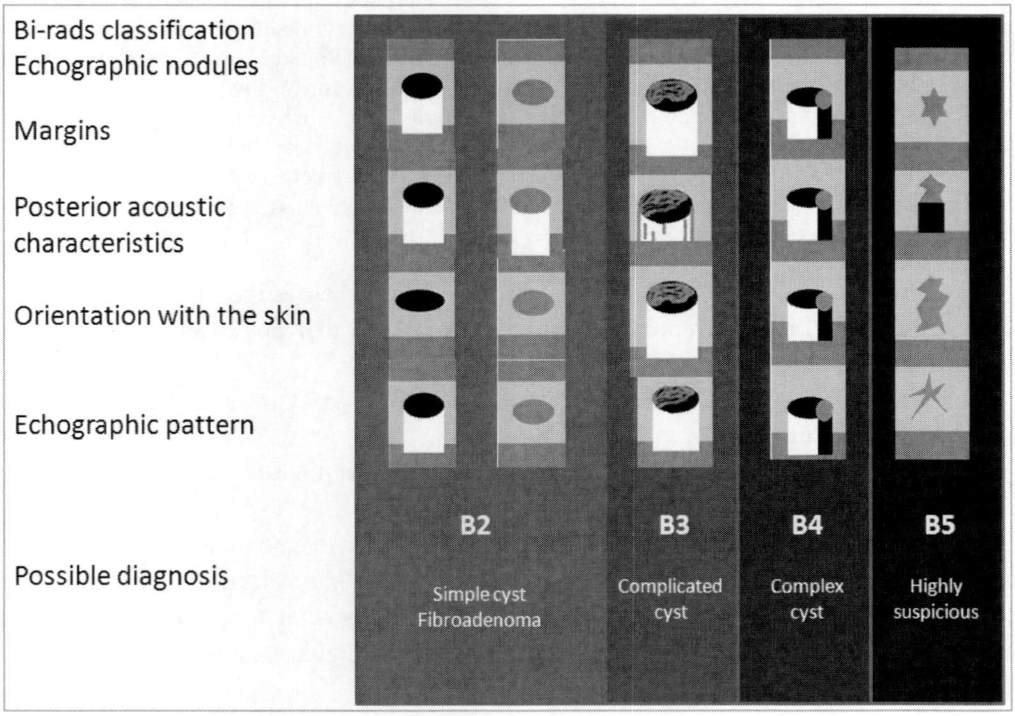

Figure 4. BI-RADS classification of nodules on sonography.

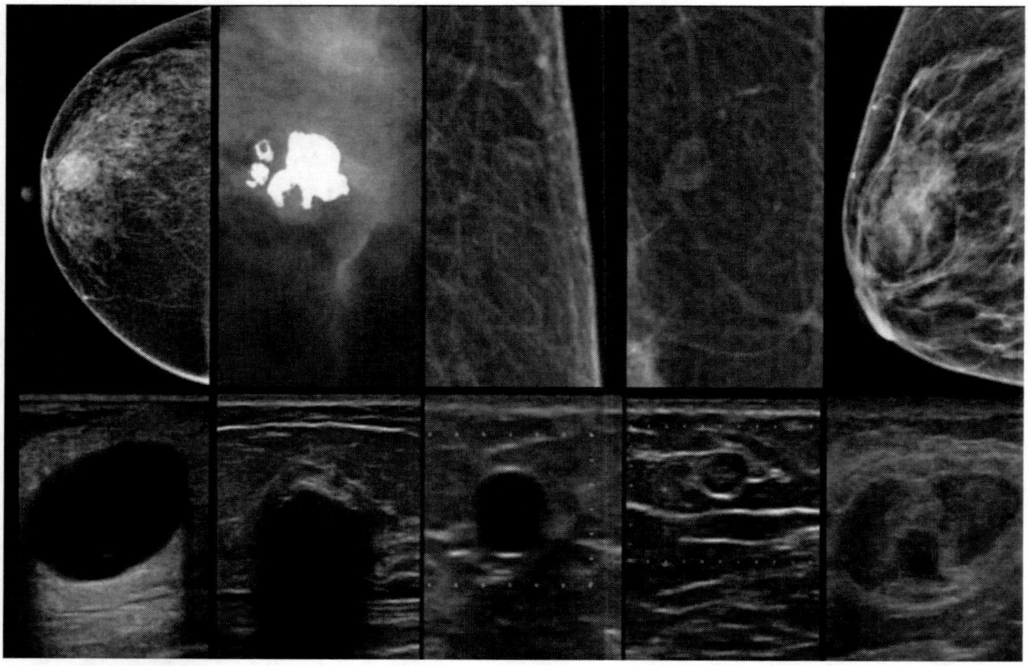

Figure 5. (a-e) Mammographic images of the most frequent benign breast lesions (upper) in correlation with Sonographic images (lower). (a) Simple cyst. Mammography shows at retroareolar level a nodule of medium density, defined with regular contours without calcifications in its interior (upper). USG shows defined anechoic nodule with regular borders with posterior acoustic reinforcement (lower). (b) Fibroadenoma. Mammography. Nodule with irregular and amorphous thick calcification, characteristic of calcified fibroadenoma (upper). On USG: appreciation of calcification with posterior acoustic attenuation (lower). (c) Oil cyst. Defined thin-walled round nodule with radiolucent center (upper). On USG: anechoic nodule without attenuation or posterior sonic reinforcement (lower). (d) Intramammary lymph node. Ovoid nodule with middle density and fatty hilum (upper). USG shows hypoechoic nodule with echogenic center and hypoechoic cortical. (e) Hamartoma. Ovoid mass, in lateral mammographic projection is localized in anterior third and middle of upper quadrant where its density is heterogeneous with radiolucent and dense areas (upper). On USG: thick-walled ovoid mass, well defined with heterogeneous echoes in its interior (lower).

The difference lies in the addition of hardware in which there is the capacity of the x-ray tubes to turn around a nearby point or in the detector and that possesses a detector with relatively rapid reading.

Tomosynthesis significantly improved the diagnostic accuracy of noncalcified lesions in comparison with additional mammographic projections [15].

Digital mammography appears to have greater sensitivity than digital tomosynthesis of the breast for the detection of calcifications [16] (Figures 11a-b).

Summarizing, the benefits of tomosynthesis include improvements in the sensitivity of the detection of breast cancer, in the evaluation of the lesion's dimensions, and in the recall. As for the evaluation of treatment response, mammography with tomosynthesis exhibited accuracy similar to that of MR and one superior to that of digital mammography alone and USG [17].

One of the points for consideration in performing tomosynthesis is that, on utilizing ionizing radiation, one should take into account that the final dose on concluding digital mammography plus tomosynthesis will increase.

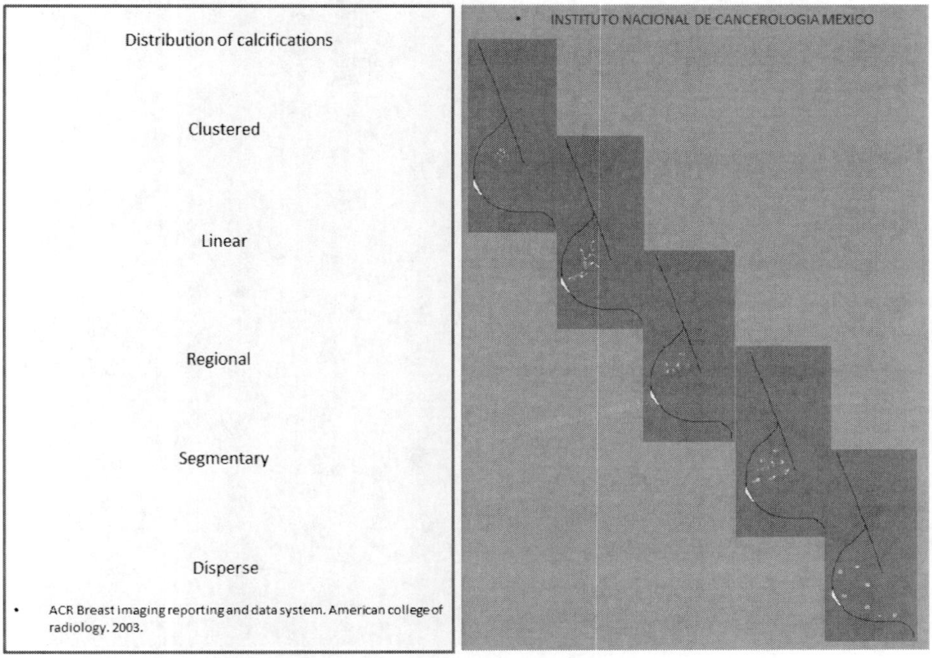

Figure 6. Calcifications. In the analysis of calcifications by mammography, their morphology, number, and distribution should be included.

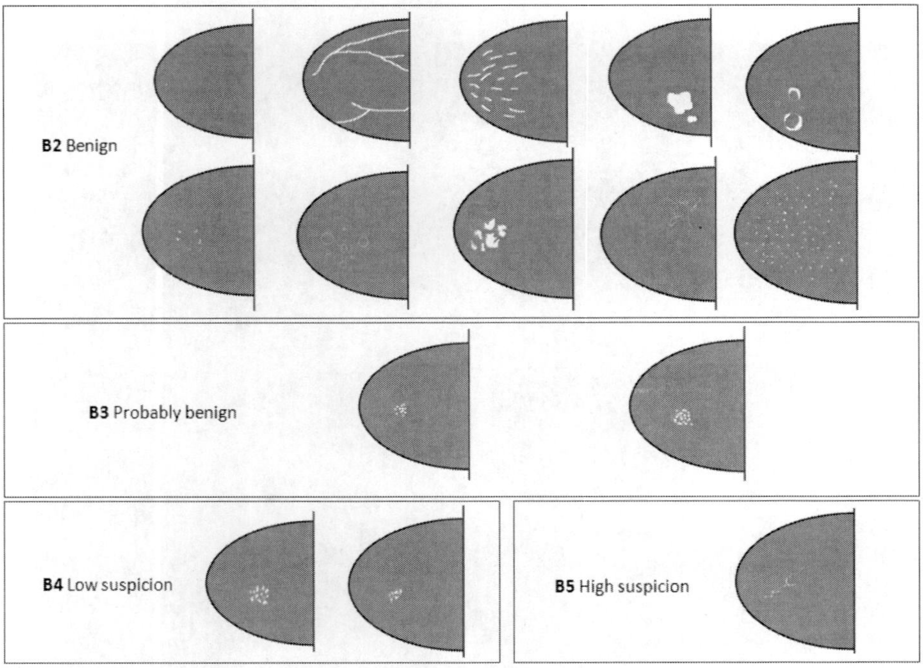

Figure 7. Evaluation of microcalcifications and their categorization. Benign calcifications are generally thick amorphous, in eggshell, or in thick lines.

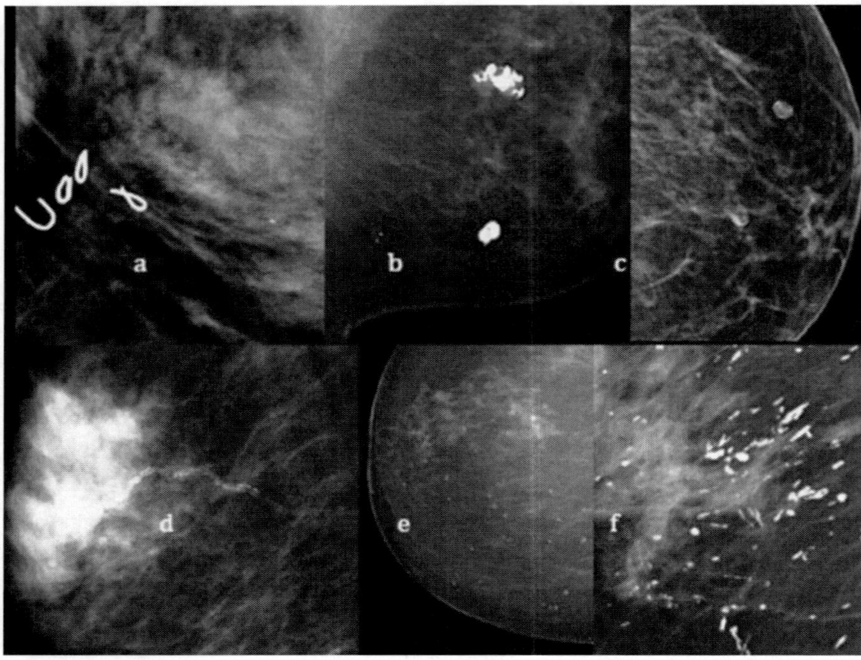

Figure 8. (a) Calcification of suture material. (b) Thick and amorphous popcorn calcifications (calcified fibroadenoma). (c) Eggshell calcification (calcified cyst wall). (d) Train-track calcification (vascular wall). (e) Round calcifications with lucent center with localization in skin. (f) Benign ductal calcifications.

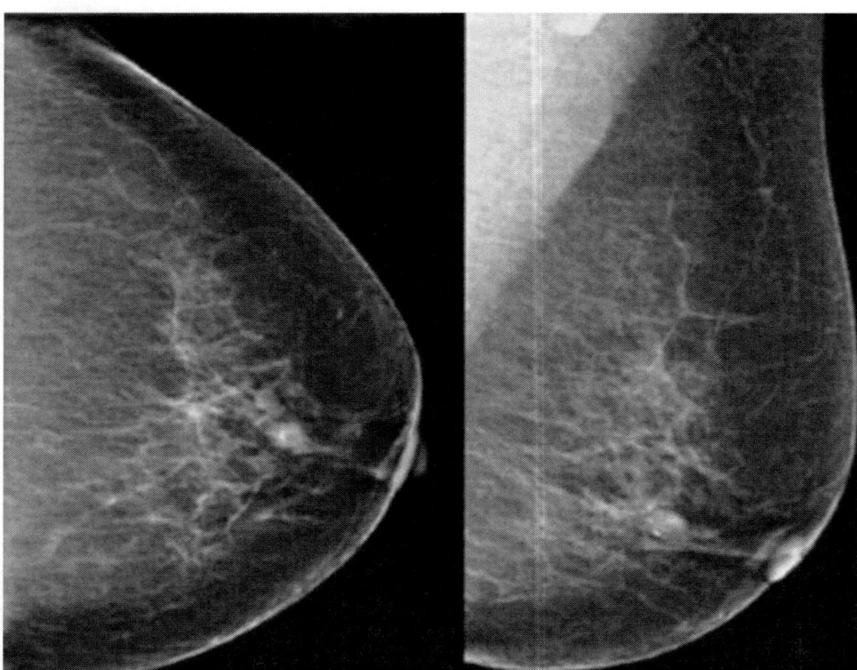

a b

Figure 9. (a) and (b). Cranial-caudal (CC) and Mediolateral-oblique (MLO) mammographic projection, as well as magnification of left retroareolar region. A nodular image is identified of median percentage of density and obscured anterior border, associated with thick calcifications.

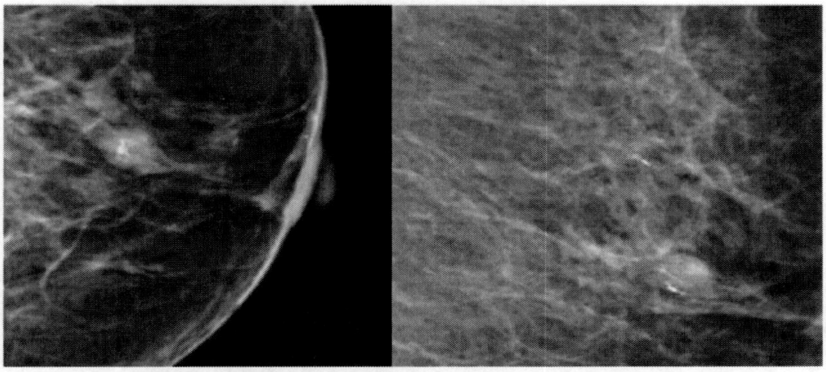

c

Figure 9. (c) Retroareolar magnification.

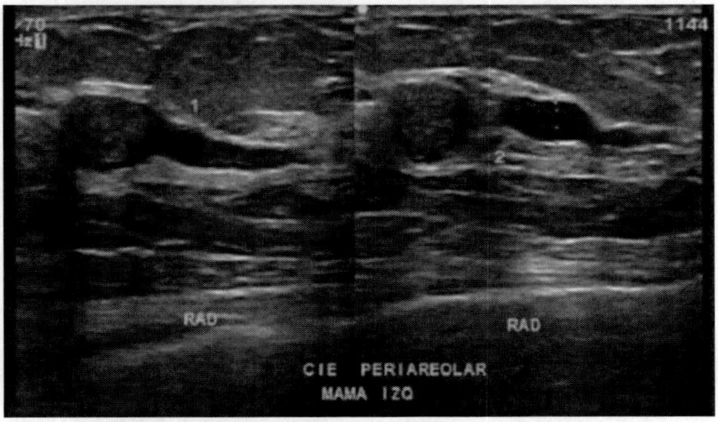

d

Figure 9. (d) Complementary USG that corroborates the presence of solid nodule at the interior of a dilated duct.

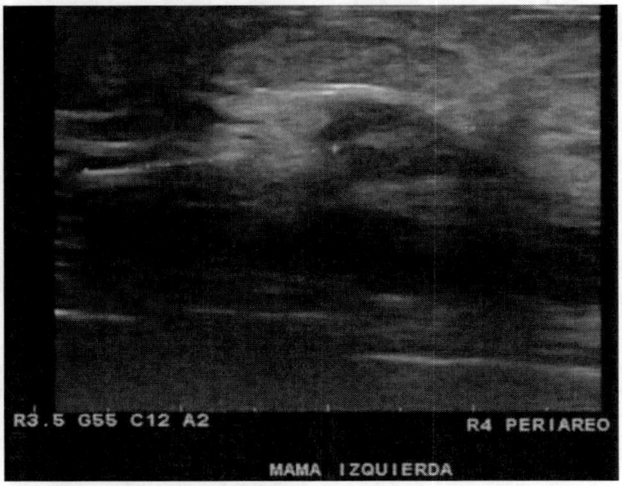

e

Figure 9. (e) Solography-guided percutaneous marking of complex nodule of left breast. Passing of needle through the nodule.

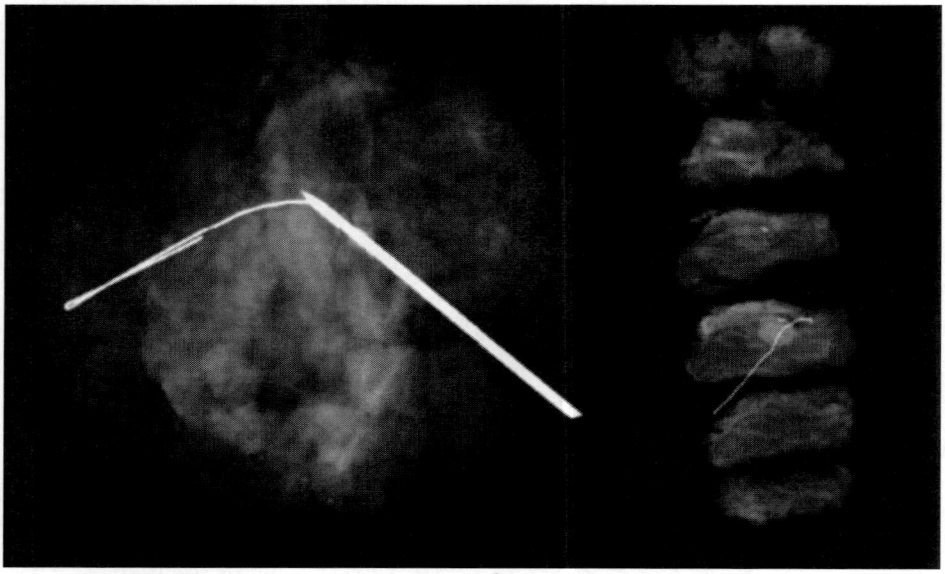

f

Histopathology report: high-grade ductal carcinoma *in situ*, intraductal papilloma, and fibrocystic changes.

Figure 9. (f) Performance of excisional biopsy. Mammographic control of surgical piece where identification of the hook wire at the center of the lesion is achieved. In image of right incision throughout surgical piece with mammographic control, achieving identification, in sample 2, of the presence of calcium deposits and in sample 3, of the separated nodule.

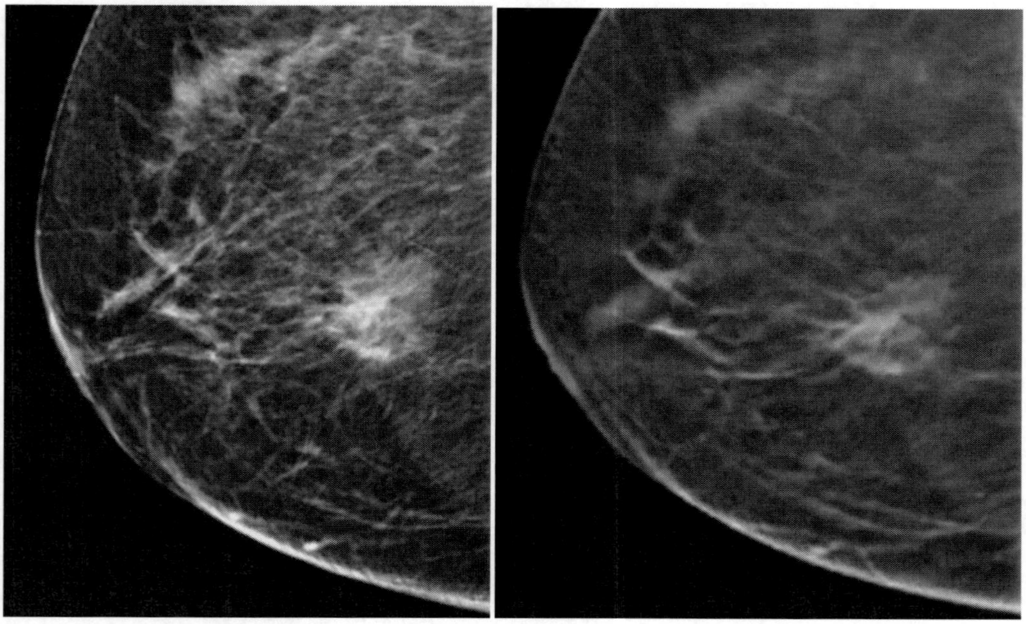

a b

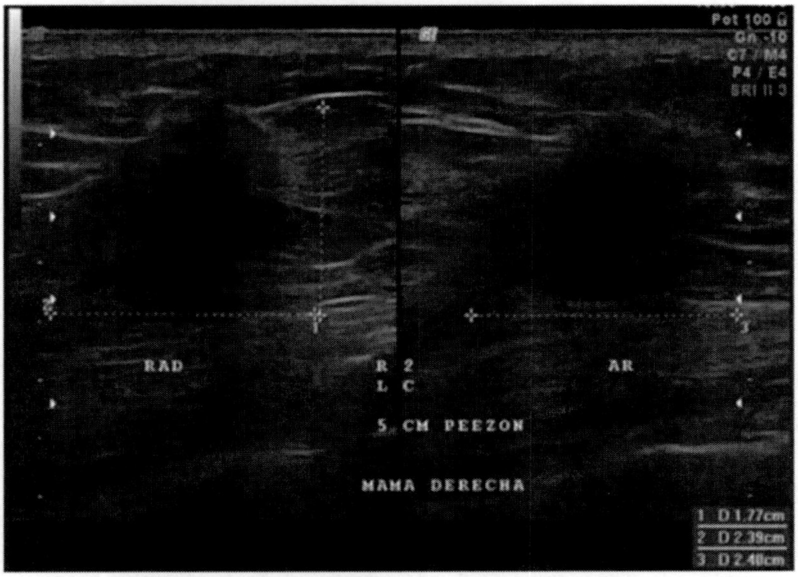

c

Figure 10. (a-c) Right digital mammography in Cranial-caudal (CC) projection, tomosynthesis, and breast USG. In the left image, a focal density zone is observed associated with localized architectural distortion localized toward the interior and posterior third quadrant and posterior third. Right image, digital mammography with tomosynthesis: density zone that achieved characterizing a nodule with spiculated borders that retracts adjacent structures. Lower image. Right breast USG, observing a hypoechoic image with posterior sonic attenuation. Irregular and poorly defined thick-walled border, BI-RADS 5, biopsy carried out, and histopathological result: ductal carcinoma.

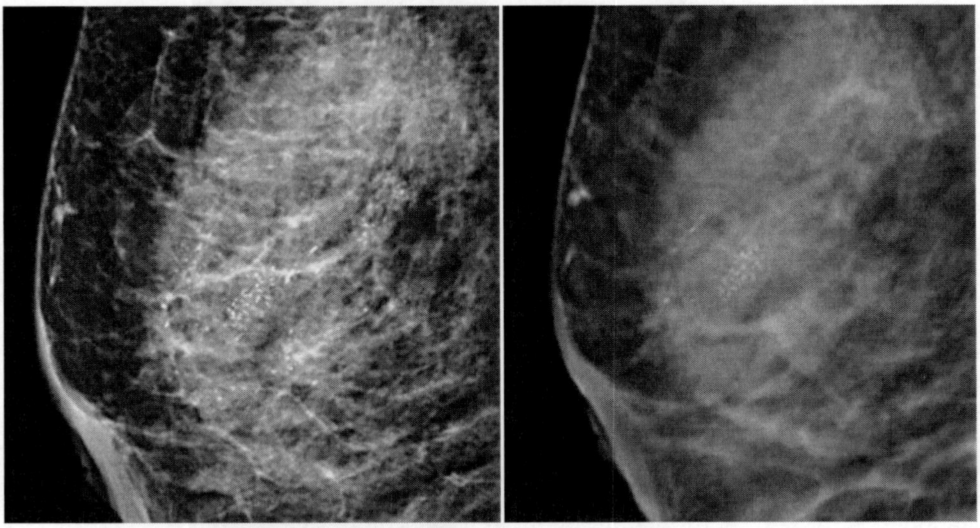

a b

Histopathology report: Invasive ductal carcinoma.

Figure 11. (a) Right MLO projection with approach to upper quadrants that shows focal asymmetry associated with polymorphic and linear microcalcifications with segmentary distribution. (b) Tomosynthesis in the same projection, it being possible to evaluate the calcifications and their distribution and extension. Short needle-aspirated, stereotactic-guided biopsy.

In reference to this, various studies have been carried out to determine the amount of radiation and the glandular dose, demonstrating that the means of these are found within the parameters established by the norm.

Despite this, the dose for performance of the tomosynthesis study increases by up to 20% of that involved with performing a digital mammography alone and therefore protocols have been established for effecting both studies simultaneously and not digital mammography and later mammography plus tomosynthesis.

This effect is due to the total glandular dose per breast would increase to 7.2 mGy, multiplying by 2-3 times the risk for cancer and the mortality increase associated with digital mammography (2.6-3.3 and 0.7 × 0.9 per 100,000 women, respectively) in women exposed at the age of 50 years [18].

In a study conducted by Skaane and colleagues in a series of 12,631 evaluated patients, it was demonstrated that the use of tomosynthesis led to a reduction in the number of false positives and to better detection of invasive carcinomas [19].

Furthermore, in a meta-analysis carried out by Lei et al., in seven studies in which digital mammography vs. digital mammography plus tomosynthesis was performed, the authors reported that tomosynthesis had 90% sensitivity and 79% specificity for diagnosing malignant lesions, while these for digital mammography were 89.0% and 72.0%, respectively, concluding that tomosynthesis exhibited greater sensitivity and specificity than digital mammography [20].

Controversially, Thibault et al. carried out a comparison among the performances of tomosynthesis, mammography, and USG, and found that conducting mammography in combination with tomosynthesis was not superior to digital mammography, and that performing mammography plus tomosynthesis plus USG was not superior to mammography plus USG, which is customarily carried out, suggesting that more clinical studies are required that determine the evaluation of the integration of tomosynthesis in evaluation of the breast as standard procedure [21].

Likewise, it must be considered that the interpretation time of tomosynthesis increases and that this must be taken into account, especially in screening programs.

Ultrasound

Breast Ultrasound (USG) demonstrates different applications and is especially utilized for differentiating cystic lesions from solid nodules with high specificity. In combination with mammography, USG contributes to the differentiating between benign and malignant solid lesions. Breast USG can be performed in mode B, compound images, and in tissue harmonic imaging for better visualization of breast lesions and for reducing imaging artifacts, Doppler application, contrast agents for measuring tumor blood flow, and elastography. Given certain tumor hardness, USG is able to aid in differentiating between benignancy and malignancy and as the method-of-choice for guiding breast biopsies and other interventional procedures. This, together with the application of BI-RADS for the characterization of nodules observed by USG, has improved diagnostic breast USG (Figure 12).

Color Doppler and Pulse-Doppler

These detect the movement of red globules in the blood flow permitting us to evaluate the vascularity of the lesions. These studies also show the direction of the flow, allowing for evaluation of neovascularization, assessment of vascular breast diseases, demonstrating inflammatory hyperemia, and permitting the evaluation of the fremitus test, which measures vibratory acoustic response in the vocal Fremitus test.

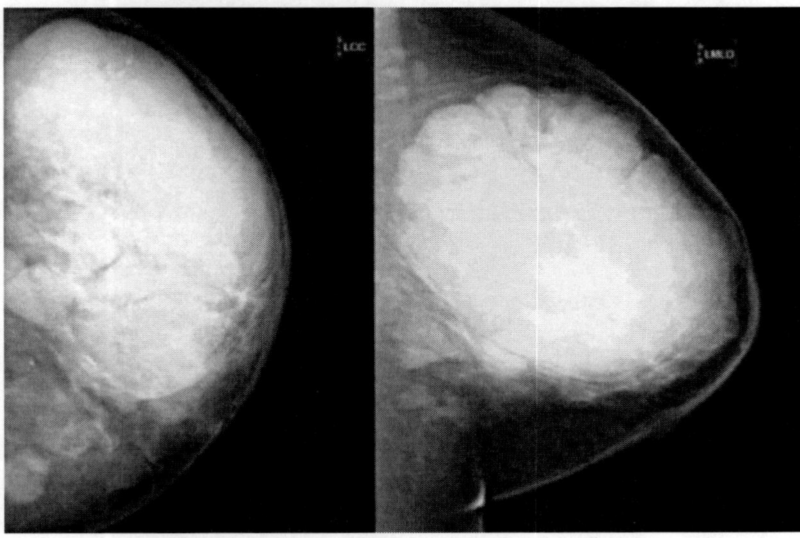

a b

Figure 12. (a-b) Extensive USG. Female aged 51 years who presents due to a mass in left breast. Left mammography in which an extremely dense breast is identified.

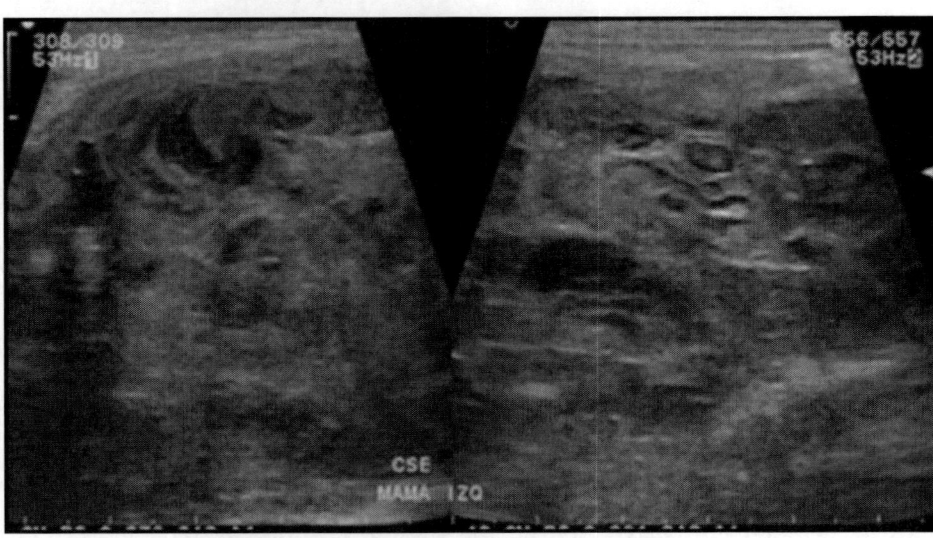

c

Figure 12. (c) On USG, the presence is identified by multiple nodular images, the largest with hypoechoic predominance with areas tending to be cystic in its interior. When lesions are large in size, compound images can be obtained.

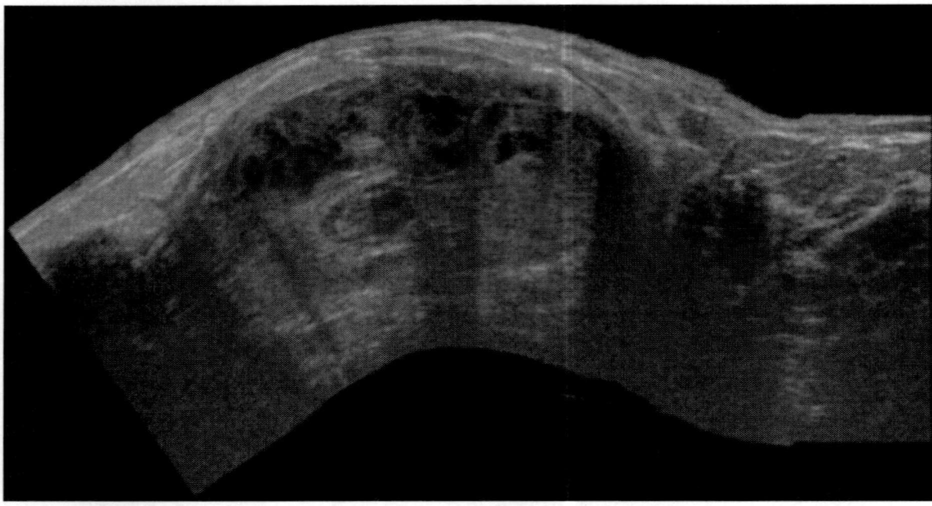

d

Figure 12. (d) Extensive scans are a USG modality that allows assessment of masses of great size or extension. This was submitted to biopsy with Histopathological report (HpR) of bilateral diabetic mastopathy. Bilateral mastectomy was carried out that corroborated diabetic mastopathy and high-grade sarcoma of the mammary stromal.

In the latter test, the patient is asked to constantly repeat a vowel. In the suspicious lesion, its behavior is assessed with color Doppler. If the lesion is benign the color box fills up, and if it is malignant there is the absence of color.

However this test has fallen into disuse given its poor sensitivity. Power Doppler is more sensitive to the presence of flows or of small vessels, and is not conditioned to the direction of the flow. When a lesion is evaluated with color Doppler and does not show increased vascularity, it mainly evaluates characteristics in grey scale for their characterization. This is because it has been demonstrated that the presence of increased vascularity can present in benign as well as in malignant lesions.

Color Doppler is a very useful tool for detecting isoechoic lesions, palpable or not, by means of the presence of adjacent neovascularity, but this datum is very nonspecific in that there is also the presence of very vascularized benign lesions [22] (Figure 13).

When neovascularization is detected in a lesion one must always question whether it will require a biopsy. I such case we should be prepared for the presence of bleeding, despite having coagulation times within the norm as a possible complication [22].

In terms of pulse-Doppler, which permits semi quantitative evaluation of blood flows by means of Resistance indices (RI) and peak systolic velocities as well as assessment of the flow spectrum, is a useful tool, specifically in breast.

However, even with the technological advances, it still is very nonspecific. It has been mentioned in diverse studies that an RI of 0.75 is equal to malignancy; nonetheless this can vary according to the menstrual cycle or to the ingestion of hormones.

Finally, if measurements are taken in central or peripheral vessels of the lesion, there can be variations among these.

Taken together, pulse-Doppler is not routinely used in the evaluation of breast lesions [22].

Elastography

Elastography is a tool that allows for evaluation of nodule hardness by means of tissue compressibility. A grey scale evaluates the nodule-of-interest while on the other hand the transducer is placed on the lesion and sustained compression is carried out, the observance of whether the lesion is elongated would indicate to us that it is a benign lesion; if on the contrary the lesion would be suspected of being malignant. Compressibility is also evaluated by means of a special filter that is superimposed on the nodule-under-study and that presents a color scale (256 colors) that extends from blue, passing through green, up to red, with the operator determining the spectrum of the latter, and the color determining the hardness, which is generally red, while the softness in the extreme opposite appears with the color blue (Figure 5).

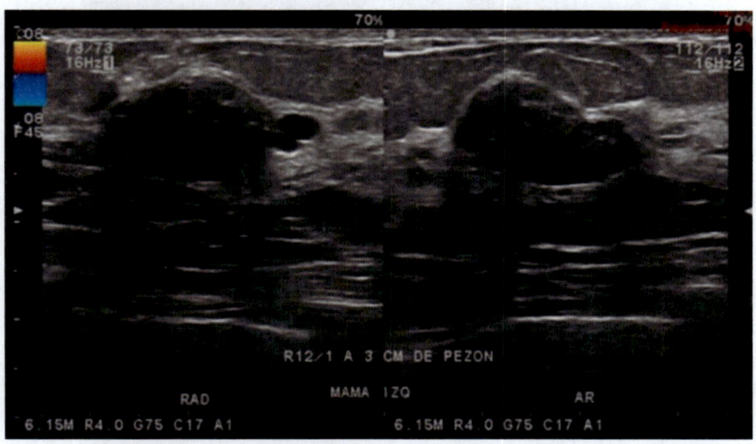

a

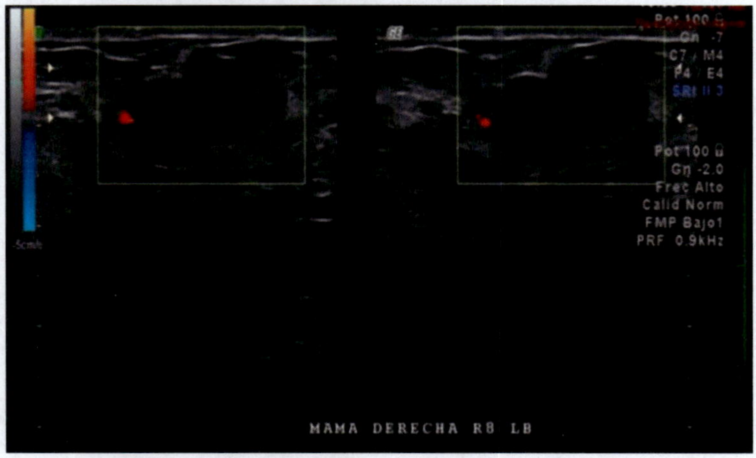

b

Figure 13. (a-b) Color Doppler USG. Two cases of fibroadenoma in two different patients: a) Female aged 50 years with the presence of a hypoechoic microlobulated nodule (upper image), partially defined, that with color Doppler does not demonstrate angiogenesis, and b) Female aged 47 years with the presence of heterogeneous macrolobulated nodule of hypoechoic predominance (lower image) with areas tending to be anechoic in their interior, but with color Doppler the increase of peripheral vascularity is identified.

However, this compressibility is operator-dependent in that the results will depend on the strengths of the explorer as the mobility of the transducer from one side to the other, with angular movements, can obtain results that will be modified.

New ultrasound equipment with elastography perform this compression directly from the transducer and thus avoid false positives and operator-dependent results [23, 24].

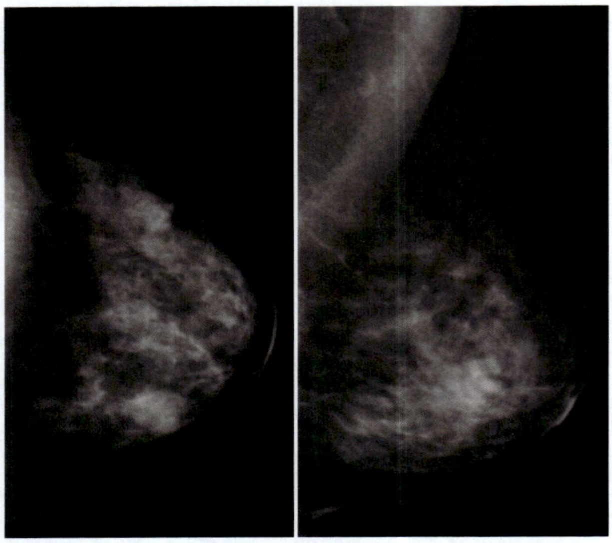

a

Figure 14. (a) Elastography. Female aged 51 years submitted to screening mammography: a) Left mammography where a radiopaque nodule is identified, macrolobulated, partially defined, localized in middle third of the internal quadrant interline of left breast.

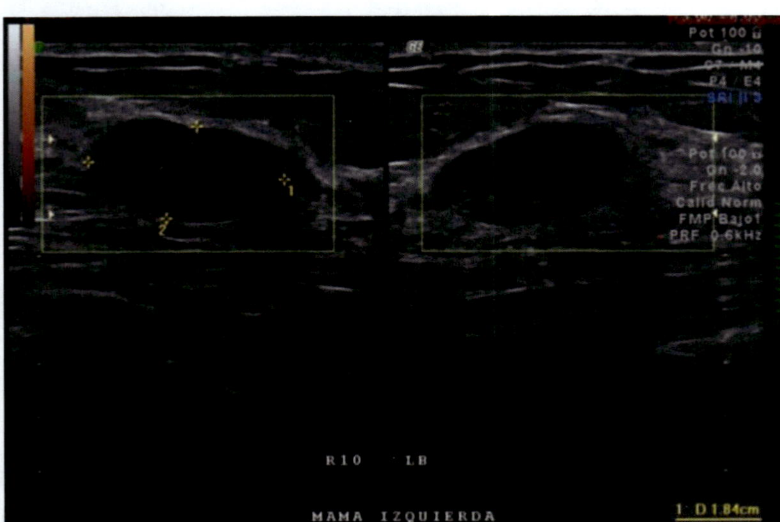

b

Figure 14. (b) On USG, the presence is corroborated of a solid nodule, macrolobulated, of 1.8 cm at its greatest axis, of hypoechoic predominance with areas tending to be anechoic in its interior and of undetermined aspect.

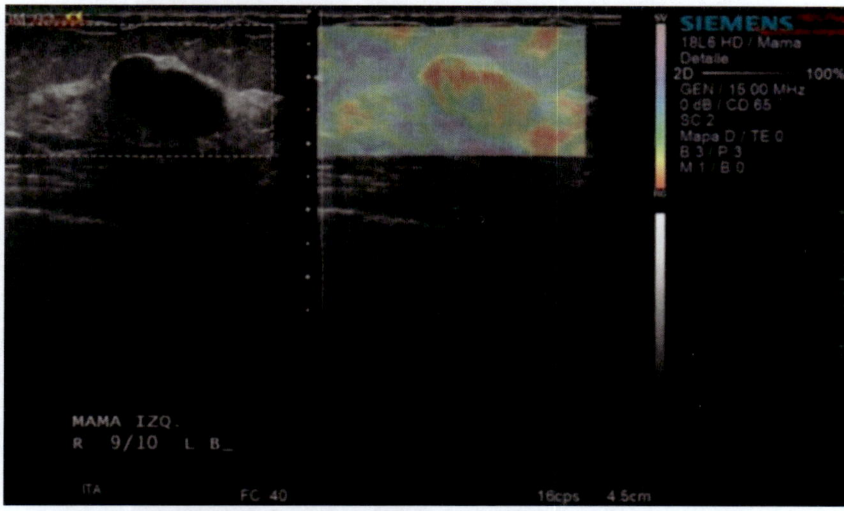

c

Figure 14. (c) Elastography is performed that shows, with the color map, areas of greater hardness in red and others of lesser hardness in greens and yellows, which could indicate to us an etiology more oriented toward benignancy. The lesion is biopsied with a histopathological report of fibroadenoma.

In some studies, mention has been made that elastography entertains the same performance of conventional USG with 86.5% sensitivity, 89.8% specificity, and 88.3% accuracy in terms of differentiation between benign and malignant nodules [25] (Figure 14).

3D Breast Ultrasound

Automatized breast echography, known as Automated breast ultrasound (ABUS), comprises USG equipment that allows evaluation of the breast in three-Dimensional (3D) images in real time. It possesses a linear transducer for evaluating the breast, in addition to having a mobile arm in which a type of plate is localized, of approximately 30 cm, which is placed on the breast and permits the acquisition of axial, coronal, and sagittal images of the breast, as well as its reconstruction in 3D. Acquisition time of the images lasts approximately 10 minutes. On encompassing the entire breast and reconstructing it in 3D the formation of images is avoided and the study is no longer operator-dependent.

However, among its limitations are when dealing with voluminous breasts, in which case images must be acquired by segment because it is not possible to add all of the segments together for carrying out an image in 3D due the software available at present.

Therefore, given the characteristics of the axilla, the latter is not assessable and therefore requires its study with the conventional transducer [26]. While the time for conducting the study is much less, evaluation of the approximately 50 images to be assessed takes much more time for the Medical Radiologist to interpret the study.

Among its advantages are that it permits us to evaluate and determine the characteristics, number, and localizations of the lesions.

It is a very useful tool for the appraisal of multifocality and multicentricity [26].

The sonographic findings that orient us in the characterization of the lesions are mentioned as follows:

Nodules: USG allows determining characteristics such as form, contour, wall, and contents of the nodules observed in mammographic studies. The findings indicate that the lesion is benign when they are rounded or macrolobulated contour with a fine wall. With regard to its echo texture, when the nodule is anechoic it indicates the presence of liquid; while if it is echogenic it indicates fatty contents, or it is hypoechoic if it refers a solid lesion. If the nodule is hypoechoic and presents posterior acoustic reinforcement, this indicates to us that the content is not very solid and that it can be gelatinous. With regards to size, the nodule tends to be higher than wider. The interface of the lesion with adjacent soft tissues is abrupt. In the case of solid nodules, these can present calcium deposits in their interior, indicating calcified fibroadenomas or calcified papillomas, or even the capsule can be calcified, in which case thinking should be directed towards calcified oil cyst, or it may even be thought that it could be fat necrosis with eggshell calcification [22, 26-28, 29].

If the sonographic finding is an anechoic image with the presence of posterior acoustic reinforcement, we should first think of treating a simple cyst. Among differential diagnoses is the galactocele, in which there is the antecedent of recent lactancy.

Breast implants also present these characteristics, but are larger in size. The hemangioma comprises another differential diagnosis where in the latter increased vascularity is identified, as well as the presence of tortuous vessels [22, 26, 28].

If the nodular image is anechoic with echogenic areas in its interior and if posterior acoustic reinforcement is present among the diagnoses, we find the hemorrhagic cyst. The intracystic papilloma is another diagnoses that can be considered and it is where we can observe that the internal echoes do not mobilize with changes in the patient's position, while with color Doppler feeder vessels can be identified of the solid portion. The abscess should also be considered and in this case the presence of heat, flushing, and edema of the adjacent tissues will orient us toward this diagnosis. However, Galactocele and fat necrosis should also be considered [22, 26, 28].

If the nodular image is anechoic or hypoechoic, with an echogenic area that can be with or without posterior acoustic reinforcement, and with discrete sonic attenuation, the analysis should take us to conclude that the lesion is an oil cyst, a galactocele, or even an abscess. The clinic and the associated findings are the tools that aid us in reaching the final diagnosis [22, 26, 28]. When we are before an anechoic nodular image occupied by fine echoes with or without liquid-liquid level and posterior acoustic reinforcement present, we should consider that it is a hemorrhagic cyst without clot present, infected cyst, abscess, sebaceous cyst, epidermal inclusion cyst, cyst with debris in its interior, or a complicated cyst. In an anechoic nodular image with septa in its interior and posterior acoustic reinforcement present, these can be observed in cases of infected hemorrhagic cyst, complex cyst, or in galactoceles [22, 26, 28]. If the nodular image is heterogeneous hypoechoic without posterior acoustic reinforcement, we should think of fibroadenomas, in which we can observe the defined contour or, on occasion, the macrolobulated contour and discrete marginal posterior sonic attenuation. Other diagnoses to consider are oil cysts or fat necrosis.

It is important to remember that during breast development the mammary bud can be observed as a retroareolar hypoechoic nodular image that develops first in one breast than in the other. This usually presents itself between 9 and 10 years of age, although formerly this took place between the ages of 11 and 12 years.

The mammary bud can be palpable and on occasion can be associated with direct trauma. On finding hypoechoic nodular images with echogenic center, these correspond to lymph nodes, which can be found within the breast at any localization, oftentimes towards the Upper outside quadrant (UOQ) [22, 26, 28]. Isoechoic lesions in adjacent tissue can be a lactating adenoma or even a fibroadenoma, although the latter is not a habitual presentation [22, 26, 28]. If the lesion is solid hypoechoic with posterior acoustic reinforcement, it can be a fat lobule, fibroadenoma, phyllodes tumor, focal fibrosis, intramammary lymph node, intracystic papilloma, or fat necrosis. When the nodular lesion is hypoechoic with areas of discrete or absent posterior acoustic reinforcement, phyllodes tumor, fibroadenoma, lymph node central necrosis, and focal fibrocystic change come to mind as possible diagnosis [22, 26, 28].

Solid hypoechoic nodular lesions with posterior acoustic shadowing can be simple cysts with calcifications on their wall, calcified oil cyst, postsurgical fibrosis, focal fibrocystic changes, radial scar, or galactocele with very thick liquid. If the nodular lesion is hypoechoic with hyperechoic areas that give rise to posterior acoustic shadowing, we should consider calcified fibroadenoma, calcified fat necrosis, or calcified axillary lymph node when there is a granulomatous lesion in the lymph node [22, 26, 28].

In hyperechoic nodular lesions without posterior sonic reinforcement or posterior sonic attenuation, the lesions are considered as lipomas, hamartomas (although generally in this diagnosis we can observe hypo- and hyperechoic areas intermixed with the presence of a fine wall), hematomas, and fibroadenomas. In the latter this is not the customary echographic characteristic and can be observed in patients with prolonged anovulatory cycles. If the solid nodular lesion is hyperechoic with posterior acoustic shadowing, we should consider a foreign body, calcified fibroadenoma, hyalinized fibroadenoma, fat necrosis, or postsurgical fibrosis [22, 26, 28]. The presence of an echogenic halo around a nodule can be a fibrous peri cystic halo in inflamed cysts or can even look like a pseudocapsule. In a malignant lesion, when an echogenic halo is present, it corresponds to the desmoplastic reaction that is formed in the adjacent tissues. When this is due to the response of normal tissue attempting to encapsulate the lesion, it speaks of a lesion of slow growth [22, 26, 28].

In the presence of dilated ducts, the latter can be unique, multiple, or grouped, and they can present at any age and during lactancy. If echoes present in their interior, these can be secondary to detritus and even more so when these are mobile. If the echoes do not show movement or if a solid intraductal nodular is observed, we should think of intraductal papilloma as the lesion. If there are various lesions, then it is papillomatosis [22, 28].

Calcium deposits: Calcifications are generally puntiform or in small groups, and if in small groups they are not able to be seen by USG, at least if they are associated with nodules or masses. Calcifications that are able to be seen are thick amorphic calcium deposits associated with fat necrosis due to a surgical event or to microtraumas, or to calcified oil cysts observed in mammographic studies that will show posterior sonic attenuations [22, 29, 27].

Non-Nodular Lesions

Among the non-nodular lesions that can be found there are zones of posterior sonic attenuation and the distorsion of breast tissue. Posterior acoustic shadowing areas without nodules can be, on occasion, the sole finding that is generally associated with malignancy.

However, there are some benign lesions that can present in this manner, and postsurgical changes, stromal fibrosis, fat necrosis, or diabetic mastopathy come to mind.

The latter presents itself in women with diabetes and without adequate control of glycemia during a prolonged period of time.

Within distorsions zones, these correspond to zones in which normal breast architecture is lost and within benign breast pathology, distorsions zones can be due to focal or diffuse fibrosis or, on occasion, to radial scar postsurgical fibrosis [22, 28-30].

Diffuse edema of the breast is observed with thickening of the skin, loss of the interface of the diverse anatomical planes of the breast, stromal prominence, and prominence of the lymphatic vessels. It can be associated with cardiac insufficiency, abscess, recent postsurgical changes, and with venous obstruction generally secondary to subclavian vein thrombosis or lymphedema [22, 28, 30].

There are dynamic tests that can be carried out in case of doubt and that are performed in real time. These are compressibility and mobility tests. Benign lesions are mobile, thus not adhered to deep planes. In terms of compressibility, whether the lesion is compressible means that it elongates, and while during a focal compression or on evaluation with elastography, it indicates to us that we have a benign lesion. However, Leucht (1992) considers that up to 50% of benign and malignant lesions are not compressible [22, 30].

For the diagnosis of benign as well as of malignant breast pathology, it is useful to know family history, pathological personal data, gyneco-obstetric antecedents, risk factors, and clinical data that can orient us toward the possible diagnoses.

Magnetic Resonance

The role of Magnetic resonance (MR) of the breast has been established as a complement of conventional diagnostic techniques such as mammography and USG.

MR of the breast permits the detection and characterization of benign lesions, primary breast cancers, recurrent, and allows evaluation of response to therapy.

The breast imaging lexicon published by the American College of Radiologists (ACR) permits a standardized and coherent description of the morphological and kinetic characteristics of breast lesions [31]. Breast lesions that are detected on MR are focused or foci (point of reinforcement with a diameter of <5 mm), mass (a three-dimensional (3D) lesion that is the occupant of space with morphology, margin, and internal reinforcement), and non mass reinforcement (uptake of an area without its defining a mass) [32]. Normal breast tissue shows posterior background reinforcement on administration of contrast. In general, it is bilateral, symmetrical, and diffuse. However, on occasion it can be focal, regional, and/or asymmetrical as it is the combination of the enhanced tissue volume as well as of the enhanced intensity. Especially in premenopausal women, it can appear as focal reinforcements, and this aspect can lead to the conclusion of false positives [33].

When the findings by MR are a mass, the margins are the most reliable characteristic for distinguishing between benign and malignant processes. The circumscribed margin is found clearly defined and is characteristic of benign lesions (Negative predictive value [NPV], 95%). Lobulated morphology, if it does not show reinforcement, is probably benign (NPV, 100%), and also if it shows moderate or marked reinforcement, NPV is 67% (Figure 1).

The absence of reinforcement has a high NPV of malignancy (88-96%), and when homogeneous reinforcement is exhibited, a Positive predictive value (PPV) of 87% has been reported for benign disease if the enhancement of these characteristics persists up to the late phase.

If the finding by MR is nonmass reinforcement, distribution has a greater predictive value of malignancy than the internal enhancement of the same. If its distribution is focal, diffuse, or in multiple regions of symmetrical and bilateral form in premenopausal women, there is a greater probability of it being conditioned for physiological parenchymatous reinforcement, and the possibility should be considered of repeating MR between days 7 and 14 of the menstrual cycle [34] (Figure 15).

If a mass is lobulated and demonstrates moderate or marked enhancement (NPV, 67%), additional evaluation may be justified to determine the lesion. The correlation between the lesion part with reinforcement and its signal intensity in the T2 sequence is useful. Signal hyperintensity in the T2 sequence in the same lesion portion that appears reinforced in T1-potentiated images is highly suggestive of benignancy, although not all masses with a high intensity signal in T2-potentiated images are benign [35].

Many benign breast lesions can appear as reinforcements, including nonproliferative lesions (hyperplasia and fibroadenomas), proliferative lesions without atypia (sclerosing adenosis, complex sclerosing lesions, moderate hyperplasia), and lobular and atypical ductal hyperplasia.

The reported MR specificity is 37-100%. This relatively low specificity is one disadvantage, and rigorous criteria have been proposed for interpretation of the images.

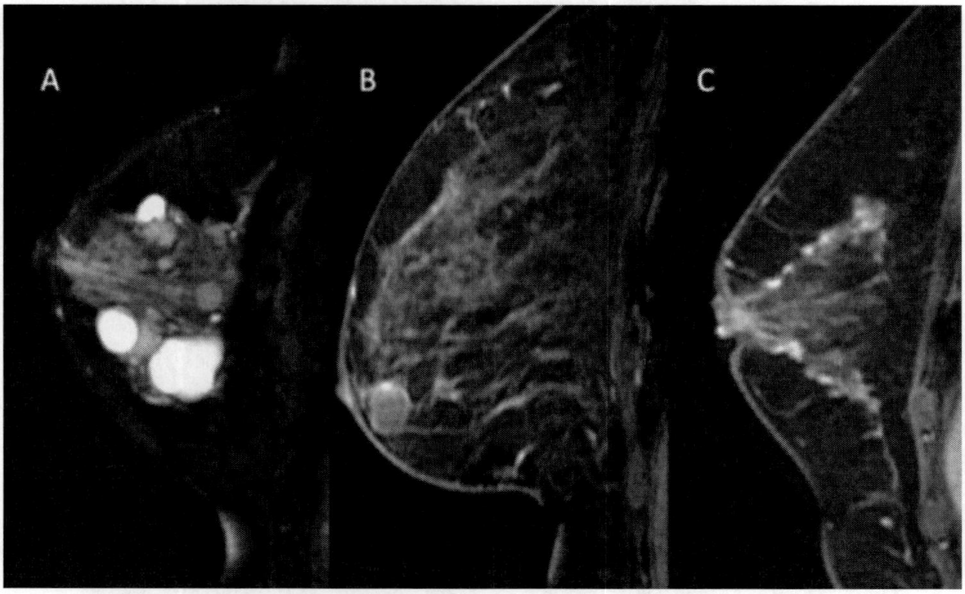

Figure 15. (A) Female aged 40 years with round, oval, and circumscribed masses that represent the presence of simple or of complicated cysts. (B) Female aged 43 years with ovoid and circumscribed mass annular reinforcement compatible with fibroadenoma. (C) Female aged 45 years with nonmass reinforcement in Upper outside quadrant (UOQ) and presence of foci distributed in diffuse form conditioned by fibrocystic changes.

This permits us to explore two concepts for improving specificity: First, detailed analysis of the morphological characteristics of the lesions with high-resolution spatial sequences; and second, we can also obtain dynamic data derived from the kinetic patterns utilizing the dynamic protocols (kinetic reinforcement curves) with the addition of molecular information (spectroscopy) and cellular density (diffusion) [36].

Kinetic Reinforcement Curves

The dynamic uptake patterns of contrast are divided into three types. Initially, these are divided into the kinetic uptake curve of Initial Phase and Late Phase.

Initial Enhancement Phase: This refers to the increase of signaling intensity during the first 2 minutes after the injection of intravenous (IV) contrast, or when the curve begins to change, according to the percentage of the signal increase. If it is increased by 50-60%, it corresponds to Slow, if by 60-100% to Medium, and of 100% or more, it corresponds to Rapid.

Late Reinforcement Phase: This refers to the signal intensity curve 2 minutes after administration of contrast or after the curve begins to change, and is described as follows: Persistent, when there is continuous increase of enhancement; Plateau, in which signal intensity remains constant after the initial peak; and Washout, which exhibits rapid washout or loss of >10% of maximal signal intensity.

The type 1 enhancement pattern is generally associated with a benign finding (83% benign, 9% malignant) (Figure 16). The type II enhancement pattern possesses 42.6% sensitivity and 75% specificity for detection of malignancy. The type III enhancement pattern is generally not observed in benign lesions and has 90.4% specificity [37].

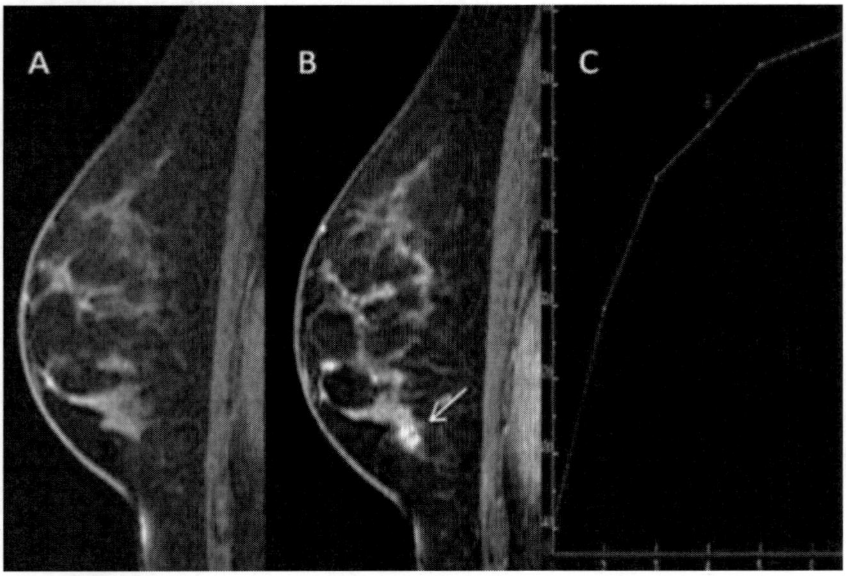

Figure 16. Female aged 47 years with diagnosis of papillomatosis. (A) T1 sequence without contrast. (B) T1 sequence with contrast that shows nonmass reinforcement in Lower inside quadrant (LIQ) of left breast. (C) Type 1 dynamic curve with slow initial phase and late persistent reinforcement.

Diffusion

This has become an important technique for distinction between benign and malignant lesions. Diffusion is based on the molecules of water in the tissues. For quantifying diffusion, the value of the Apparent diffusion coefficient (ADC) is utilized. The computer calculates the ADC of each pixel of the image and exhibits it as a parametric map in color or in grey scale.

Manually it is possible to draw a Region-of-interest (ROI) above the image, thus obtaining the numerical ADC value for a determined tissue.

At present, there is no numerical standard for each value because there is no consensus on technical parameters [38]. Many studies have demonstrated an inverse correlation between the cellularity of breast cancer and the value of ADC with numerical values $>1.2 \times 10^{-3}$ in benign lesions.

Cysts, fibroadenomas, and fibrocystic disease exhibit high signal intensity or are isointense in the T2- potentiated sequence.

Abscesses and mastitis have low ADC values, similar to those of malignant tumors. However, the low ADC value area within the absence in general has high signal intensity in T2-potentiated images, which indicates a high water and viscosity content. Thus, the findings obtained during physical exploration should be considered, simplifying this mode of radiologic diagnosis (Figure 17).

Intraductal papilloma is one of the breast lesions that can be poorly diagnosed as a malignant tumor due to a low ADC value and therefore it is important to correlate this with other imaging methods.

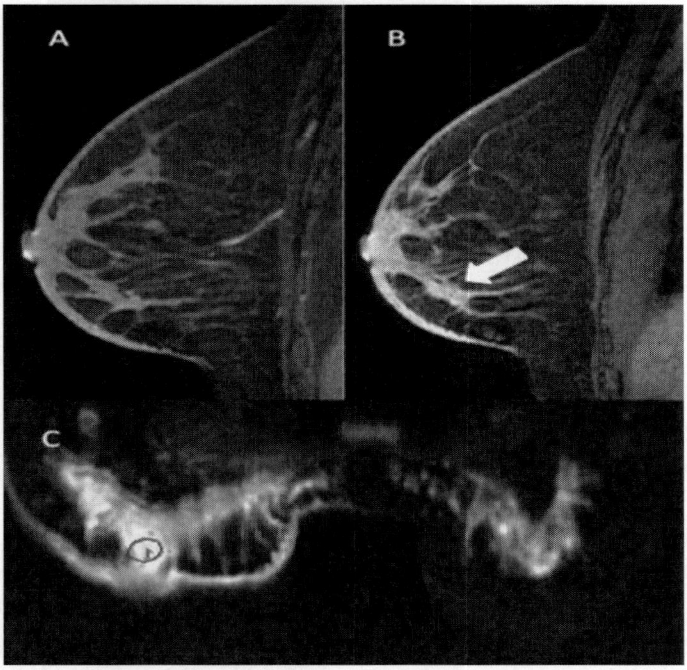

Figure 17. Female aged 53 years with diagnosis of xxxx in Lower outside quadrant (LOQ) of right breast. (A) T1 sequence without contrast. (B) T1 sequence with contrast that shows segmentary reinforcement associated with thickening of the skin. (C) Diffusion with restriction and ADC of 1.8×10^{-3}.

Hematomas that contain intracellular components, such as intracellular oxyhemoglobin, deoxyhemoglobin, or methehemoglobin, significantly demonstrate reduced diffusion in comparison with hematomas that contain smooth blood cells (extracellular methehemoglobin). Some hematomas have high signal intensity in precontrast T1-potentiated images and therefore T1-potentiated images should be evaluated together with the potentiated images in diffusion, thus avoiding erroneous diagnoses [39].

Spectroscopy

On MR information on the lesion's chemical composition can be evaluated with spectroscopy, which provides biochemical information on the tissue being appraised. The value is based on the detection of high levels of choline derivatives, which together are denominated TCho, a tumor marker whose presence and increase in the concentration of the metabolite present in breast cancer and that behaves like a rising chemical displacement with a percentage change of (3.2 ppm, parts per million) on its graphic registration [40].

Spectroscopy improves the specificity of MR, aids in better differentiating benign and malignant lesions, and diminishes the number of unnecessary biopsies without compromising the diagnosis of breast cancer. It presents 70-96% sensitivity and 67-100% specificity. Benign breast lesions have exhibited a total absence of detectable choline compounds [41] (Figure 18), although choline signals have been documented in groups of lactating breasts favoring false positives [42].

Other Studies

To date the fundamental purpose of breast imaging studies has been the detection of nonpalpable lesions on imaging, which has been adhered to for various decades thanks to mammography.

However, currently there exists the requirement of searching for ever smaller lesions, utilizing one or various imaging methods, given that each passing day is witness to more interesting findings of precursor lesions of cancer. Mammography continues to be the imaging method-of-choice for screening in breast, with sensitivity of detecting breast cancer of 70.8% in patients aged 40-44 years and of 84.5% in patients aged 75-89 years.

One limitation of mammography is its being a biplanar study, even when the target organ is three-dimensional or volumetric, which results in tissue superimposition. As previously mentioned another limitation is dense breasts, which has given rise to the advent of new imaging techniques or tools [43], such as the case of digital mammography, tomosynthesis, computed tomography (CT), different USG techniques, nuclear medicine studies, including Single-photon emission computed tomography (SPECT), Positron-emission tomography (PET), PET/Computed tomography (PET/CT), Positron-emission mammography (PEM), and Magnetic resonance (MR).

These are studies that permit obtaining different type of information in a simultaneous manner: the former provides anatomical information, while nuclear medicine studies provide functional information, and MR provides a combination of both [44].

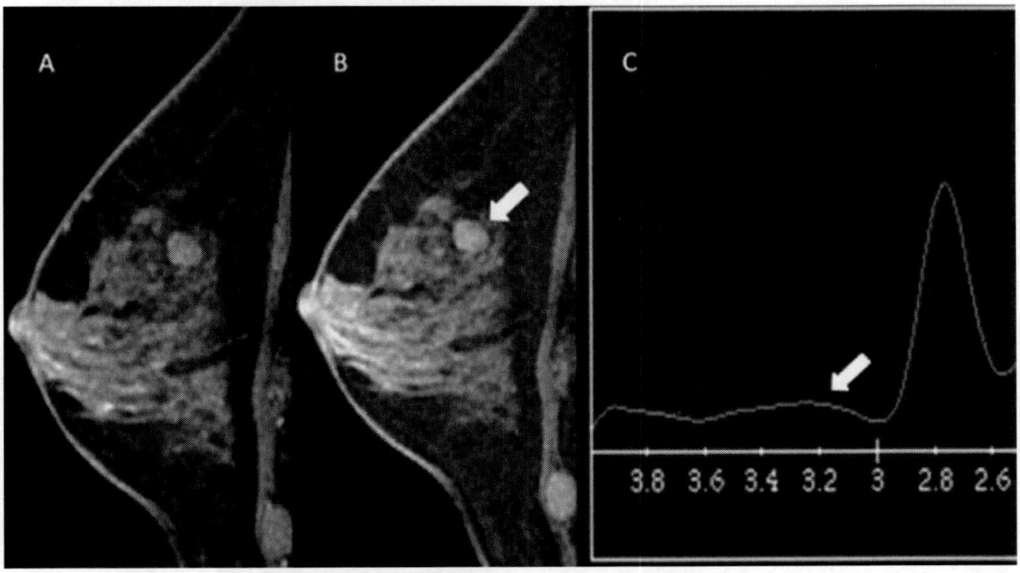

Figure 18. Female aged 48 years with diagnosis of fibroadenoma. (A) T1 sequence without contrast and with presence of hypointense ovoid mass. (B) Mass with homogeneous reinforcement in Upper outside quadrant (UOQ) of right breast. (C) Spectroscopy with negative choline peak.

Bioelectrical Impedance

Analysis of bioelectrical impedance is a noninvasive and painless, easy-to-apply method that has demonstrated good correlation with classical techniques for the study of body composition when the physiological and hydration conditions of the individual are not modified.

Thus, bioelectrical impedance has a growing application in the health sciences. The practice and development of this technique is based on measurement of the impedance or the response that the biological tissues present in terms of their properties, with the passing of an alternate electrical current with very low voltage intensity. This is a tool that is utilized within the hospital ambit in the following cases: to estimate body composition in 2 or 3 compartments (fat mass and fat-free mass) or fat mass, cellular mass, and extracellular mass; to monitor cellular wear or deterioration; to evaluate the level and distribution of water in the body; and to observe the fluctuation of body fluids. Different medical specialties, such as Endocrinology, Nephrology, and Pediatrics, and diverse pathological situations can be benefited by this method. The unique and main contraindication for this technique is application in patients who are carriers of internal metallic prostheses.

There are also multiple works that report of the use of this technique in AIDS, hemodialysis, obesity, nutritional alterations, cancer, and diabetes, among others [45].

Halley and colleagues apply bioelectrical impedance for the management of breast cancer-associated lymphedema, which demonstrates an impedance of 2-83%. The most frequently employed measurement methods for lymphedema are bioelectrical impedance, volume displacement, and perimetral measurements.

Hayes et al. (2008) refer that lymphedema was not detected in 40-60% of patients measured with self-evaluation or perimetral instruments.

Furthermore, diagnosis was false in 12% of patients with perimetral instruments and in 40% of those employing self-evaluation instruments [46]. Berlit et al. (2013) refer to 85.7% sensitivity and 97.4% specificity in the prediction of lymphedema, with a PPV of 54.6% and a NPV of 97.4% [47].

Electrical Impedance

This is also known as Electrical Impedance Scanning (EIS) or Electrical Impedance Tomography (EIT).

It is a diagnostic technique by means of which breast imaging, noninvasive and in real time is employed since the decade of the 1980s, which consists of mapping the different dielectric properties of normal breast tissue with respect to malignant tissue, all based in terms of impedance and electrical conductivity.

In normal tissue there are variations of impedence that allow for the determination of the different tissue types. A malignant tumor typically undergoes a substantial increase of capacitance and of conductivity compared with neighboring tissues.

During the procedure the patient is in decubitus position and holds a metallic cylinder, or a patch is placed on the patient's arm. The electrical source sends a 1-2.5-volt electric signal to the patient. To complete the circuit, a catheter is employed with which the impedence is measured. The electrical signals are recovered and are reproduced on a computer screen. Cancerous cells possess lower impedance than healthy cells and this translates into a brilliant spot on the screen.

This device exhibits a physiological (functional) image of the breast with respect to a morphological (anatomical) image. The procedure lasts approximately 15 min. and there is no known contraindication. Its main indication is in patients with mammographic findings of BI-RADS categories 3 or 4 of the American College of Radiologists (ACR), in that it attempts to diminish the number of unnecessary biopsies and nonconclusive mammographies.

This device is not intended to be a screening device for breast cancer. Its employment in detecting and evaluating lesions not identified by other modalities has not yet been completely studied, although the use of this technique has been approved for commercialization by the US Federal Drug Administration (FDA) in 1999, in Greece (1997), in Russia, Korea, and in China (1998).

In three reviews published in 2004, 2009, and 2011 that incorporate more clinical studies, this technique continued to be considered under experimentation given the results of contradictory clinical studies with regard to the possible advantage of the diagnosis of images classified as doubtful (BI-RADS 3/4) [48]. After the date of publication of the last review, a validation study of diagnostic tests has been identified that included 808 patients who presented an abnormality in breast mammography and/or echography and on whom a study with electrical impedence was practiced.

Compared with the result of the biopsy, electrical impedance demonstrated 87% sensitivity and 85% specificity in the diagnosis of breast cancer, results which ere similar to those presented by echography associated with mammography [49].

Some of the proposed applications include monitoring lung function, detection of skin cancer and localization of epithelial foci. Currently all of these applications are considered experimental [50].

Dedicated Breast Computed Tomography (DBCT)

This study is an excellent tool for the diagnosis of thoracic and abdominal pathology and therefore its use is common. Also, due to anatomical concerns, the mammary glands are included in the images obtained. This technique has been approved for the analysis of benign as well as for malignant lesions, and this method is not the method-of-choice as unique method. Sometimes mammary lesions are better visualized by tomography, above all if the breasts are dense or if they present lesions that are localized adjacent to the thoracic wall or in axilla [51].

The applications of multislice Computed tomography (CT) in breast are for the detection of breast cancer and its differentiation from benign lesions, lesion extension, axillary lymph node affectation, or distal, evaluation of residual tumor after neoadjuvant chemotherapy or of excision, tumor recurrence, and as a guide for interventionist procedures (Figure 19). Among its advantages we find that DBCT exhibited excellent spatial resolution, permitting reconstruction with excellent quality in images and in less time than MR. The patient is found in supine decubitus position, which provides the patient more comfort.

It also possesses excellent spatial resolution, allowing for reconstruction with excellent imaging quality. Three-dimensional (3D) images for surgical planning and the use of contrast medium allow simultaneous evaluation of lymph node chains and the thoracic cage, among others. However, it also has disadvantages, such as the case of exposure to radiation, and for this reason MR is preferred [52].

Findings in the breast that can be observed on tomography include the following: Benign: fibroadenomas, phyllodes tumor, hematomas, seromas, inflammatory or granulotomatous diseases, fat necrosis, and cysts; and Malignant: primary or secondary carcinomas, metastasis, and iatrogenic carcinomas [53]. Miyake et al. suggest the usefulness of DBCT in differentiating between benign and malignant breast lesions with high sensitivity [54].

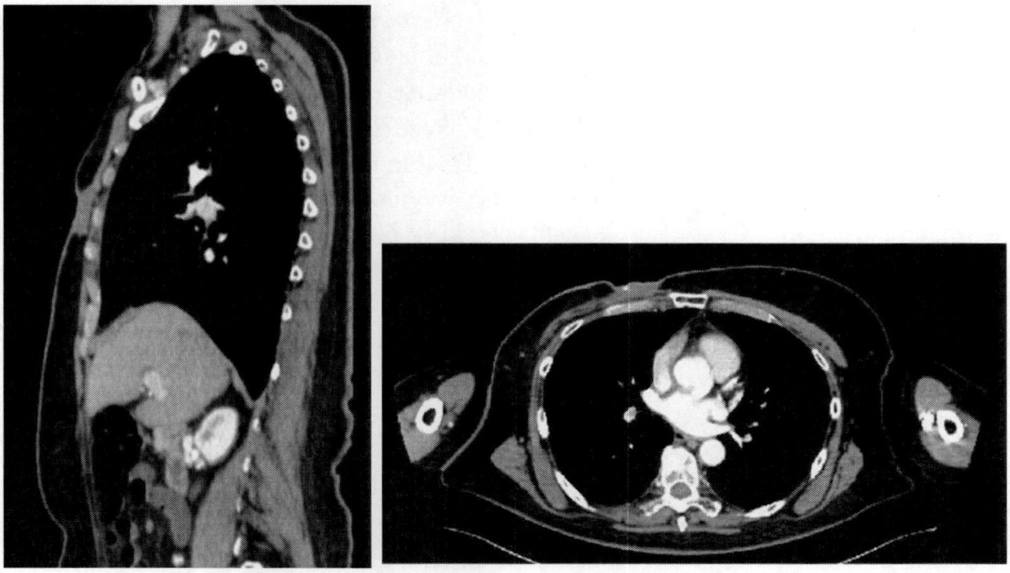

Figure 19. Tomographic images. Evaluation for observing site postmastectomy recurrence. Female 51 years with background of right and diagnosis was infiltrating ductal carcinoma. After a 15-year follow-up, ulcerated lesion in scar is present, histopathological report of infiltrating ductal carcinoma.

In conclusion, this study is not considered a method of evaluation of breast lesions. The study is, rather, the emergence of a novel imaging technique that permits fusion between morphological and functional studies such as PET/CT, which has been a point of reference for the diagnosis and follow-up of diseases such as cancer, and widely utilized in head and neck tumors, individual pulmonary nodules, lung cancer, cancer of the esophagus, colorectal cancer, lymphoma, melanoma, and breast cancer, among others [55].

Positron-Emission Tomography-Computed Tomography (PET-CT)

Positron-emission tomography (PET) is the imaging technique that has had the greatest impact on the management of the oncological patient in the last decade.

The radiopharmaceutical that has allowed this advance in the clinic has been f-Fluorodeoxyglucose (FDG).

Advantages of PET: the possibility of studying the whole body in a sole exposure, which allows establishing a distal extension of malignant tumors and high sensitivity and high resolution of contrast, which permit the identification of certain lesions with greater ease. Its disadvantage lies in its anatomical information.

Thus, in 1998 PET/CT emerged that permitted, in a sole exploration, the obtaining of anatomical and metabolic information where the final images are shown as fused [45].

Metabolic activity offers additional information about the biology of the tumor and can be utilized to differentiate between benign and malignant tumors to identify early-stage metastasis, to stage the disease, and to appraise disease extension and treatment response.

In the study of breast cancer, whole-body PET/CT is extremely useful in tumor staging. However, one limitation is its low spatial resolution (less discernible distance between two objects), which allows for sensitivity and specificity of 80 and 76%, respectively, for the study of the primary tumor [55].

More than 90% of PET studies are utilized to evaluate oncological problems, and only 10%, for neurological, cardiological, infectious, and inflammatory problems [56].

Correction of image attenuation provides quantitative information on the concentration of the radiopharmaceutical in the tissue. Standard uptake value (SUV) is a calculation that allows for a semiquantitative quantification of 18 FDG in the tissues, which derives from the amount of FDG by dividing by the patient's weight and multiplying it by the dose administered [43].

Diverse causes are known of falsely negative results, such as the following: lesions measuring 4-8 mm (systemic resolution); patients with hyperglycemia at the moment of injection of the radiopharmaceutical; lesions localized in physiological high-uptake zones; and conditions inherent to the tumor (poor mitotic activity, low proliferative potential, and prolonged duplication time). Because glucose uptake is not exclusive to tumor cells, it is also present in recently formed granulation tissues and in macrophages. Tuberculosis, silicosis, histoplasmosis, abscesses, sarcoidosis, and cicatricial granulation tissue are potential causes of false-positive results [56].

There is physiological uptake in brain, myocardium, urinary tract and, to a lesser degree, in liver, spleen, bone marrow, and gastrointestinal tract.

Other less frequent uptake sites comprise the endometrium, the salivary glands, and the brown fat localized in the supraclavicular and paraspinal region.

Dense breasts can take up a moderate amount of 18 FDG (SUV, <1 nl). During lactancy, uptake rises and can be demonstrated asymmetrically, although these changes revert after 3 or 4 weeks after the end of lactancy.

FDG Uptake in Benign Pathology

Recent postsurgical and radiotherapy changes tend to increase the uptake of the radiopharmaceutical across the margins of the scar or the radiated area.

This is due to the infiltration of leukocytes in the granulation tissue that is associated with the local inflammatory process. There can also be uptake of the radiopharmaceutical by the axillary lymph nodes as a response to an inflammatory or infectious process, or secondary to a recent biopsy, which can originate false-positive results.

18 FDG can accumulate in the areas affected by pathologies such as proliferative processes (hyperplasia with or without atypia, and benign neoplasms, adenomas or fibroadenomas). Post-traumatic changes, such as hematoma, take up 18 FDG in rings during various weeks, as well as fat necrosis, acute or chronic inflammatory processes of the subcutaneous cellular tissue, mastitis, abscesses, tuberculosis, and sarcoidosis, among others.

After chemotherapy, it is expected to observe a diffuse and uniform increase of bone marrow, which resolves after two months of the conclusion of the treatment [43].

PET/CT with 18 FDG can detect increased metabolic activity before structural changes are produced. However, its capacity to detect lesions <1 cm in diameter is limited, due to its low spatial resolution (approximately 4-8 mm) (43). Some studies report 90% specificity for differentiating between benign or malignant lesions. The standard value that is utilized for effecting this differentiation is between 2 and 2.5 SUV.

Sensitivity will depend on tumor size as some report 25% for lesions <1 cm, 84% for tumors 1-2 cm, and 100% for lesions >5 cm [55].

Initial results show that sensitivity levels are approximately 93%, similar to those of Magnetic resonance imaging (MRI). These results convert this technique into a promising study, with applications in surgical planning, follow-up, and neoadjuvant treatment response and recurrence. However, there are some disadvantages related with cost and difficulty in radiopharmaceutical management techniques [55].

Positron-Emission Mammography (PEM)

This method integrates a conventional mammography system and 18 FDG emission images with better spatial resolution than PET and low doses of the radiopharmaceutical (3-5 milliCuries, mCi), short uptake time (approximately 10 min), and better compression than that of the mammography. This consists of a set of 12 images for each breast in CC and MLO projections, equivalent to those obtained by mammography. Narayanan et al. suggest the management of a lexicon similar to that utilized by the ACR for mammography, USG, and MR for reports [19].

In 2007, Schilling reported that PEM presented 92.3% sensitivity for detection of malignant lesions, while PET presented one of 39%, and MRI one of 89.7%.

At present, multiple radiopharmaceuticals that are different from FDG are being developed that will exert a great impact on the molecular biology of breast cancer. This in turn will permit, in the future, personalization of each patient's treatment and the improvement of his or her prognosis [44]. It is noteworthy that the calculation method of Standard uptake value (SUV) in this study is not standard. It is quantified by comparing the degree of uptake in the tumor in relation to breast or glandular tissue fat, which does not render it comparable with the method on which whole-body PET is based. However, values of <1.5 suggest benign lesions and values between 1.5 and 2, suspicious lesions [57].

In conclusion, PEM will be a more useful complement for conventional breast imaging, providing the following advantages: it permits the visualization of tumors of <1 cm; it does not depend on the presence of microcalcifications for the identification of ductal carcinoma *in situ;* and it aids in surgical planning, suggesting size of resection and/or probable re-excision of margins because it has the potential of accurately establishing disease extension (Figure 20).

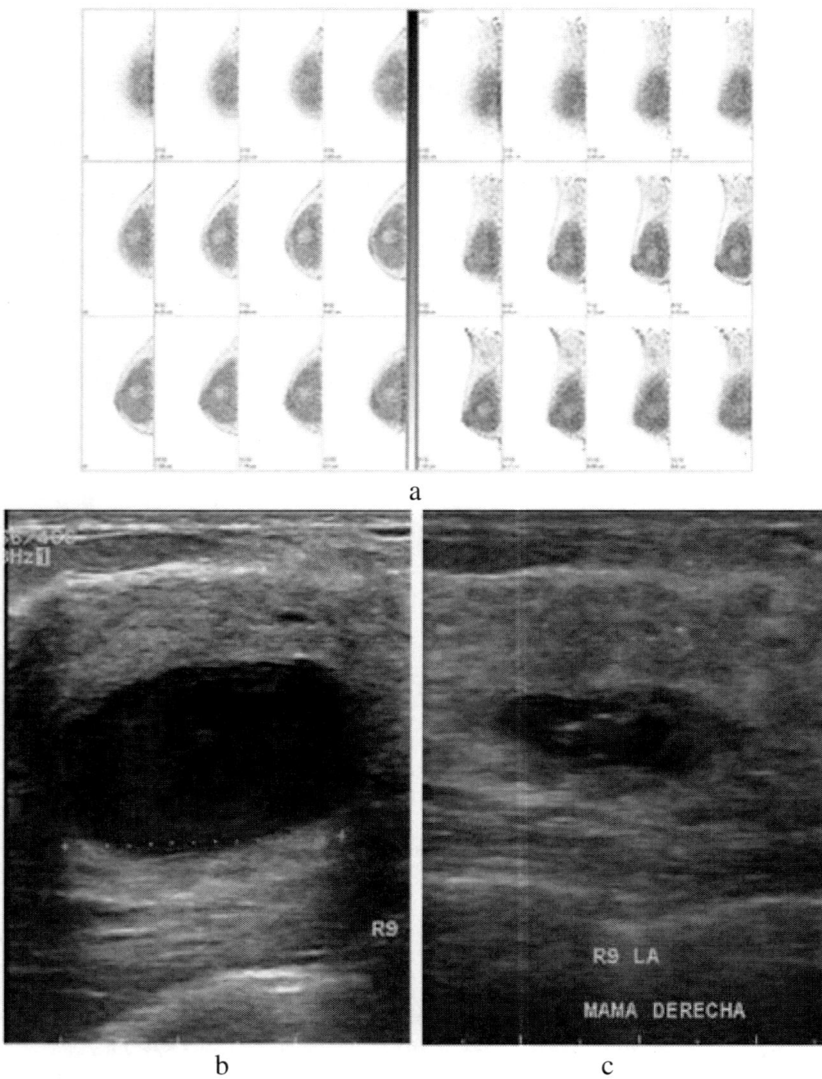

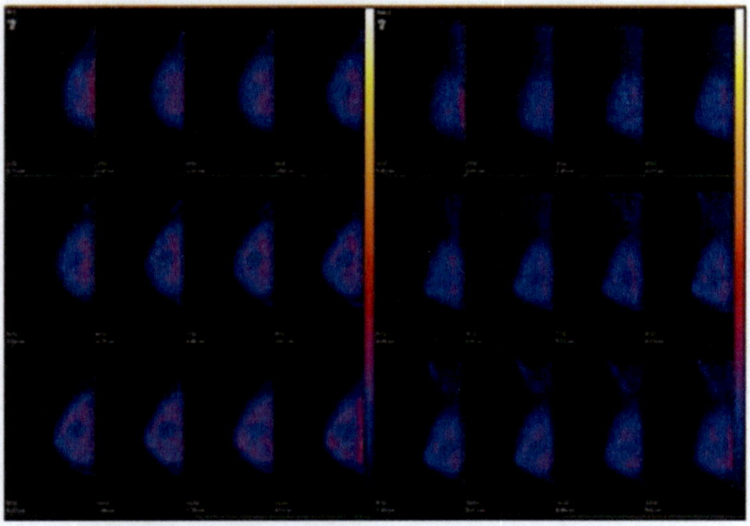

d

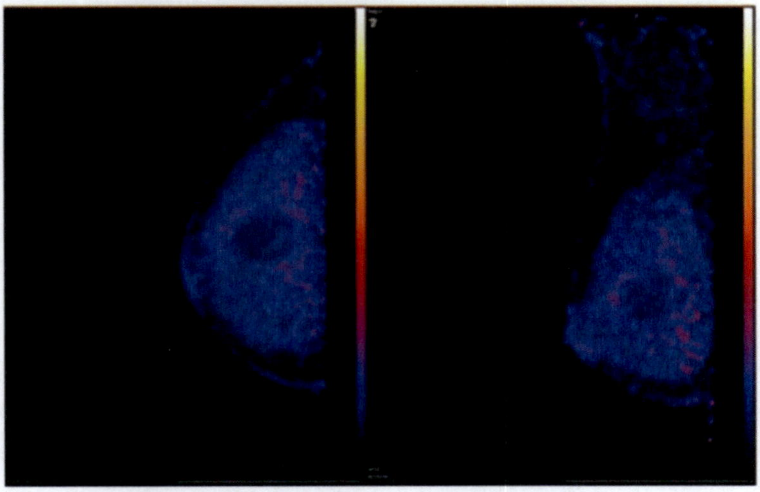

e

Figure 20. Female patient aged 35 years with breast USG and PEM with ^{18}f-FDG of right breast. Images on the left in upper and lower plane of PEM in Cranial-caudal (CC) and Mediolateral-oblique (MLO) projections of right breast, observing a nodular zone that well defines the absence of metabolism localized in the middle third and posterior of the Upper outside quadrant (UOQ) that correlated with nodule of anechoic oval morphology by USG compatible with simple cyst (upper right images).

The advances and continuous improvement of imaging technologies, such as digital mammography, Computer-aided diagnosis (CAD), Magnetic resonance imaging (MRI), and Positron-emission mammography (PEM), have improved sensitivity in the detection and diagnosis of breast cancer, but each modality provides greater benefits when it is utilized according to the individual characteristics of each patient, such as age, risk factors, and breast density. The clinic should be aware of the benefits and weaknesses of each of the technologies with the purpose of appropriately applying each of the latter [56].

Digital Infrared Thermal Imaging (DITI)

This is an accurate, quantifiable diagnostic technique, without contact, and noninvasive that permits the examiner visualization and quantification of changes in skin surface temperature with the use of angiogenesis-based infrared cameras.

Medical research has proven that DITI is a useful tool in the investigation and is effective in the diagnosis of breast cancer, nervous system disorders, metabolism, head and back problems, pain syndromes, arthritis, vascular disorders, and soft-tissue lesions, among others [44].

Kontos et al. (2012) carried out a study with thermography in 63 women who would later be submitted to surgery or excisional biopsy due to the clinical suspicion in mammary gland, finding 25% sensitivity and 85% specificity, 24% PPV, and 86% NPV. Despite its being a noninvasive and nonpainful method, its use is not recommended in the primary evaluation of symptomatic patients or for screening [58]. The US Federal Drug Administration (FDA) has authorized DITI as an auxiliary or additional tool for detecting breast cancer.

It has been widely utilized as a tool in the diagnosis of breast cancer, but has not had full acceptance due to the high incidence of false positives. The combination of mammography and thermography increases sensitivity to 93% and on possessing three methods (clinical examination, mammography and thermography), 98% sensitivity is considered [59] (Figure 21).

Other Techniques Exist during an Experimentation Phase, Such As

A. Photoacoustic tomography: method capable of detecting vascularized tumors of approximately 1-2 mm (47).
B. Magnetic resonance electrical impedance tomography (MREIT): novel modality that allows reconstructing images according to the electrical conductivity of the tissues, based on the greater conductivity of cancerous tissues. It can provide a new noninvasive method for detecting the first stages of cancer [60].
C. Laser mammotomography: usefulness in blood perfusion studies, oxygenation of tissues, and neovascularization of the brain, breasts, and limbs [44].
D. Diaphonography or transillumination: technique based on the use of infrared light on tissues which generates different grades of attenuation of light, degenerating shadows that can be processed to unfold as images. This modality produces a high number of false positives and negatives in relation to mammography and USG, accounting for its not having achieved great clinical acceptance [44].

Biopsy

When a patient is diagnosed with a breast lesion by clinical evaluation and/or by imaging studies, it is not always possible to determine its benign nature accurately, or there can be a suspicion of breast cancer. In such cases a cytological or histological biopsy becomes necessary (Figure 22).

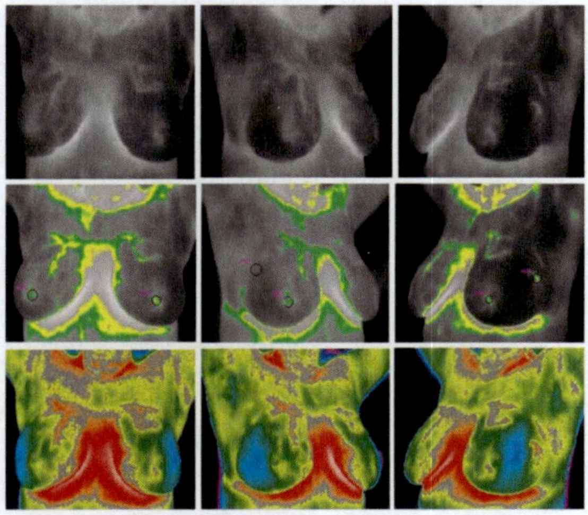

a

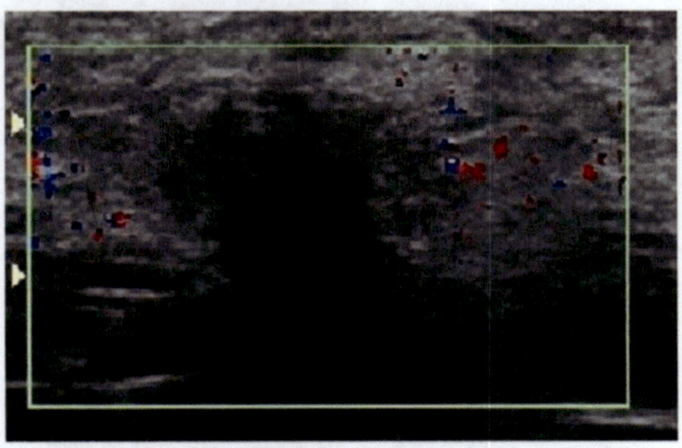

b

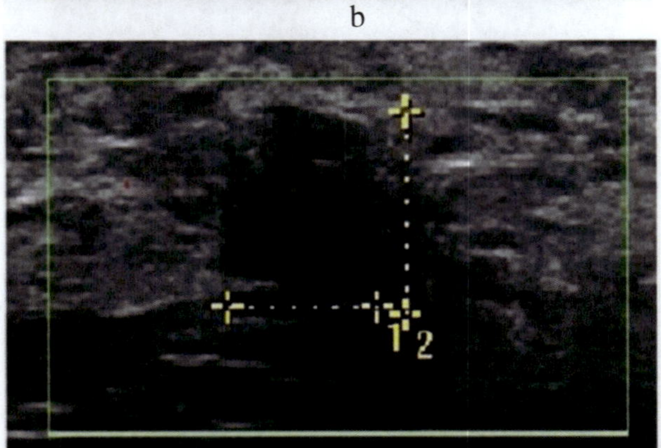

c

Histopathological report (HpR): fibrocystic changes with scarce glandular formations with cellular atypias. There is no radiological-thermographic diagnostic correlation in addition to the presence of atypias in the HpR. Proceeding to prior marked excision, obtaining as diagnosis (dx), Definitive infiltrating ductal carcinoma SBR 4(1-2-1) with component of low-grade carcinoma *in situ*. Tumor of 2 × 2 cm. Negative sentinel lymph node.

Figure 21. Patient aged 66 years with MG and breast USG BI-RADS category 5 in left breast by focal asymmetry on Upper outside quadrant (UOQ), which by USG corresponds to spiculated hypoechoic nodule <1 cm localized in r1. Prior to carrying out Tru-cut biopsy (bx), thermography is performed with a report of benign findings and bilateral thermographic activity.

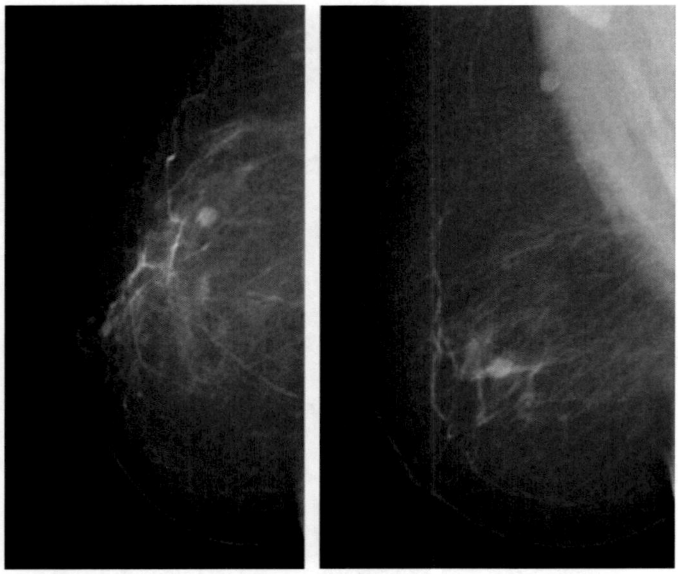

a

Figure 22. (a) Mammography in Mediolateral-oblique (MLO) and Cranial-caudal (CC) projections of right breast. Nodule identified of median percentage of density localized at the interline of the external quadrants. Its contours are irregular and partially defined without calcium deposits in its interior. Vascular calcification and presence of intramammary and axillary lymph node (tail of Spence) of benign appearance.

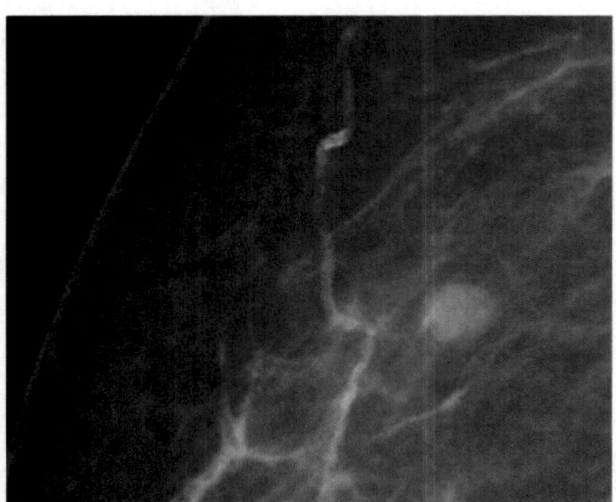

b

Figure 22. (b) Complementary mammographic projection. Magnification in right breast external quadrant. Characterization achieved of described nodule and its anterior border showing discrete spiculation.

Figure 22a-d Woman aged 47 years with antecedent of left mastectomy 3 years previous. Right breast screening mammography.

There are some benign breast lesions that become a diagnostic challenge, such as abscesses, hematomas, radial scars, postsurgical scars, diabetic mastopathy, focal fibrosis, sclerosing adenosis, granular cell tumor, extra-abdominal desmoid tumor, medial insertion of the major pectoral muscle, the sternal muscle and axillary adenopathies (due to HIV-associated infection, collagen-related vascular lesions, tuberculosis lesions, and bacterial lymphadenitis).

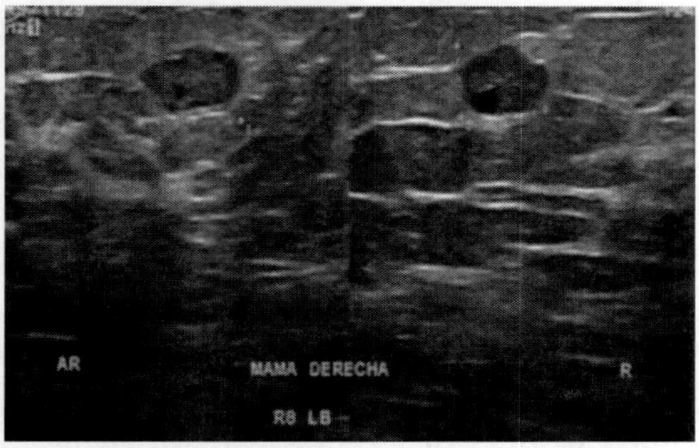

c

Figure 22. (c) Right breast USG with the presence of heterogeneous hypoechoic nodule, of lobulated contour and apparently defined, mixed echoes in its interior, without attenuation or posterior sonic reinforcement.

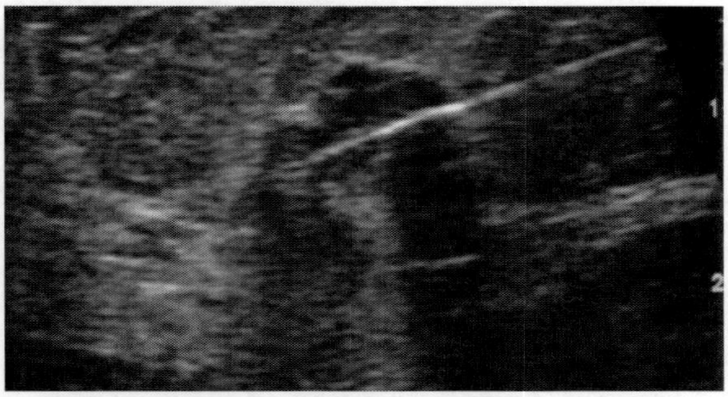

d

Histopathological report: Atypical ductal hyperplasia. Percutaneous needle localization for excisional breast biopsy. Histopathological report on excisional biopsy: High-grade ductal hyperplasia *in situ* with foci suggestive of invasion.

Figure 22. (d) Sonograph-guided and fine-needle biopsy of nodule in right breast. The described nodule is identified and the needle is at the center of the lesion.

It is of great importance to know the imagenological characteristics of these, as well as the patient's clinical antecedents, and frequently requires their confirmation through biopsy given that it is very difficult to differentiate these from malignant neoplasms of the breast [61].

At some clinical centers, there is a preference for performing fine-needle cytology as initial diagnosis. Despite its being a rapid method, it presents errors and limitations in the diagnosis [62].

Surgical diagnosis is the 'gold standard' for diagnosis; possessing as its main limitations its high cost, cosmetic damage, increase morbility and interference with the surgical procedure for cancer treatment. Therefore today it is not the initial method-of-choice in the diagnosis of breast cancer [63].

Imaging-guided percutaneous Core-needle biopsy (CNB) limits the previously mentioned potential problems. Whenever possible, CNB should be carried out under USG-guidance, avoiding ionizing radiation with comfort for the patient and visualization in real time.

The accuracy of CNB is very similar to that reported for excisional biopsy. Sensitivity is around 96%. The rate of false negatives is between 0 and 12% [64].

Although USG-guided CNB comprises an accurate diagnostic alternative, it is indispensable to possess radiological-pathological correlation and adequate follow-up of benign lesions in order to avoid an erroneous diagnosis.

High-risk lesions and ductal carcinoma *in situ* diagnosed by CNB require excision with the purpose of avoiding underestimation [65].

When the mammographic and pathological findings are discordant or when a high-risk lesion is found, this can be associated with a malignant tumor or with an invasive tumor [66].

Histological underestimation after a CNB (13.5%), especially in high-risk proliferative breast lesions (Figure 23) (radial scar, atypical lobular hyperplasia, lobular carcinoma *in situ*, and papillary lesions), requires excision of the lesion because in the particular case of lesions of risk. This means that these lesions can contain a cancer in some patients or can become cancer at some moment of the patient's life.

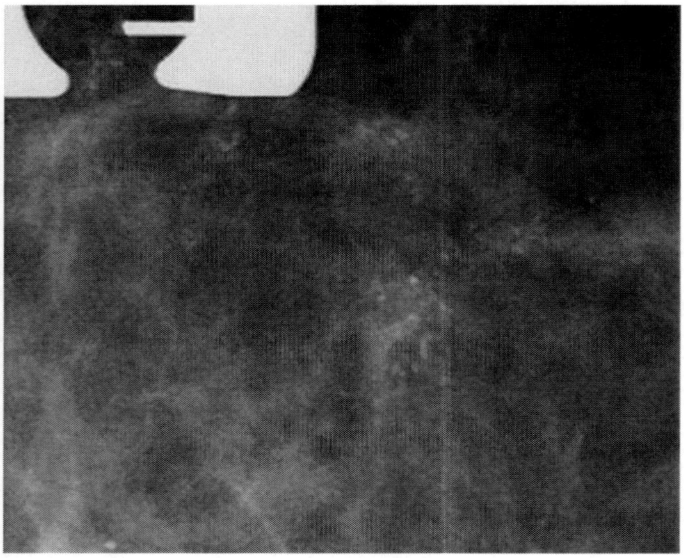

a

Histopathological report: Columnar cell hyperplasia with architectural and cytological atypia.

Figure 23. (a) Female aged 47 years, asymptomatic with detection mammography. a). Mammographic projection of localization for stereotactic-guided biopsy with Fine-needle aspiration (FNA). Very-low-density linear and ramified pleomorphic calcifications.

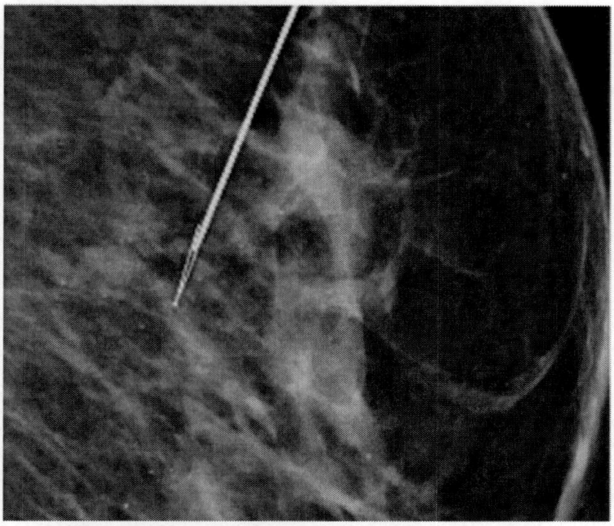

b

Figure 23. (b) Given the histopathological report, excisional biopsy was carried out with prior percutaneous hook wire marking. In the mammographic projection, the hook wire is localized at the center of the cluster of the calcium deposits described.

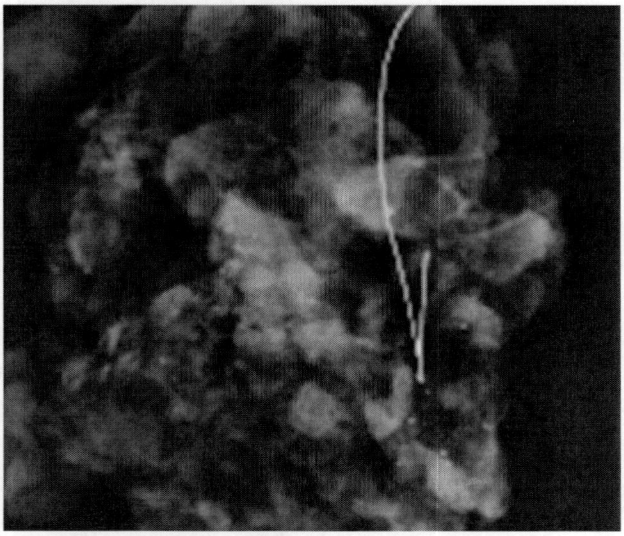

c

Histopathological result: Columnar cell hyperplasia with architectural atypia and cytology with multiple foci of high-grade ductal carcinoma. Intraductal papillomatosis.

Figure 23. (c) Control mammographic image of the divided surgical piece, observing the presence of the harpoon and calcium deposits very near the surgical border; thus, the surgical margins are amplified.

When there is low suspicion of malignancy on imaging and where adequate histological samples have been taken for the pathology report and where the final report does not show atypia, follow-up and close surveillance is recommended. There are multiple publications that recognize vacuum-assisted biopsy, and while it can diminish underestimation, in reality it cannot replace surgery in this group of lesions [67].

References

[1] Morrow, M. The evaluation of common breast problems. *Am. Fam. Physician.* 2000 Apr.15;61(8):2371-2378.

[2] American College of Radiology. Mammography. Breast Imaging Reporting and Data System, *Breast Imaging Atlas*, 4th ed. Reston, VA, US: American College of Radiology; 2003.

[3] Shapiro, S., Venet, W., Strax, P., Venet, L., Roeser, R. Ten- to fourteen-year effect of screening on breast cancer mortality. *J. Natl. Cancer Inst.* 1982;69(2):349-355.

[4] Tabár, L., Fagerberg, C. J., Gad, A., et al. Reduction in mortality from breast cancer after mass screening with mammography: randomised trial from the Breast Cancer Screening Working Group of the Swedish National Board of Health and Welfare. *Lancet.* 1985;1(8433):829-832.

[5] Tabár, L., Vitak, B., Chen, H. H., Yen, M. F., Duffy, S. W., Smith, R. A. Beyond randomized controlled trials: organized mammographic screening substantially reduces breast carcinoma mortality. *Cancer.* 2001;91(9):1724-1731.

[6] Tabár, L., Vitak, B., Chen, H. H., et al. The Swedish Two-County Trial twenty years later: updated mortality results and new insights from long-term follow-up. *Radiol. Clin. North Am.* 2000;38(4):625-651.

[7] Tabár, L., Vitak, B., Chen, T. H., et al. Swedish Two-County Trial: impact of mammographic screening on breast cancer mortality during 3 decades. *Radiology.* 2011;260(3):658-663.

[8] Bird, R. E., Wallace, T. W., Yankaskas, B. C. Analysis of cancers missed at screening mammography. *Radiology.* 1992;184(3):613-617.

[9] NCI-funded Breast Cancer Surveillance Consortium co-operative agreement, *"Performance Measures for 1,960,150 Screening Mammography Examinations from 2002 to 2006 by Age - based on BCSC data as of 2009."* November 15, 2011. (http:// breastscreening.cancer.gov/data/performance/screening/2009/perf_age.html).

[10] Kerlikowske, K., Grady, D., Barclay, J., Sickles, E. A., Ernster, V. Effect of age, breast density, and family history on the sensitivity of first screening mammography. *JAMA.* 1996;276:33-38.

[11] Humphrey, L. L., Helfand, M., Chan, B. K., Woolf, S. H. Breast cancer screening: a summary of the evidence for the US Preventive Services Task Force. *Ann. Intern. Med.* 2002;137(5 Part 1):347-360.

[12] Carney, P. A., Miglioretti, D. L., Yankaskas, B. C., et al. Individual and combined effects of age, breast density, and hormone replacement therapy use on the accuracy of screening mammography. *Ann. Intern. Med.* 2003;138(3):168-175.

[13] Pisano, E. D., Gatsonis, C., Hendrick, E., et al. Diagnostic performance of digital versus film mammography for breast-cancer screening. *NEJM.* 2005;353(17):1773-1783.

[14] Taourel, P., Merigeaud, S., Aubert, E., Millet, I., Curros Doyon, F., Lacroix, J., Prat, X., Pujol, J. Tomosynthesis: luxury or necessity? *J. Radiol.* 2009 Dec.;90(12):1813-1821.

[15] Zuley, M. L., Bandos, A. I., Ganott, M. A., Sumkin, J. H., Kelly, A. E., Catullo, V. J., Rathfon, G. Y., Lu, A. H., Gur, D. Digital breast tomosynthesis versus supplemental diagnostic mammographic views for evaluation of noncalcified breast lesions. *Radiology.* 2013 Jan.;266(1):89-95.

[16] Spangler, M. L., Zuley, M. L., Sumkin, J. H., Abrams, G., Ganott, M. A., Hakim, C., Perrin, R., Chough, D. M., Shah, R., Gur, D. Detection and classification of calcifications on digital breast tomosynthesis and 2D digital mammography: a comparison. *AJR Am. J. Roentgenol.* 2011 Feb.;196(2):320-324. doi: 10.2214/AJR.10. 4656.

[17] Luparia, A., Mariscotti, G., Durando, M., Ciatto, S., Bosco, D., Campanino, P. P., Castellano, I., Sapino, A., Gandini, G. Accuracy of tumour size assessment in the preoperative staging of breast cancer: comparison of digital mammography, tomosynthesis, ultrasound and MRI. *Radiol. Med.* 2013 Oct.;118(7):1119-1136.

[18] Chevalier del Rio, M. Nuevas tecnologías en mamografía y su impacto en los valores de dosis. *Radiología.* Dec. 2013. (http://dx.doi.org/10.1016/j.rx.2013.09.004).

[19] Skaane, P., Bandos, A. I., Guillén, R., Eben, E. R., Ekseth, U., Haakenaasen, U., Izadi, M., Jebsen, I., Jahr, G., Krager, M., Niklason, L. T., Hofvind, S., Gur, D. Mammography alone and digital mammography plus in a population based screening program. *Radiology*. 2013 Apr.;267(1):47-56.

[20] Lei, J., Yang, P., Zhang, L., Wang, Y., Yang, K. Diagnostic accuracy of digital breast tomosynthesis versus digital mammography for benign and malignant lesions in breasts: a meta-analysis. *Eur. Radiol.* 2013 Sep. 13.

[21] Thibault, F., Dromain, C., Breucq, C., Balleyguier, C. S., Malhaire, C., Steyaert, L., Tardivon, A., Baldan, E., Drevon, H. Digital breast tomosynthesis versus mammography and breast ultrasound: a multireader performance study. *Eur. Radiol.* 2013 Sep.;23(9):2441-2419.

[22] Stavros, T. A., Rapp, C. L., Parker, S. H. *Ecografía de Mama*. Edit. Marbán; 2006. pp. 1-107, 877-946.

[23] Jung Min Chang, Moon, W. K., Cho, N., Kim, S. J. Breast mass evaluation: factors influencing the quality of US elastography. *Radiology.* 2001 Apr.;259(1):59-64.

[24] Berg, W. A., Sechtin, A. G., Marques, H., Zhang, Z. Cystic breast masses and the ACRIN 6666 experience. *Radiol. Clin. North Am.* 2010 Sep.;48(5):931-987.

[25] Itoh, A., Ueno, E., Tohno, E., et al. Breast disease: clinical application of US elastography for diagnosis. *Radiology.* 2006;239(2):341-350.

[26] Cho, N., Moon, W. K., Cha, J. H., Kim, S. M., Han, B. K., Kim, E. K., Kim, M. H., Chung, S. Y., Choi, H. Y., Im, J. G. Differentiating benign from malignant solid breast masses: comparison of two-dimensional and three-dimensional US. *Radiology.* 2006 Jul.;240(1):26-32.

[27] Nunes, V., de Pace, S., Medicis, N. *Mama Diagnostico por Imagen*. Vol. 2. Editorial Amolca; 2010. pp. 453-504.

[28] Correira de Rocha, D., de Pace Bauab, S. *Tratado de Imagenología de la Mama*. 2ª. ed. Editorial Amolca; 2006. pp. 2-28.

[29] Joo Hee, Moon, W. K., Cho, N., Kim, S. M., Park, S. H., Han, B. K., Choe, Y. H., Park, J. M., Im, J. G. Characterization of benign and malignant solid breast masses: comparison of conventional US and tissue harmonic imaging. *Radiology*. 2007(1); 242: 63-69.

[30] Fernández Cid, A., Fernández Cid, M. *Mastología*. 2ª ed. Editorial Masson; 2006. pp. 489-511.

[31] Macura, K. J., Ouwerkerk, R., Jacobs, M. A., Bluemke, D. A. Patterns of enhancement on breast MR images: interpretation and imaging pitfalls. *RadioGraphics*. 2006;26: 1719-1734.

[32] American College of Radiology. *Breast imaging-reporting and data system (BI-RADS)*. 4th ed. Reston, VA, US: American College of Radiology; 2003.

[33] Camps Herrero, J. Resonancia magnética de mama: estado actual y aplicación clínica. *Radiología*. 2011;53(1):27-38.

[34] Agrawal, G., Min-Ying Su, Nalcioglu, O., Feig, S. A., Jeon-Hor Chen. Significance of breast lesion. Descriptors in the ACR BI-RADS MRI Lexicon. *Cancer*. 2009;115:1363-1380.

[35] Malich, A., Fischer, D. R., Wurdinger, S., et al. Potential MRI interpretation model: differentiation of benign from malignant breast masses. *AJR Am. J. Roentgenol*. 2005; 185:964-970.

[36] Tozaki, M., Fukuma, E. 1H MR spectroscopy and diffusion-weighted imaging of the breast: Are they useful tools for characterizing breast lesions before biopsy? *AJR*. 2009; 193:840-849.

[37] Erguvan-Dogan, B., Whitman, G. J., Kushwaha, A. C., Phelps, M. J., Dempsey, P. J. BI-RADS–MRI: a primer. *AJR*. 2006;187:152-160.

[38] El Khouli, R. E., Jacobs, M. A., Mezban, S. A., Peng Huang, Kamel, I. R., Macura, K. J., Bluemke, D. A. Diffusion-weighted imaging improves the diagnostic accuracy of conventional 3.0-T breast MR imaging. *Radiology*. 2010;256:63-74.

[39] Woodhams, R., Ramadan, S., Stanwell, P., Sakamoto, S., Hata, H., Ozaki, M., Kan, S., Inoue, Y. Diffusion-weighted imaging of the breast: principles and clinical applications *RadioGraphics*. 2011;31:1059-1084.

[40] Kim, J. K., Park, S. H., Lee, H. M., et al. *In vivo* 1H-MRS evaluation of malignant and benign breast diseases. *Breast*. 2003;12(3):179-182.

[41] Tse, G. M. K., Cheung, H. S., Lai-Man Pang, Chu, W. C. W., Law, B. K. B., Kung, F. Y. L., Yeung, D. K. W. Characterization of lesions of the breast with proton MR spectroscopy: comparison of carcinomas, benign lesions, and phyllodes tumors. *AJR*. 2003;181:1267-1272.

[42] Bartella, L., Wei Huang. Proton (1H) MR spectroscopy of the breast. *RadioGraphics*. 2007;27:241-252.

[43] Stoopen, M., García Mónaco, R., et al. Avances en diagnóstico por imágenes, mama. *Colegio Interamericano de Radiología (CIR)*. 2010;109-119.

[44] Wolbarst, A. B., Heende, W. R. Evolving and experimental technologies in medical imaging; *Radiology*. 2006 Jan.;238(1):16-39.

[45] Avril, N., Adler, L. P. F-18 fluorodeoxyglucose-positron emission tomography imaging for primary breast cancer and loco-regional staging. *Radiol. Clin. North Am.* 2007 Jul.; 45(4):645-657.

[46] Cheifetz, O., Haley, L. Secondary treatment for lymphedema, a breast cancer. *Can. Fam. Physician*. 2010;56:1277.

[47] Xia, W., Piras, D., van Hespen, J. C., van Veldhoven, S., Prins, C., van Leeuwen, T. G., Steenbergen, W., Manohar, S. An optimized ultrasound detector for photoacoustic breast tomography. *Med. Phys.* 2013 Mar.; 40(3):032901. doi: 10.1118/1.4792462.

[48] Jausoro, A. *Nuevas Técnicas de Diagnóstico por Imagen del Cancer de Mama: Mamografía Digital, Impedancia y Conductividad Eléctrica*. Vitoria-Gasteiz, España: Departamento de Sanidad, Gobierno Vasco; 2000.

[49] Raneta, O., Ondruš, D., Bella, V. Utilisation of electrical impedance tomography in breast cancer diagnosis. *Klinonkol.* 2012;25(1):36-41.

[50] Assenheimer, M., Laver-Moskovitz, O., Malonek, D., Manor, D., Nahaliel, U., Nitzan, R., Saad, A. The T-scan technology: electrical impedance as a diagnostic tool for breast cancer detection. *Physiol. Meas.* 2001;1. doi:10.1088/0967-3334/22/1/301.

[51] Sun Mi Kim, Park, J. M. Computed tomography of the breast, abnormal findings with mammographic and sonographic correlation. *J. Comp. Assist. Tomogr.* 2003;27(5):761-770.

[52] Kyoungkang, D., Kim, M. J., Jung, Y. S., Yim, H. Clinical application of multidetector row computed tomography in patient with breast cancer. *J. Comp. Assist. Tomogr.* 2008;32:583-598.

[53] Metz, C., et al. Incidental breast lesions on chest CT with ultrasound and mammographic correlation. *Contemp. Diagn. Radiol.* 2012;35(22):1-5.

[54] Narayanan, D., Madsen, K. S., Kalinyak, J. E., Berg, W. A. Interpretation of positron emission mammography: feature analysis and rates of malignancy. *AJR Am. J. Roentgenol.* 2011 Apr.;196(4):956-970.

[55] Páez, G., et al. Positron emission tomography: a new paradigm in cancer management. *Rev. Colomb. Cancerol.* 2007;11(1):5-12.

[56] Berman, C. G. Recent advances in breast-specific imaging. *Cancer Control*. Oct. 2007, 14:4.

[57] Schilling, K., et al. Positron emission mammography in breast cancer presurgical planning: comparisons with magnetic resonance imaging. *Eur. J. Nucl. Med. Mol. Imag.* 2011;38:23-36. doi: 10.1007/s00259-010-1588-9.

[58] Kontos, M., et al. Digital infrared thermal imaging (DITI) of breast lesions: sensitivity and specificity of detection of primary breast cancers. *Clin. Radiol.* 2011 Jun.;66(6): 536-539. doi: 10.1016/j.crad.2011.01.009.

[59] Eddie, Y., et al. Computer simulation in conjunction with medical thermography as an adjunct tool early detection of breast cancer. *BMC Cancer*. 2004:4:17.

[60] Sadleir, R. J., Sajib, S. Z., Kim, H. J., Kwon, O. I., Woo, E. J. Simulations and phantom evaluations of magnetic resonance electrical impedance tomography (MREIT) for breast cancer detection. *J. Magn. Reson.* 2013 May;230:40-49. doi: 10.1016/j.jmr.2013.01.009.

[61] Pojchamarnwiputh, S., Muttarak, M., Na-Chiangmai, W., Chaiwun, B. Benign breast tumors mimicking carcinoma at mammography. *Singapore Med. J.* 2007 Oct.;48(10): 958-968.

[62] Dennison, G., Anand, R., Makar, S. H., Pain, J. A. A prospective study of the use of fine-needle aspiration cytology and core biopsy in the diagnosis of breast cancer. *Breast J.* 2003;9:491-493.

[63] Ishman, J. E., Milikowski, C., Ramsinghani, R., Velásquez, M. V., Aviram, G. US-guided core-needle biopsy of the breast: how many specimens are necessary? *Radiology*. 2003;226:779-782.

[64] Schueller, G., Jaromi, S., Ponhold, L., et al. US-guided 14-gauge core-needle breast biopsy: results of a validation study in 1352 cases. *Radiology*. 2008;248:406-413.

[65] Londero, V., Zuiani, C., Furland, A., Nori, J., Bazzocchi, M. Role of ultrasound and sonographically guided core biopsy in the diagnostic evaluation of ductal carcinoma *in situ* (DCIS) of the breast. *Radiol. Med*. 2007;112:863-876.

[66] Rungruang, B., Kelley, J. L. 3rd. Benign breast diseases: epidemiology, evaluation, and management. *Clin. Obstet. Gynecol.* 2001 Mar.:54(1):110-124.

[67] Zuiani, C., Londero, V., Bestagno, A., Puglisi, F., Di Loreto, C., Bazzocchi, M. Proliferative high-risk lesions of the breast: contribution and limits of US guided core biopsy. *Radiol. Med.* 2005 Nov. Dec.;110(5-6):589-602.

In: Benign Disease of the Breast
Editors: J. de la Garza Salazar, C. Arce Salinas et al.
ISBN: 978-1-63321-624-2

Chapter 14

Benign Breast Diseases: Current Pathological and Molecular Concepts

Hector Aquiles Maldonado-Martinez, Victor Manuel Perez-Sanchez, Claudia Haydee Caro Sanchez, Paula Juarez-Sanchez and Abelardo Meneses-Garcia
Pathology Department
Instituto Nacional Cancerologia-Mexico, Mexico City, DF, Mexico

Abstract

BBD of the breast are much more common than malignant lesions. The spectrum of Benign breast disease (BBD) includes a large number of physiopathological lesions of the different components of the breast (epithelial, stromal, adipocytes, or vascular). Breast tissue is under a complex system of influence by systemic factors, particularly hormones, as well as a number of local factors. This interrelationship results in different clinical manifestations for which a clear-cut clinical and histopathological separation between the physiologic and pathologic changes may not be always possible. This situation has led to a great deal of confusion, particularly in certain entities, with different nomenclatures for the same lesion , and unfortunately for many of them, the lack of a unique, unequivocal and commonly accepted definition. In the academic field, the consequence of this situation has been that benign breast disorders have been the subject of a relatively few isolated and unconnected studies, frequently ignoring earlier related work. Hence, it is even more difficult, to find in the literature, complete and broad scope data concerning the mechanisms involved in the development of such disorders.

From a practical point of view, much of the interest in BBD focuses on its relationship with the subsequent development of carcinoma. Breast lesions that do not increase the risk of breast cancer should be distinguished from those that confer a small or a moderate increase in risk, and this stratification should be reflected in BBD classification.

Taking all of this into account, in this chapter, benign lesions of the breast are summarized to include: inflammatory lesions, fibroepithelial lesions, stromal lesions, benign epithelial proliferations/fibrocystic changes, and benign epithelial neoplasms.

Finally, the study of BBD with current molecular methodologies suffers from the same limitations stated previously. However some insight in the biology and classification of BBD has been gained through their application. Such evidence is of importance and is commented on each of the sections of this chapter when available.

Introduction

Benign breast diseases (BBD) include physiopathological disorders of the different components of the breast (epithelial, stromal, adipocytes, or vascular).

BBD of the breast are much more common than malignant lesions, although their true incidence is difficult to estimate [1,2]. In fact, they are at least 10 times more common than breast cancer in the West [3]. Up to 30% of women who suffer from BBD will require treatment at some time in their lives [4].

Broadly summarized, breast tissues are under a complex system of control by systemic factors, particularly hormones, acting through their respective receptors, as well as a number of local factors. These include paracrine hormones, released by one type of cell to influence the adjacent cells of similar or differing function, juxtacrine factors, situated on the surface of the producing cell to influence adjacent cells by direct contact, and autocrine hormones, which act on the same cell by intracellular or surface receptors. All of these hormones interact, as is true for systemic hormones, by influencing locally derived factors—cell adhesion-related proteins, as well as autocrine and paracrine hormones—to produce signal pathways that finally result in cell regulation and stimulation [5]. Estrogen mediates the development and elongation of ductal tissue, progesterone facilitates ductal branching and lobuloalveolar development, and prolactin regulates the production of milk protein. At puberty, estradiol and progesterone levels increase to initiate breast development. A complex tree-like structure results, comprising 5–10 primary milk ducts that originate at the nipple, 20–40 segmental ducts, and 10–100 subsegmental ducts, whose endpoints are glandular units denominated terminal-duct lobular units [6].

In the adult breast, cyclic changes occur during the menstrual cycle that result in an increased rate of cell proliferation during the luteal phase. An increase in breast size by up to 15% may occur during this phase. At menopause, the total number of lobules diminishes [7].

In women, adolescence, and in the mid-20s, the lobules and stroma in the breast may respond to hormonal stimuli in an exaggerated fashion with the development of single and multiple palpable fibroadenomas. In the third and fourth decades of life, the degree of diffuse palpable nodularity may increase. In histologic terms, this increase represents adenosis, that is, enhancement of the amount of normal lobular tissue. The stroma may also undergo hypertrophy, resulting in palpable areas of ill-defined fullness, frequently in the axillary tail. In women between the middle of the fourth decade of life and menopause, glandular tissue may undergo further hypertrophy in association with an increase in stromal tissue. A higher prevalence of cyst formation is associated with late menopause [8]. At the morphological level, the result of the interaction along time of the breast tissue with systemic and local influence of the milieu is what we call "fibrocystic changes". This designation is now preferred over previous ones, since in up to 50–60% percent of women without breast disease, this histologic pattern may be evident. Also, the term "fibrocystic changes" implies that women with lumpy breasts or breasts with nondiscrete nodules do not have breast disease. The fibrocystic changes detected clinically entail no increased risk of breast cancer.

Classification of BBD is controversial due to lack of clear-cut clinical and histopathological separation between physiological and pathological changes in the breast [9]. Much of the controversy concerns the relationship between BBD and the subsequent development of carcinoma.

There have been two classifications of great importance in the understanding and classification of the benign disorders. The first represents the histological classification based on the work of Dupont and Page [10], which was adopted at the consensus meeting of the College of American Pathologists (CAP) in 1985. The concept of benign epithelial proliferative disease encompasses histological characteristics of BBD that have a cancerous potential. Derived from this fact, three groups of BBD have been specified; nonproliferative lesions; proliferative lesions without atypia, and lesions with atypical hyperplasia [5].

The second corresponds to the Aberrations of Normal Development and Involution (ANDI) classification of BBD, which provides an overall framework for benign conditions of the breast encompassing both pathogenesis and degree of abnormality. This classification states that breasts are under endocrine control and show a wide range of appearances during reproductive life. However, some authors think that the ANDI classification causes confusion due to a lack of clarity in distinguishing between normal physiological and pathologic changes [5].

Table 1. Classification of benign breast lesions on histologic examination, stratified by associated risk of invasive carcinoma*

Risk	Proliferation	Histologic Findings
No increase	Minimal	Fibrocystic changes; simple fibroadenoma; and miscellaneous (lobular hyperplasia, juvenile hypertrophy, and stromalhyperplasia)
		Benign tumors: hamartoma, lipoma, benign phyllodes tumor, solitary papilloma, neurofibroma, giant adenoma, and adenomyoepithelioma
		Traumatic lesions: hematoma, fat necrosis, and lesions caused by penetration by a foreign body
		Infections: granuloma and mastitis
		Sarcoidosis
		Metaplasia: squamous and apocrine
		Diabetic mastopathy
Small increase (Relative risk [RR] <2.0)	Proliferative without atypia	Usual ductal hyperplasia, complex fibroadenoma, papilloma or papillomatosis, radial scar, and blunt duct adenosis
Moderate increase(RR, >2.0)	Proliferative with atypia	Atypical ductal hyperplasia and atypical lobular hyperplasia

In a practical classification, breast lesions that do not increase the risk of breast cancer should be distinguished from those that confer a small increase in risk (Relative risk [RR], <2.0) or a moderate increase (RR, >2.0) [7] (Table 1).

Unlike invasive breast cancer, the molecular alterations that comprise the underpinnings of the development and progression of breast cancer precursors are less well established. The main reasons for the limited molecular data on these lesions are their limited size and the limited availability of fresh/frozen samples, coupled with the challenges posed for modeling cancer progression from *in situ* to invasive stages using *in vitro* or *in vivo* models [11]. Numerous proliferative lesions of the breast have been reported as associated with increased risk of breast cancer development, either in the same or in the contralateral breast. Some of these risk indicators have been shown to be clonal, neoplastic proliferations and to have histological, immunohistochemical, and molecular features identical to those of matched invasive breast cancers, either synchronous or metachronous. Lesions that comply with these criteria are considered breast cancer precursors. Given that the chances of one of these precursors progressing to invasive breast cancer rarely, if ever, equate to 100%; these lesions are, in fact, nonobligate precursors. [11].

In this chapter, benign lesions of the breast are summarized to include inflammatory lesions, fibroepithelial tumors, mesenchymal tumors, myoepithelial-epithelial/myoepithelial lesions, benign epithelial proliferations/fibrocystic changes, benign epithelial neoplasms, and tumors of the nipple.

Inflammatory and Related Lesions

A variety of inflammatory and reactive changes can be observed in the breast. While some of these changes are the result of infectious agents, others do not have a well-understood etiology and may represent local reaction to a systemic disease or a localized immune response to an as-yet-unidentified antigen. For the majority of the entities reviewed in this section, and as previously stated, the central physiopathological events appear to be those derived from the immune response and inflammatory reaction. In some others, however, the cause lies in mechanical or other factors for which one of the main effect responses will be an inflammatory reaction.

Acute Mastitis

Acute mastitis usually occurs during the first 3 months postpartum (75–95% of cases) in breastfeeding mothers. Also known as puerperal or lactating mastitis, this disorder comprises a cellulitis of the interlobular connective tissue within the mammary gland, which can result in abscess formation and septicemia.

Because of wide differences in breastfeeding methods and support, which are intimately related with acute mastitis risk factors, its incidence varies widely across populations: 9.5–33% in lactating women [12], or 7.8–11.1 cases per 10,000 deliveries [13]. Acute mastitis presents with equally frequency in the right and left breasts [14].

Risk factors fall into two general categories: a) improper nursing technique, leading to milk stasis and cracks or fissures of the nipple, which may facilitate the entrance of microorganisms through the skin, and b) stress and sleep deprivation, both of which lower the mother's immune status and inhibit milk flow, thus causing engorgement [15]. Breastfeeding baby factors, such as attachment difficulties for breastfeeding, cleft palate, or short frenulum, are also important [12].

The diagnosis of acute mastitis is based on clinical symptoms and signs indicating inflammation, usually accompanied by acute systemic reaction. Patients typically present with localized, unilateral breast tenderness and erythema, fever, malaise, fatigue, body aches, and headache [12]. The role of milk culture is controversial. Because lactating mastitis is a process of subcutaneous cellulitis and the detection of pathogens in breast milk may not always be possible: positive cultures can result from normal bacterial colonization, and negative cultures do not rule out mastitis [15–18]. Even more so, although with a reduced frequency in healthy breastfeeding mothers, the same microorganisms are recovered from patients with mastitis and control women [19]. Culture has been recommended when the infection is severe, unusual, or hospital-acquired, or if it fails to respond to 2 days of treatment with appropriate antibiotics [12]. Despite the low level of evidence due to the low number of studies, study limitations, and culture difficulties, *Staphylococus aureus* is considered the main infectious agent. Some authors also report *Staphylococus epidermidis*, Group B *Streptococci*, or some Gram-negative bacteria as other possible infectious agents [19–21], with coagulase-negative *Staphylococcus* possibly being even more important than *Staphylococcus aureus* [20].

Because diagnosis is made on a clinical basis, there is little information about histopathological data and its role, if any, in the diagnosis and management of acute mastitis. Its role is only marginal and limited, mainly in the cytological examination of fluid from abscess drainage. The findings in such cases are thick cellular smears, with acute inflammation with or without fat necrosis, macrophages, multinucleated giant cells, and cell debris [21]. In the rare occurrence of surgical treatment with resection, the histological appearance of specimens from these lesions depends on the chronicity of the process, varying from acute inflammation that may be accompanied by focal necrosis, to organized chronic abscesses [22].

Because the duration of symptoms before starting treatment is found to be the only independent risk factor for abscess development, early diagnosis and early management of mastitis is of value [23]. However, there is little consensus on the type or duration of antibiotic therapy and when to begin antibiotics. Breast emptying with frequent nursing or manual pumping and starting empirical antibiotic therapy appears to be the most appropriate approach [12,23,24]. When puerperal mastitis-associated abscess occurs, incision and drainage are usually recommended; however, suitable patients assessed by ultrasonography can also be treated without surgery by needle aspiration and antibiotics, with excellent cosmetic results [21,15,12].

In contrast to acute lactating mastitis, nonpuerperal acute mastitis usually corresponds to abscess formation and infection, due to a variety of distinct inflammatory breast disorders, such as granulomatous mastitis [15,25], duct ectasia [26], complications of surgery or trauma, or autoimmune disease-related mastitis. The microorganism spectrum differs from that of acute puerperal mastitis, although *Staphylococci* are also the main pathogens [21]. Treatment should be with abscess drainage, either through Ultrasound (US)-directed needle aspiration or surgical incision. The possibility of associated carcinoma should be ruled out in these cases [21].

Plasma Cell Mastitis/Mammary Duct Ectasia

Mammary duct ectasia and periductal mastitis are two morphological aspects of a distinctive clinical entity that can mimic invasive carcinoma [15] and that continue to be considered separate entities by some authors [22,27]. The main differences upon which such a distinction rests are its association with tobacco consumption, age at presentation, natural history of the lesions (single events vs. previous clinical symptoms), and histopathological findings. Some of these disparities have been explained as two different stages of the same pathological process in which the initial clinical manifestations, at an earlier age, would correspond mainly to inflammatory changes (plasma cell mastitis, also called periductal mastitis). Accordingly, later stages, at a more advanced age, would manifest as chronic reparative changes (mammary duct ectasia). Conflicting results have been found in relation to natural history [27,28], while tobacco consumption appears to be related only with periductal mastitis [27,29]. Further studies should help clarify the uncertainties regarding the singularity or inter-relationships of the main elements- dilated ducts, periductal inflammation, bacterial infection, and nipple retraction. In the meantime, we present here the data corresponding to these two conditions under the concept of two stages of the same entity.

Plasma cell mastitis/mammary duct ectasia is an infrequent disease comprising 1–2% of symptomatic breast conditions [30]. It primarily affects middle-aged to elderly parous women, who usually present with nipple discharge and palpable subareolar mass with or without inflammation; some other less frequent symptoms include noncyclical mastalgia, nipple inversion or retraction, subareolar abscess, mammary fistula, or axillary lymph nodes [15,30,26]. Late stages, with predominance of duct ectasia, are usually asymptomatic, and the lesion is detected mammographically due to microcalcifications [15].

The pathogenesis and the etiology of the disease continue to be debated. Smoking has been implicated as an etiologic factor, particularly in early stages, in young women with inflammatory component (plasma cell mastitis) [27,29]. While bacteria can be isolated in cases with abscess, they also appear to play some role in cases without abscess but with inflammation [30,31]. In support of the two-stage concept of this entity, some authors have proposed inflammatory duct damage as the cause leading to duct dilatation [32].

The most important histological features in the early inflammatory stage are a marked, diffuse, plasma cell infiltrate surrounding the ducts (Figure 1), as well as some lobules, with lymphocytes and neutrophils variably present but not in sufficient numbers to obscure the plasmacytic reaction. A histiocytic reaction, sometimes with granulomatous features to desquamated epithelium and lipid material in the ducts, is responsible for areas that appear grossly to be xanthomatous or comedo-like [33].

In the late stage, dilatation of major ducts in the subareolar region dominate the histological picture; the ducts contain eosinophilic, granular secretions and foamy histiocytes within both the duct epithelium and the lumen [15]. The inspissated luminal secretions may undergo calcification [15]. Inflammatory reaction is less abundant but still present. Lymphocytes and smaller numbers of plasma cells, neutrophils, and histiocytes are found circumferentially throughout the thickness of the dilated ducts and in the periductal stroma. Eventually, the duct epithelium becomes atrophic, flat, and inconspicuous, and the duct becomes encased in a thick laminated rim of fibrosis and hyperelastosis that leads to mural thickening [22]. In some instances, the sclerotic process includes actively proliferating granulation tissue and hyperelastosis, which narrows and may totally occlude the ducts [22].

The latter configuration has been termed mastitis obliterans [34]. Occasionally, a more intense periductal reaction resulting in abscess formation may result from disruption of ducts and discharge of stasis material into the surrounding tissue [32].

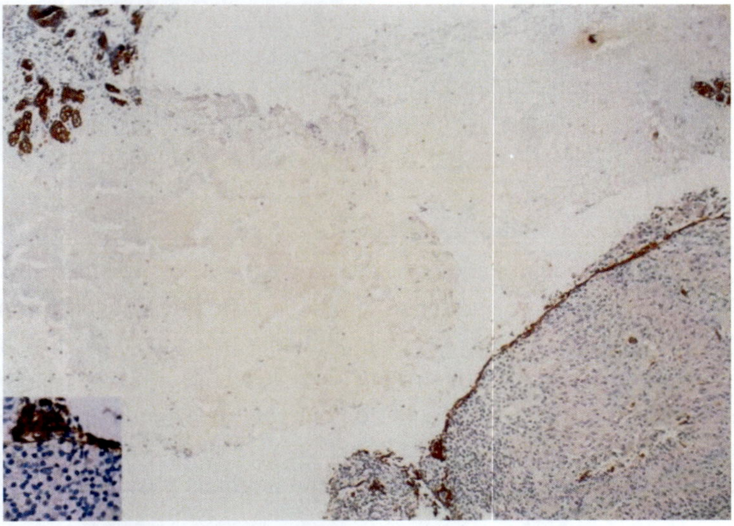

Figure 1. Ductal ectasia/Plasma cell mastitis. Abundant inflamation with numerous plasma cells (Inset) underneath the epithelium of a fragmented specimen from a patient with ductal ectasia/plasma cell mastitis. Inflammatory reaction affecting the ducts may obscure the epithelium linning them, cytokeratin immunoreaction makes evident the epithelial lining (100X).

Treatment in symptomatic cases with evident inflammatory component includes antibiotic therapy; surgery with excision of the central mammary tissue and larger ducts has also been employed, particularly for cases with abscess or fistula [36,26,35]. In the late stage, particularly if asymptomatic, mammary duct ectasia generally does not require surgery and should be managed conservatively [37]. There is no evidence in the literature indicating that mammary duct ectasia is associated with an increased risk for breast cancer. In some patients, clinical presentation and mammographic findings may suggest malignancy, and biopsy may be required to exclude it [15].

Granulomatous Mastitis

Granulomatous reactions resulting from an infectious etiology, foreign material, or systemic autoimmune diseases such as sarcoidosis and Wegener's granulomatosis can involve the breast. Identification of the etiology requires microbiologic and immunologic testing, in addition to histopathological evaluation. In addition, in some other entities as plasma cell mastitis/mammary duct ectasia or fat necrosis, a subset of cases may develop chronic granulomatous inflammatory reaction, although not as a characteristic feature. In cases with infectious etiology, different types of organisms have been reported to cause granulomatous mastitis, the most important of these being *Mycobacterium tuberculosis* and *Corynebacterium* spp. [15,33,38].

Tuberculous Mastitis

Tuberculosis of the breast is a very rare disease. However, both clinical and radiological features of tuberculous mastitis are not diagnostic and can easily be confused with either breast cancer or pyogenic breast abscess as diagnosed by clinicians.

Bearing in mind the fact that traveling from one place to another in the global world has been increasing and that the prognosis for complete cure with appropriate antituberculous drug therapy is excellent, this entity should also be taken into consideration. Definitive diagnosis of the disease is based on identification of typical histological features under microscopy or detection of tubercle bacilli with mycobacterial culture [39].

Idiopathic granulomatous mastitis (IGM)

IGM is a lobule-centered granulomatous lesion without an identifiable etiology. This diagnosis can be made only on the presence of such a histopathological pattern of response after excluding other possible causes of granulomatous lesions. IGM has been described worldwide in all races, the majority of patients with IGM are at child-bearing age, and the process is usually unilateral and involving more than one breast quadrant [40]. Because of its association with breastfeeding [25], an autoimmune localized response to retained and extravasated fat and protein-rich secretions in the duct has been postulated [15].

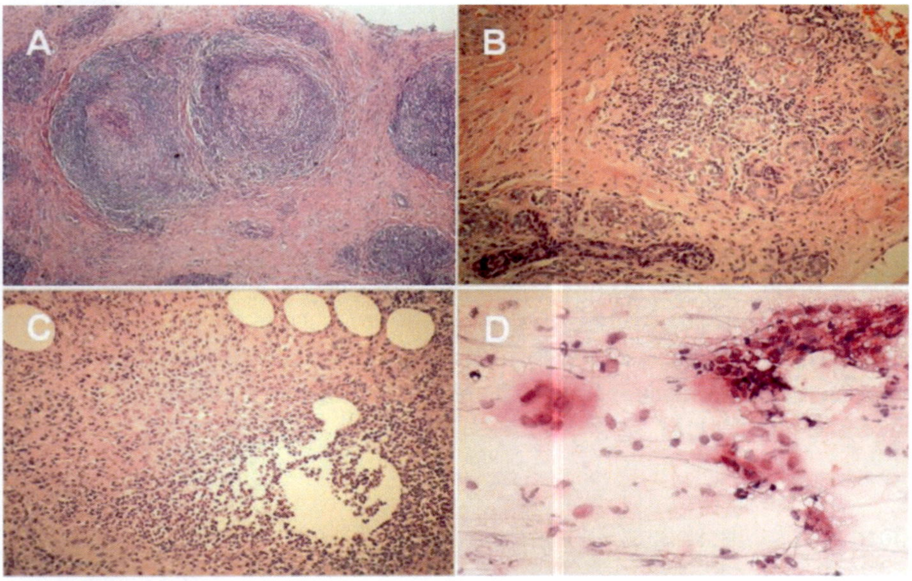

Figure2. Granulomatous mastitis. Evident granulomas in a breast tissue core (A 40X HE), with predominant lobular involvement, sparing ducts (B 200X HE). Microabscess formation is a common feature(C200X HE). Fine needle aspiration biopsy shows numerous epitelioidhistiocytes and multinucleated giant cells (D400X HE).

However, despite this association and some others, such as hormonal contraception and smoking [40], the etiology of the disease remains largely unknown [41]. Histologically, the characteristic features are chronic non-caseating granulomatous inflammation centered on mammary lobules, frequently with multinucleated giant cells and microabscess formation [40, 42]. Another frequent feature is the presence of clear lipoid spaces, particularly in necrotic foci [25] (Figure 2). No standard treatment has been defined. While some series solely describe clinical observation, others have used steroids or antibiotics. Some authors propose complete surgical resection whenever possible as the recommended therapy [15]. The persistence, recurrence, and complications such as abscess formation, fistulae, and chronic suppuration are encountered in about 16–50% of cases; thus, long-term follow-up is necessary in these patients [25,41,43].

Fibroepithelial Tumors

Fibroepithelial lesions are a heterogeneous group of entities, some neoplastic and others hyperplastic, with the common presence of glandular and stromal components, which currently include conventional Fibroadenoma (FA), myxoid fibroadenoma, the fibroadenoma variant, Phyllodes tumor (PT), hamartoma, and Pseudoangiomatous stromal hyperplasia (PASH). In the latter entity, some pathologists would not usually consider fibroepithelial lesion, but PASH can create a well-defined nodule containing both stroma and glands, resembling both FA and PT.

Fibroadenoma (FA)

Fibroadenoma accounts for the vast majority of benign breast tumors. Clinically, FA usually occurs in younger women, aged 20–30 years, but may also be observed in postmenopausal-age groups. They are slow-growing tumors, <3 cm in size, except for rare giant fibroadenomas. The overall risk of developing breast carcinoma in patients with a history of fibroadenoma is low, ranging from 1.5–2.6-fold compared with control patients in different studies, and it may be higher in women with a familial history of breast cancer or in women carrying the *BRCA1* gene mutation, justifying excision of complex fibroadenoma in women at high risk for developing cancer. The incidence of carcinoma arising within a fibroadenoma is reported to be from 0.1–0.3%. Although ductal and lobular carcinomas *insitu* occur with equal frequency, the majority of invasive carcinomas are reported to be lobular-type [44–47].

FA on gross examination, and appears to be well. Circumscribed and firm in consistency, with a white tan-to-gray homogenous, smooth-cut surface (Figure 3).

Microscopically, fibroadenomas show biphasic growth with ductal and stromal proliferation; the latter may exhibit a predominant intracannalicular or pericannalicular growth pattern with varying degrees of cellularity. Histological stromal patterns in fibroadenoma include diffuse myxoid change, hyalinization, and increased cellularity, as in cellular fibroadenoma; less frequently, foci of smooth muscle differentiation may be observed in fibroadenoma, in addition to other stromal alterations such as foci of pseudoangiomatous stromal hyperplasia [48].

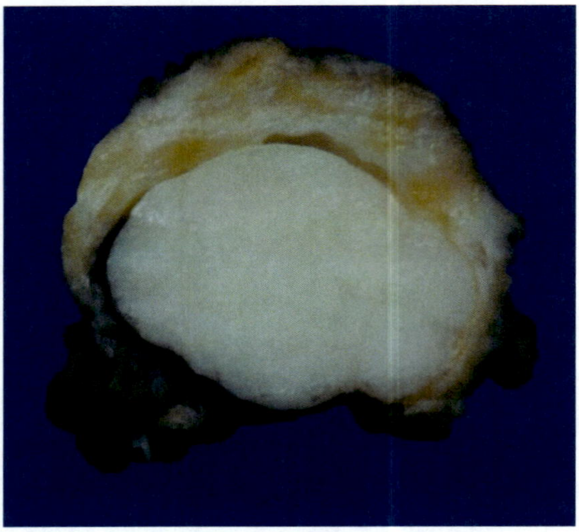

Figure 3. Macroscopy of fibroadenoma, tumor well circumscribed, white, homogenous, smooth-cut surface.

These stromal variations are important to keep in mind when evaluating such lesions in small Core-needle biopsy (CNB) because myxoid stroma may at times mimic colloid (mucinous) carcinoma, especially in fragmented biopsies. Cellular fibroadenoma with intracannalicular growth pattern can closely mimic benign PT. The distinction is based on overall, diffuse stromal cellularity, which is sometimes accentuated around epithelial clefts in PT. In CNB specimens, this distinction can be challenging, but it is critical because of the different behavior and clinical management for these two entities. In such cases, surgical excision for better classification is recommended.

Epithelial alterations within fibroadenoma include squamous and apocrine metaplasia and various degrees of hyperplasia, including atypical ductal and lobular hyperplasia.

Giant fibroadenoma (GFA)

GFA accounts for 0.5–2% of all cases of fibroadenomas [49] and is more frequent in young and Black patients. This subtype is characterized by its large size and rapid growth [49]. Giant breast tumors are rapidly growing breast masses with diameters exceeding 5 cm and/or weights of >500 gr [50–53]. They rarely grow to immense proportions, resulting in congestion and ulceration of skin by centrifugal pressure. Such an enlargement of the breast can be due to giant fibroadenoma, cystosarcoma, PT, or virginal hypertrophy, which occur in that order of frequency [50].

Myxoid fibroadenoma (MFA)

MFA consist of distorted glands embedded in fibrous connective tissue that contains abundant pale, blue-gray extracellular matrix.

MFA tend to arise in women in the fifth or sixth decade of life, but also arise in younger women. Mammography does not appear to detect MFA as consistently as it discloses conventional MFA; thus, many MFA present as palpable masses or as lesions detected by Magnetic resonance imaging (RMI) but are not observed on a mammogram. MFA occurs in the familial condition Carney syndrome, which comprises cardiac and cutaneous myxomas, melanocytic schwannomas, pigmented cutaneous lesions, and proliferations of endocrine tissues. The majority of patients with MFA do not present the remaining lesions associated with Carney syndrome [54, 55].

Macroscopic examination shows a well-defined nodule, sometimes lobulated, that is composed of tissue often described as mucoid, shiny, or translucent.

Accumulation of myxoid material in the specialized stromal compartment, dissection of myxoid material into the stroma, and distortion of the entrapped glands in irregular patterns characterize MFA. Conventional FA with especially myxoid stroma display a proliferation of fibroblasts not observed in MFA. The glands do not show apocrine metaplasia or adenosis in conventional FA.

PT with myxoid stroma usually form obvious fronds, and other regions of the tumor demonstrate proliferation of stromal cells. On CNB, myxoid stroma may at times mimic colloid (mucinous) carcinoma, especially in fragmented biopsies [56].

Cellular fibroadenoma (CFA)

CFA is conventional FA with highly cellular, homogeneous stroma, but there is no atypia or mitosis. Cellular fibroadenoma with intracanalicular growth pattern can closely mimic benign phyllodes. The distinction is based on overall, diffuse stromal cellularity, which is sometimes accentuated around epithelial clefts in the PT [48]. In CNB specimens, this distinction can be challenging, but it is critical because of the different behavior and clinical management for these two entities. In such cases, surgical excision for better classification is recommended.

Juvenile fibroadenoma (JFA)

JFA is a rare, distinctive type of fibroepithelial tumor that is observed most commonly, but not exclusively, in adolescent girls. This entity is characterized by extracellular matrix that typically consists of collagen rather than myxoid ground substances. The stromal cells grow in a pericannalicular pattern instead of in the intracannalicular configuration. The ductal epithelium usually displays florid, conventional ductal hyperplasia.

Complex fibroadenoma (CFA)

In 1994, Dupont et al. introduced the term “complex fibroadenoma“, and it is applied if any of the following features are present:

1. Cysts >3 mm in diameter
2. Sclerosing adenosis
3. Epithelial calcifications
4. Papillary apocrine change.

Patients with CFA have a 3-fold higher likelihood of developing invasive breast cancer than women without such tumors [44].

Fibroadenoma with multinucleated stromal giant cells

A very rare histological finding is the presence of multinucleated giant cells throughout the stroma of a benign fibroadenoma. Cells of this type, which are more commonly found incidentally within the interlobular stroma of breast tissue, are benign and should not be mistaken for malignant cells on microscopic examination.

Unfortunately, lack of awareness of this pathological entity can lead to diagnostic confusion among pathologists, resulting in multinucleate giant cells being mistaken for highly mitotic cells and consequently, the fibroadenoma being mistaken for a malignant lesion. This may have serious implications for subsequent management of the patient. The presence of this unusual cell type in the stroma does not alter the prognosis of the otherwise benign lesion [57].

Immunohistochemistry of FA

The stromal component shows vimentin and focal Sm-actin expression, but does not show Ck5/14. The majority of fibroadenomas express the progesterone receptor, whereas the estrogen receptor is expressed in a minority of tumors [58–60]. The estrogen receptor is mainly confined to the epithelial component, whereas the progesterone receptor is located in both the epithelial and stromal compartments [58,61,62].

It appears that the levels of sex hormone receptors in fibroadenoma tissue vary during the menstrual cycle. CD34 and bcl-2 staining is more abundant in the stroma of fibroadenoma than in normal breast [63].

Immunohistochemical evaluation of the MIB1 index can discriminate between the majority of fibroadenomas and PT. The distinction between fibroadenoma with high MIB1 index and benign PT remains problematic [64].

Genetics of FA

Cytogenetic studies of fibroadenomas show that 10–40% of tumors appear to display clonal chromosomal aberrations [65–67]. The majority of authors were unable to assign a specific abnormality to fibroadenomas, i.e., no preferential involvement of a chromosomal region or specific breakpoint has been recorded. A study found that the majority (84%) of fibroadenomas is characterized by 6q alterations [68]. Because a similar high frequency of 6q alterations is found in premalignant lesions and in carcinomas of the breast, the authors conclude that genes located on 6q are among the earliest events in the pathogenesis of cancer.

Phyllodes Tumor

On gross examination, Phyllodes tumor (PT) is also as well-delineated and circumscribed as fibroadenoma, but the cut surface exhibits cleft-like spaces with interspersed nodular stromal growth, and the color varies from tan-to-yellowish gray (Figure 4).

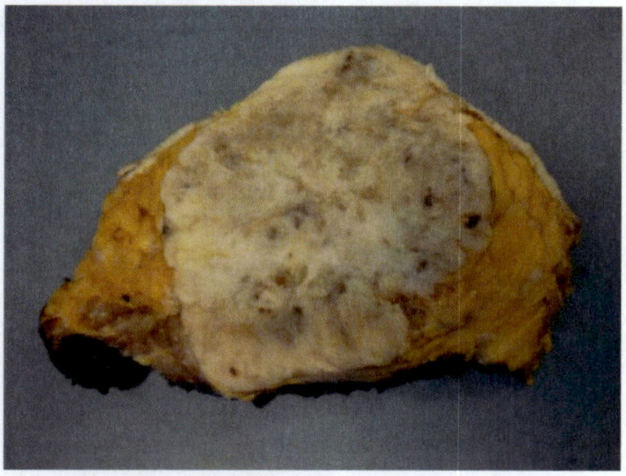

Figure 4. Macroscopy of phyllodes tumor with cleft-like spaces, interspersed nodular stromal growth, white to gray color change.

Large tumors may show areas of hemorrhage and necrosis, and malignant PT may have a fleshy, sarcoma-like cut surface that is softer in consistency than that of a fibroadenoma or benign PT. Histologically, PT are classified into different grades to predict their prognosis and clinical behavior by the World Health Organization [69]. These include benign, borderline, and malignant PT based on histological parameters including stromal cellularity, nuclear atypia, and degree of pleomorphism, mitotic activity, tumor margin/border (pushing or infiltrative), and stromal overgrowth. In a recent study by Tan et al. [70], only three histological features (cellular Atypia, Mitosis, and Overgrowth of Stroma) and surgical margins (together denominated "the AMOS criteria''), but not stromal hypercellularity or tumor border, were independent predictive factors of clinical behavior in PT (Figure 5). There are significant differences in the treatment modalities between PT and fibroadenomas. The mainstay of treatment for PT is surgical resection with wide margins, whereas close follow-up or enucleation is acceptable for the treatment of fibroadenomas. The local recurrence rate of PT is 10–18%, with negative and positive resection margins, respectively [71]. In one study, a higher local recurrence rate was also associated with marked stromal proliferation and necrosis, but not with tumor grade [71]. However, association of local recurrence rate with tumor grade was observed in other studies, showing that recurrence occurred in 8–10% of benign, in 14–20% of borderline, and in 29–50% of malignant PT [70,72]. In addition to its tendency toward local recurrence, PT have a malignant potential and are capable of systemic spread. Overall, 9–27% of malignant PT can metastasize to distant organs through the lymphovascular route and are associated with increased risk of mortality [72–74]. Benign PT may transform into a higher grade and recur as borderline or malignant PT.

Immunohistochemistry

Epithelial cell layers show Ck5/14 and Ck8/18/19 positivity, and Carcinoembryonic antigen (CEA) immunoreactivity is present in the majority of phyllodes tumors [75]. Expression of Estrogen receptors (ER) and Progesterone receptors (PR) in the epithelial cells of Phyllodes tumors (PT) has been shown as increased compared with that in normal breast epithelium. Further, an inverse relationship between epithelial PR and ER expression and degree of malignancy was found [76]. Stromal expression of PR and ER is uncommon observed. PR appears to be expressed more frequently in PT as compared with ER [76].

Expression of the androgen receptor appears to be low [76], although others have concluded the complete opposite.

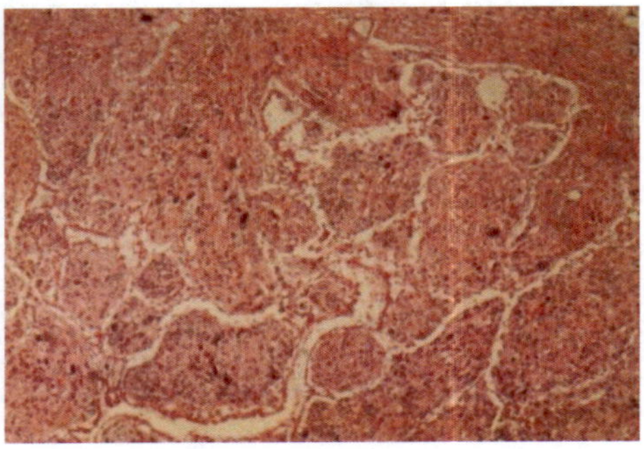

Figure 5. Microscopy of phyllodes tumor with stromal overgrowth showing marked nuclear pleomorphism (200 X HE).

The basic immunoreaction of the stroma is with vimentin; depending on the metaplasias present, additional markers are expressed such as Sm-actin in myoid differentiation [77–79]. In contrast with malignant adenomyoepithelial tumors, PT are Ck5/14-negative; thus, this may aid in distinguishing difficult cases.

Excess perivascular deposition of type IV collagen has especially been observed in the stroma of malignant PT, and tenascin is more diffusely present in the stroma of PT than in that of normal breast and fibroadenomas.

Ki67 expression is used for recording PT and possesses prognostic value.

P53 accumulation is more often observed in borderline and malignant tumors, is associated with increased proliferation, and has exhibited prognostic value in some studies. The stromal component of PT displays an increasing level of cell cycle deregulation with higher tumor grade. On the other hand, cell cycle aberrations are not found in the epithelial compartment.

CD34 and bcl-2 staining in stroma is more conspicuous than in normal breast and tends to be decreased adjacent to the epithelium in contrast with the normal breast. CD34 was observed as more frequent in benign than in malignant PT. C-kit (CD117) and Sm-actin are more frequent in the stroma of malignant PT [80]. Likewise, Sawyer et al. found stromal c-kit and c-myc expression more frequently in malignant PT [81].

Genetics

No allelic loss of 3p was found in one study [82]. However, another study found that 10 of 42 PT showed allelic imbalances in one or more markers on 3p and 14 of 46 on chromosome 1q. Five tumors had changes in both the epithelium and stroma, and eight tumors had changes only detectable in stroma and eight changes in the epithelium only. Three tumors exhibited low-level microsatellite instability in the epithelium, but not in the stroma. The authors raise the possibility that in some PT, the epithelium may be neoplastic [84].

Cytogenetic studies have uncovered complex and varying karyotypic changes in benign and malignant PT[83–85]. The gain of 1q and structural changes of10q emerged as frequent chromosomal changes in one study [86]. Mutations in the juxtamembrane region of the proto-oncogene c-kit (CD117) have been found in two malignant PT [80].

Mutation of p53 has been found occasionally as well [87]. In a study applying comparative genomic hybridization [88]. PT showed no evidence of genomic amplification, but frequent changes comprised gain of 1q (7/18) and loss of 3p (6/18), followed by gain of 7q (4/18) and loss of 6q (4/18) and 3q (3/18). Gain of 1q material was significantly associated with histologically defined stromal overgrowth. All cases with gain of 1q and without 1p gain had a clinical history of recurrence; therefore, gain of 1q might be an indicator of local aggressiveness, thus requiring more radical treatment. A study confirmed that gain of 1q is frequently found, but the authors failed to relate this with clinical behavior or tumor grade [89].

Role of Core Needle Biopsy in Diagnosis of Fibroepithelial Tumors

Our practice has demonstrated that a cellular fibroepithelial lesion on Core-needle needle biopsy (CNB) that is difficult to classify as fibroadenoma or PT is best completely excised for accurate classification.

Hamartoma of the Breast (HB)

Diagnosis of hamartoma is defined as a tumor-forming mass of disorganized but well-differentiated cells autochthonous to their place of origin. Hamartoma of the breast (HB) was first described in 1971 by Arrigoni et al. in a study of 10 patients whose breast tumors clinically and grossly resembled fibroadenomas [90]. HB are also known as fibroadenolipomas, lipofibroadenomas, or adenolipomas. The reported incidence of BH is 0.7% of all benign breast tumors in females [91]. Macroscopically, HB are typically well-demarcated, occasionally lobulated lesions with smooth contours and an often rubbery grayish-white to yellow cut surface, resembling a fibroadenoma or a lipoma [15,92]. There are two common variants of HB: adenolipoma and chondrolipoma [93]. Macroscopically, adenolipomas are soft, circumscribed, occasionally lobulated masses bordered by a thin fibrous pseudocapsule. The cut surface reveals a variegated pattern of fat and fibrous breast parenchyma. Lesions with abundant fat resemble lipomas [93].

Originally, Arrigoni et al. macroscopically identified 'mammary glandular tissue with a prominent lobular arrangement, fibrous stroma and fat in variable proportions'[90]. However, later studies have observed fibrocystic disease, adenolipoma, fibroadenoma with fat and fibroadenoma with lobules, and heterologous elements identified as cartilage and smooth muscle [94]. This circumscribed mass of breast tissue may reveal fibrocystic and atrophic changes; pseudoangiomatous hyperplasia is frequently observed [95]. The lesion generates the impression of a 'breast within a breast' [92,95]. Usual ductal hyperplasia, apocrine metaplasia, calcification, stromal giant cells, and adenosis may be associated with hamartoma [92]. Lobular intraepithelial neoplasms and ductal intraepithelial neoplasms have also been reported to occur within the hamartoma in rare cases [92,96]. Although hamartomas are usually benign, malignant transformation is possible [91,97]. Myoid (muscular) hamartoma of the breast is a rare, benign tumor-forming lesion composed of differentiated mammary glandular and stromal structures, fatty tissue, and areas of smooth muscle [98,99].

Mesenchymal Tumors

Pseudoangiomatous Stromal Hyperplasia (PASH)

Pseudoangiomatous stromal hyperplasia, more commonly known as PASH, is a well-recognized but poorly understood entity. Pseudoangiomatous stromal hyperplasia was first described by Vuitch et al. [100] in 1986. The authors described the histological and ultrastructural features of tumorous PASH in nine premenopausal women. Each of these presented with a palpable, unilateral breast mass. There had been 150 reported cases of PASH up to 2010, while recently, in 2012, a series of 24 cases was reported [101]. Pseudoangiomatous stromal hyperplasia (PASH) is a benign myofibroblastic proliferation of nonspecialized mammary stroma. Its clinicopathological spectrum ranges from incidental, microscopic foci to clinically and mammographically evident breast masses [15, 102].

Originally, hormonal stimulation (particularly with progesterone) was suggested in the etiology of PASH, on the basis of observations that this disease is most frequently observed in premenopausal women or in elderly women taking hormone-replacement therapy, and because similar histological findings are observed in normal mammary stroma during the luteal phase of the menstrual cycle. However, the lesion has since been found in men and in women not taking hormone therapy, and only a small percentage of PASH cases are positive for ER or for PR [15].

Macroscopic features

The size of tumorous PASH ranges from 0.6–12 cm [103–105]. The largest size of tumorous PASH documented in the literature is that of 20 cm in a 36-year-old woman [106]. Grossly, the excised mass is round-to-oval, well-circumscribed, and rubbery. The outer surface is usually smooth and unencapsulated. The cut surface reveals a homogenous solid lesion with gray-white color and occasional cysts [107]. Necrosis and hemorrhage are rare [108] (Figure 6).

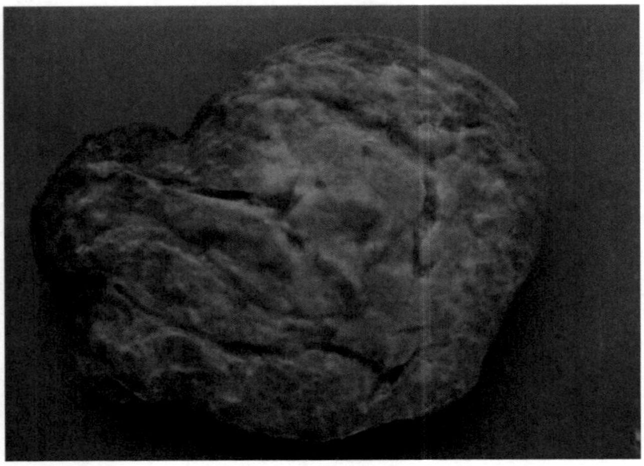

Figure 6. Macroscopy of PASH, the cut surface is homogenous, white, fibroustissue, with slit-like cystic spaces.

Microscopic features

PASH can occur as an isolated mass or may coexist with any breast lesion. Ibrahim et al. [103] demonstrated at least one microscopic focus of PASH in 23% (46 of 200) of consecutive breast biopsies and mastectomy specimens. PASH has been described in the breast stroma in association with gynecomastia in males. Milanezi et al. [104] described the presence of PASH in 23.8% of breast biopsies from men with gynecomastia. The typical lesion is composed of complex anastomosing, slit-like empty spaces in a dense, fibrous stroma. These spaces are lined with a discontinuous layer of flat, benign spindle cells. No mitosis or nuclear atypia is observed. The stromal hyperplasia may involve perilobular as well as intralobular stroma (Figure 7).

Expansion of intralobular stroma may cause effacement of terminal duct–lobular units. Isolated involvement of perilobular stroma is more common than that of intralobular stroma. The epithelium of lobules and ducts may be unremarkable or may show ductal hyperplasia and/or apocrine metaplasia. Proliferative lesions show variable cellularity, ranging from increased stromal cellularity to formation of cellular bundles in a dense collagenous background, and these lesions show a lobulocentric growth pattern. In proliferative lesions, the stromal cells may be larger and have conspicuous nuclei, but cytologic atypia is rare [103]. More florid areas may exhibit the formation of fascicles with obliteration of spaces. The cells in fascicular foci show oval nuclei with indistinct cytoplasmic borders. One study [104] found the fascicular growth pattern in 31% of cases of tumorous PASH.

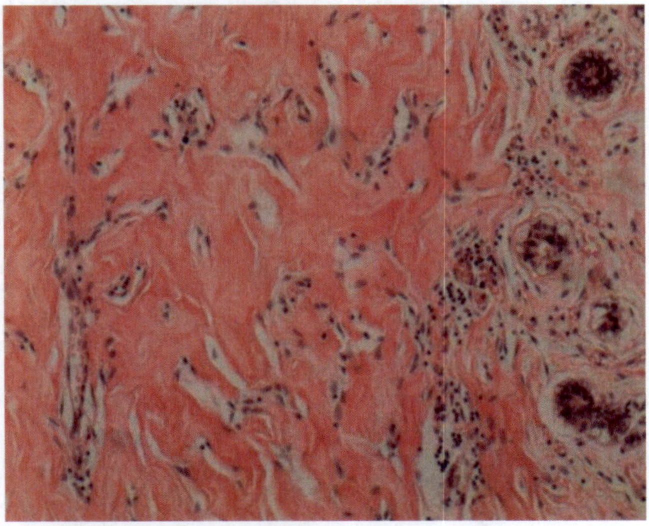

Figure 7. Microscopy of PASH with slit-like empty spaces in a dense, fibrous stroma. These spaces are lined with a discontinuous layer of flat, benign spindle cells (200X HE).

Immunohistochemistry

The spindle cells that line the slit-like spaces are positive for myofibroblastic markers including CD34, vimentin, and SMA [100,103]. They are negative for cytokeratin, S100, and endothelial markers, such as von Willebrand factor antigen and CD31. Fascicular areas may show expression of desmin. Stromal cells show nuclear positivity for PR (Figure 8). ER expression may be present but is focal and may exhibit faint positivity.

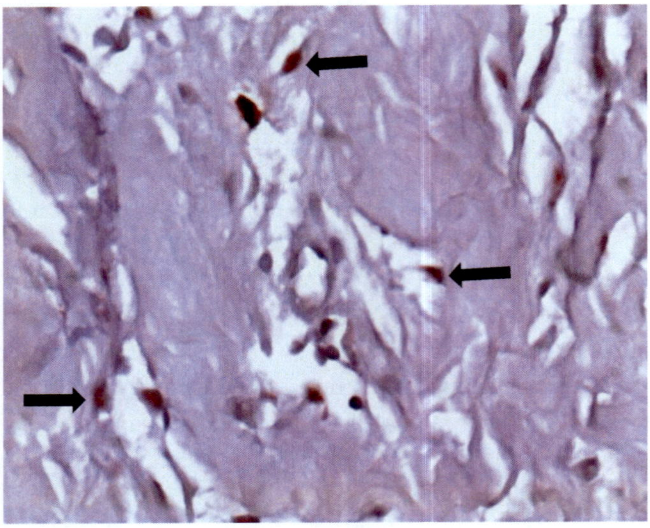

Figure 8. Microscopy of PASH, the nuclei of the stromal cells are positive for progesterone receptor (400X).

Ultrastructural studies

Spindle cells exhibit myofibroblastic features. The spaces are lined by an incomplete layer of spindle cells with elongated cytoplasmic processes [100]. The cytoplasm contains well-developed Golgi apparatus and abundant endoplasmic reticulum. The cells are joined together by rudimentary cell junctions or, very occasionally, tight junctions [108].

Differential diagnosis

Differential diagnoses include low-grade angiosarcoma, myofibroblastoma, fibroadenoma, and mammary hamartoma. The most important differential diagnosis is angiosarcoma, and it must be distinguished from PASH.

Myofibroblastoma (MFB)

MFB of the breast is an unusual benign tumor that belongs to the family of the "benign spindle-cell tumors of the mammary stroma." Myofibroblastoma was originally described as an atypical tumor occurring in the breast of adult males. Subsequently, several cases were also documented in females, suggesting that it can occur in both genders [109–116]. It is likely that the increased incidence of MFB reported in women in the last two decades could be due to increased mammographic screening. Currently, it is believed that MFB occurs mainly in older men and in postmenopausal women, and there are sporadic cases in adolescents and young adults.

Tumor size ranges from a few mm to 11 cm. On gross examination, MFB is generally a well-circumscribed, firm, and rubbery, unencapsulated, round-to-oval mass. The cut surface usually reveals a solid lesion, with a smooth or lobulated external surface, pale white-to-grayish in color, with an avariably whorling appearance [109,115,117,118].

Classic-type MFB comprises an unencapsulated tumor with a pushing, lobulated growth pattern that is usually composed of bland-looking, slender, spindle-shaped cells, closely packed in short, straight, haphazardly intersecting fascicles or in clusters of cohesive cells, interrupted by thick, hyalinized collagen bundles. A minority of cases may exhibit invasive margins with a small amount of entrapped mammary glands (Figure 9).

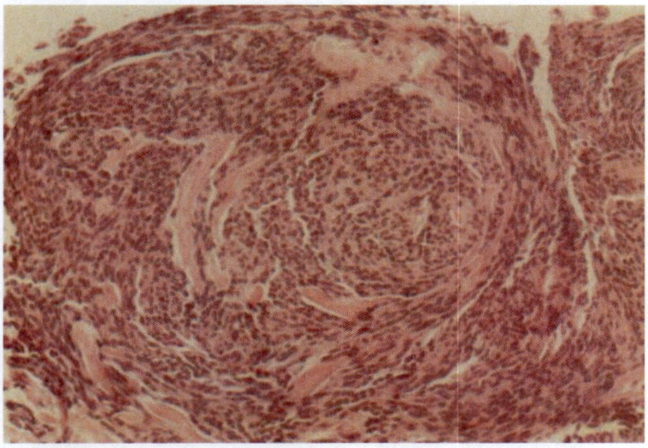

Figure 9. Microscopy of myofibroblastoma showing a fascicular tumor with pushing borders and numerous interspersed thick, hyalinized collagen bundles (200X HE).

Morphologic variant

Cellular MFB. The cellular variant is characterized by a dense proliferation of spindle-shaped cells, focally showing nuclear overlapping, with interspersed hyalinized collagen bundles, usually smaller in size than those observed in classic MFB.

Infiltrating MFB. Occasionally, MFB exhibits an extensive invasive growth pattern, entrapping fat and/or mammary glandular structures.

Epithelioid MFB. Classic-type MFB may contain a minority of epithelioid cells [110,111,114,119–121], either isolated or in clusters. Accordingly, the term "epithelioid MFB" should be reserved for tumors composed exclusively or predominantly (50%) of epithelioid cells [110, 112,119].

Deciduoid-like MFB. Recently, one case of MFB composed exclusively of cells that adopt a deciduoid-like morphology, was recognized [122].

Lipomatous MFB. Myofibroblastoma may contain a variable amount, with generally small foci, of adipose tissue as integral tumor component [109,110,117,119,123–125]. However, only cases that are composed predominantly (75% of the entire neoplasm) of a fatty component merit the name of lipomatous MFB.

Collagenized/Fibrous MFB. In the collagenized or fibrous variant, the spindle cells are distributed in a highly collagenous stroma [110, 111].

Myxoid MFB. Focal myxoid stromal changes are common in MFB.

Immunohistochemistry

The majority of cases of MFB are typically positive for vimentin, desmin, and CD34 [109–111,113,114,124,126]. Immunoreactivity for smooth muscle actin, bcl-2, and CD99 is frequently obtained, but with a variable extension in different tumors and also in indifferent areas of the same tumor [109–111,123,127]. CD68 and Factor XIIIa immunoreactivity has been documented in some cases [111,121]. Recently, MFB has also been shown to be positive for CD10.66A, and focal expression of h-caldesmon can be encountered in scattered cells

[125]. Interestingly, the majority of MFB are stained with ER, PR, and Androgen receptors (AR) [109,110,128,129]. Cytokeratins, EMA, S100 protein, HMB-45, and c-kit (CD117) are consistently negative. Immunohistochemistry is extremely helpful in confirming the diagnosis of unusual variants of MFB (Figures 10-13).

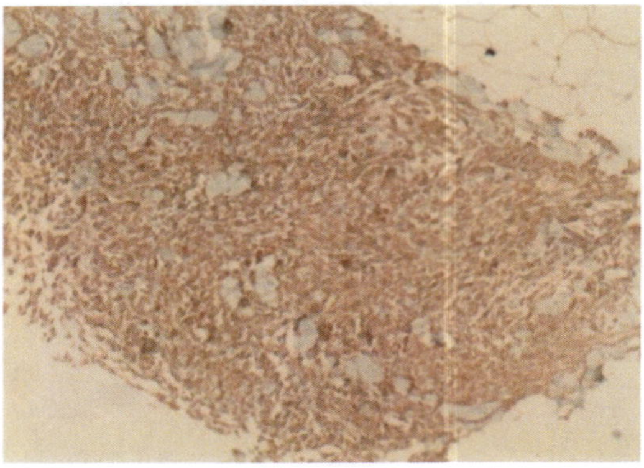

Figure 10. Microscopy of myofibroblastoma, the cells are positive for bcl-2 (200X).

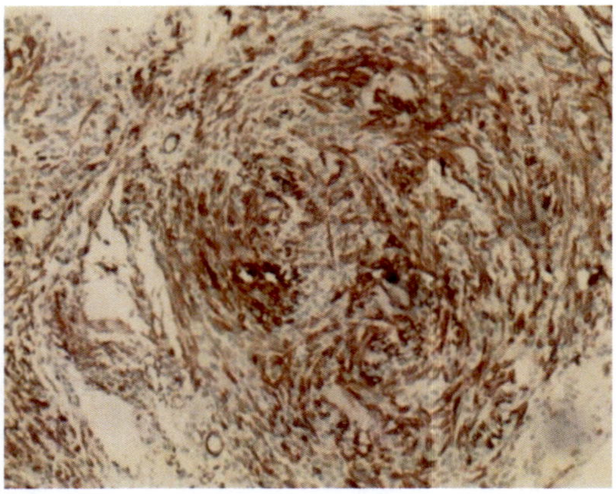

Figure 11. Microscopy of myofibroblastoma, the cells are positive for α-smooth muscle actin (200X).

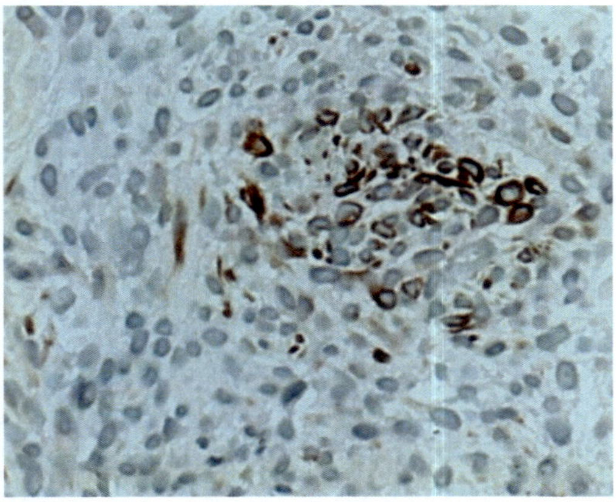

Figure 12. Microscopy of myofibroblastoma, the cells are positive for desmin (400X).

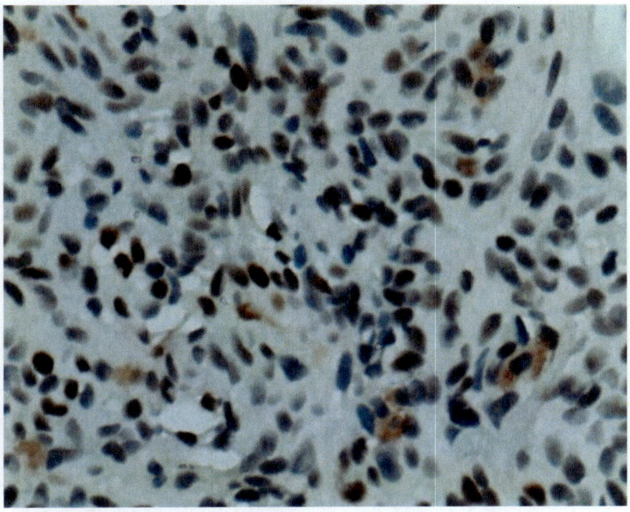

Figure 13. Microscopy of myofibroblastoma the nuclei of the cells are positive for progesterone receptors (200X).

Ultrastructural studies

The electron microscopy studies that have been performed in some cases of MFB have shown a variable admixture of undifferentiated mesenchymal cells, fibroblasts, myofibroblasts, and smooth muscle cells. Generally, myofibroblasts are represented by cells rich in organelles (rough endoplasmatic reticulum, Golgi complexes) and contain bundles of myofilaments forming focal densities, basal lamina-like materials focally identified in association with the cell surface. Fibronectin fibrils (the so-called microtendons) and fibronexus junctions, features typically observed in myofibroblasts isolated from granulation tissue of healing wounds, only take place occasionally.

Genetics

Some cytogenetic studies have shown chromosome13 rearrangements associated with the loss of the13q14 chromosomal region in two cases of mammary MFB[130] and in one case of soft-tissue MFB [131]; in one of the mammary cases, partial loss of 16q.7 was also documented.

Granular Cell Tumor

Granular cell tumor (GCT) was first reported by Abrikossoff [132] and was denominated granular cell myoblastoma. One of its characteristics is that eosinophilic granules are contained in the cytoplasm of the cells. Because the positive rates for S-100 protein and neuronspecific enolase are high, it is currently thought that this tumor originates from Schwann cells. They account for an incidence of 0.5% among soft-tissue tumors, and it has been reported that GCT primarily occur in or beneath the skin, or in the submucosa of the tongue, throat, chest wall, or bronchus.

This tumor is commonly found in those aged 10–50 years and is occurs more often in women than in men [133–137]. Granular cell tumor of the breast is largely a disease affecting women, as with other breast malignancies, but it has also been described in men, accounting for 6.6% of granular cell tumor of the breast [138]. Sonobe and colleagues [139] divided malignant granular cell tumors into two groups: those that are malignant both histologically and clinically, and those that are histologically benign but clinically malignant. The most common metastasis sites of malignant granular cell tumor are the lymph nodes, followed by the lungs.

About 2% of all granular cell tumor cases are malignant [139–142]. A tumor 3 cm or less in size can be regarded as benign. However, if the tumor grows rapidly and forms an ulcer, malignancy should be suspected.

From a histopathological perspective, Fanburg-Smith and colleagues [141] proposed the following six criteria for determining whether a tumor is malignant or not: 1) the presence of necrosis; 2) the emergence of spindle cells; 3) a vacuolar nucleus with an enlarged nuclear body; 4) an increase in nuclear division (two mitoses/10HPF); 5) an increase in the nucleoplasmic ratio, and 6) polymorphism. If none of these diagnostic criteria are met, the tumor is considered to be benign. If one or two criteria are met, the tumor is considered to be atypical, and if three or more criteria are met, the tumor is considered to be malignant.

Although there is considerable overlap in the Ki-67 proliferative index among histologically benign, atypical, and malignant GCT [135,138], statistical analysis reveals a correlation between the Ki-67 proliferative index and the malignant classification. A score of >10% for the Ki-67 index was significantly correlated with malignancy and unfavorable prognosis.

Lipoma

Lipoma is one of the most common benign neoplasms derived from fatty tissue. Its incidence accounts for approximately 16% of all mesenchymal tumors [143]. Twenty percent are located in the chest wall [144]. The breast is a common site for this pathology [145].

Macroscopy

Lipomas are well-circumscribed nodules, with an average diameter of 2.5–10 cm; however, some cases have been reported of giant lipomas measuring 24 × 20 cm [146].

Microscopy

Lipomas are composed of mature adipose tissue surrounded by a thin capsule. Variants include angiolipomas [147], and a rare example of angiomyolipoma has been reported [148].

Prognosis

Lipomas are benign and excisional biopsy is the treatment.

Vascular Proliferations of the Breast

Hemangiomas

The Perilobular hemangioma (PLH) is a microscopic benign vascular lesion that is not evident mammographically or on gross examination and that is detected during microscopic examination as an incidental finding [149]. They are microscopic in size and have been defined as measuring <2 mm; however; a few of these measuring between 2 and 4 mm have been reported [150]. They may be multiple or bilateral [151,152]. Microscopically, despite of their name, they involve the intralobular stroma, although some may be found in extralobular stroma, sometimes in proximity to ducts [152]. The lesion is a defined collection of small, thin, delicate, distinct vascular channels arranged in mesh-work fashion. It rarely may have ill-defined borders. The vessels vary in caliber, and anastomosing channels may be observed, but these are not conspicuous. Some lesions have cytologically atypical endothelial cells with prominent, hyperchromatic nuclei [149]. No treatment is required for these lesions.

In contrast to the perilobular subtype, hemangiomas of the breast are sufficiently largeto be clinically palpable or detected by mammography [149]. They present at any age [150,153,154].

The mammographic appearance is usually that of a well-defined lobulated mass that may have fine or coarse calcifications [155,156]. Grossly, hemangiomas tend to be well-circumscribed lesions without predilection for any particular location in the breast, and they measure between 0.3 and 2.5 cm.

Microscopically, these lesions are characterized by proliferation of well-differentiated, most frequently nonanastomosing vessels of varying size, located in the extralobular stroma. Sometimes, some vessels in the border of the lesion may blend with the surrounding breast parenchyma [150] (Figure 14). Thrombosis with secondary endothelial hyperplasia can occur [153]; however, endothelial papillary proliferation and mitotic activity are not observed [150].

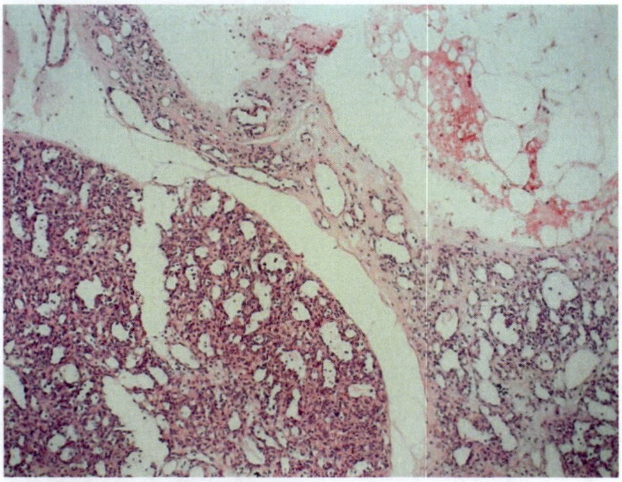

Figure 14. Capillary hemangioma of the breast, the lesion is composed of thin-walled vessels devoid of atypia or architectural complexity (100X HE).

Cavernous hemangiomas can also present in the breast. They are macroscopically evident as a dark-red or brown circumscribed mass that may appear spongy. Microscopic examination reveals dilated vessels congested with red blood cells, with few if any architectural or cytological differences from the remaining types of hemangiomas already described, except for the size of the lumina of the vessels. As is noteworthy, however, in many cavernous hemangiomas, the vascular channels mingle with the fatty parenchyma at the periphery, becoming smaller. This is also a feature of some well-differentiated angiosarcomas, but should not lead to confusion in the absence of the rest of the histological criteria for angiosarcoma [150].

Angiomatosis

Angiomatosis is a very rare vascular lesion with only a few case reports in the literature. It is a diffuse proliferation of benign vessels that infiltrates breast tissue in contiguous fashion but that does not disrupt lobular structures [157]. The vessels in angiomatosis are evenly distributed throughout the lesion and lack the microscopic cytological and architectural criteria for angiosarcoma [158].

Atypical Vascular Proliferations

Atypical vascular lesions of the breast are proliferative vessel forming lesions that do not affect mammary gland tissue but that do develop in the skin after radiation therapy for breast cancer. They involve superficial or deep dermis and are characterized by variably sized vessels that branch and may anastomose. Endothelial atypia and nuclear enlargement can be observed; however, they also lack the rest of the cytological and architectural criteria for angiosarcoma (Figure 15). Atypical vascular lesions may be precursors of angiosarcoma [159,160].

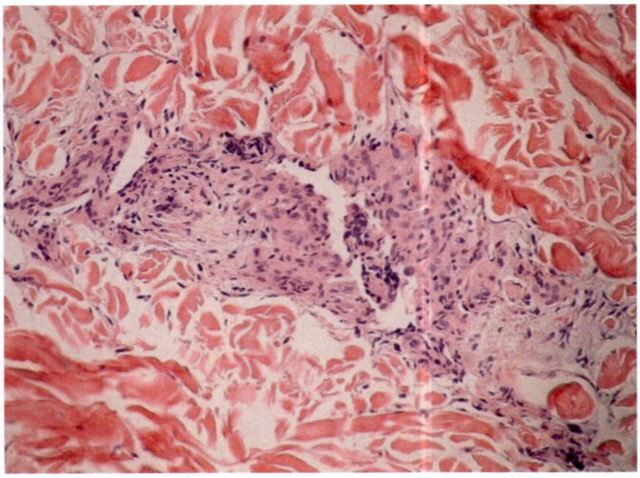

Figure 15. Radiation related atypical vascular lesion showing irregular vessels involving the dermis, that display some pleomorphic and hyperchromatic endothelial cell nuclei (200X HE).

Myoepithelial and Epithelial–Myoepithelial Lesions

Myoepithelial Lesions

Myoepithelial lesions are defined as those consisting of a pure or predominant myoepithelial cell population, myoepithelial hyperplasia, collagenous spherulosis, and we will include benign myoepithelioma [161].

Myoepitheliosis (MEP)

MEP was defined in 2003 [162] as a multifocal, microscopic proliferation of spindle-to-cuboidal myoepithelial cells growing into and around small ducts and ductules. MEP was further subdivided into intraductal and periductal varieties, depending on whether myoepithelial cells proliferatedinto, or around, ducts and ductules, respectively [162–164].

Collagenous Spherulosis (CS)

CS is a condition that consists of myoepithelial cells arranged around cribriform spaces filled with pink spherules of basement membrane material. Immunohistochemical staining with myoepithelial markers confirms the myoepithelial origin of cells encircling the rounded spaces.

The cribriform architecture is composed of purely myoepithelial cells residing within a duct/lobular unit that can be affected by a variety of proliferative changes, including usual ductal hyperplasia, intraductal papilloma, sclerosing adenosis, lobular neoplasia, and adenomyoepithelioma [165–167].

Benign Myoepithelioma

Only rare examples of benign mammary tumors showing pure myoepithelial cell differentiation have been reported [168,169].

Epithelial–Myoepithelial Lesions

Epithelial-myoepithelial lesions are composed of the dual participation of luminal epithelial and myoepithelial cells, pleomorphic adenoma, and adenomyoepithelioma [161].

Pleomorphic Adenoma (PA)

PA of the breast is a benign mixed tumor histologically similar to its salivary gland counterpart [170,171]. It consists of epithelial cells occurring as cohesive and irregular nests and tubules accompanied by dispersed myoepithelial cells immersed in a chondromyxoid matrix. PA was first reported in 1906 by Lecene [172,173], who described a case with cartilaginous and osseous metaplasia in the breast. Only 70 cases of PA of the human breast (PAB) have been documented in the world literature [174,175]. At the Instituto Nacional of Cancerología, Mexico, one case has been reported [176]. Women are more commonly affected than men (female-male ratio, 10:1), and patients can range in age from 23–78 years (mean, 61 years). Tumors range from 0.7–20 cm in diameter (3) and are most commonly located in the periareolar area [177] or in the upper outer quadrant. PA is benign, but excisional biopsy with negative margins is required for the treatment.

Adenomyoepithelioma (AME)

AME is a biphasic neoplastic proliferation of luminal and myoepithelial cells that was first described by Hamperl in 1970 [178]. Macroscopically, the size of AME ranges from 0.3–7 cm, with an average size of 2.5 cm. The tumors have been described as round-to-lobulated, well-circumscribed or discrete, and firm. The cut surface reveals pink-white to gray-tan tissue with focal-to-diffuse translucency. Hemorrhage and focal necrosis have also been reported [179]. Microscopically, the AME tumor has a biphasic nature and is composed of cuboidal-to-columnar, epithelial-lined tubules surrounded by myoepithelial cells. Three variants of AME were described by Tavassoli [163]. The first, the tubular pattern, is characterized by a balanced proliferation of rounded tubules, as well as unusually prominent and hyperplastic myoepithelial cells. The second variant is the spindle cell type, which is composed of a predominantly spindled myoepithelial cell proliferation admixed with a few columnar, epithelial-lined tubules. The third variant exhibits a lobular pattern composed of solid nests of myoepithelial cells proliferating around compressed tubules; the tumor's solid nests are then surrounded by fibrous connective-tissue septa of varying thicknesses. The majority of AME have a papillary configuration; thus, they have been considered a variant of intraductal papilloma by some authors or of morphologic evolution from intraductal papilloma.

The interplay between epithelial and myoepithelial cell elements is highlighted by immunohistochemical staining with antibodies specific for these two components. Epithelial cells uniformly react with antibodies to cytokeratins, such as cytokeratin AE1/3, CK7, and CAM 5.2. The myoepithelial component is highlighted by p63, smooth muscle myosin heavy chains, CK5, CD10, calponin, actin, and S100 [179]. Immunostaining for estrogen is either negative or weakly positive in a patchy pattern [164]. Progesterone receptor and Her2neu have been consistently reported as negative in all of the published studies [164,180].

Differential diagnosis includes papilloma, pleomorphic adenoma, microglandular adenosis, nipple adenoma. adenoid cystic carcinoma, and clear cell carcinoma. When the tumor predominantly displays a spindle cell component, it may be mistaken morphologically for a myoid hamartoma or a leiomyoma.

The majority of AME can be treated by local excision, but local recurrences have occurred 8 months to 5 years after initial excision. In the Tavassoli [163] study, the majority of tumors with recurrence were of the tubular lesion type, extending into, and blending with, the adjacent normal ducts. The recurrent lesions lacked an aggressive morphologic appearance or noticeable mitotic activity. Although the majority of AME are benign, malignant transformations of tumors have been reported in the literature [179,163].

Benign Epithelial Proliferation/ Fibrocystic Changes

Fibrocystic Changes

Fibrocystic changes (FCC) constitute the most frequent benign disorder of the breast. Such changes generally affect premenopausal women between the ages of 20 and 50 years [1,181,182]. Although many other names have been used to describe this entity over the years (including fibrocystic disease, cystic mastopathy, chronic cystic disease, mazoplasia, Reclus disease), the term "fibrocystic changes" is now preferred, because this process is observed clinically in up to 50% and histologically in 90% of women [7,183,184]. FCC may be multifocal and bilateral. The most common presenting symptoms are breast pain and tender nodularities in the breasts. Although the exact pathogenesis of the entity is not clear, hormonal imbalance, particularly estrogen predominance over progesterone, appears to play an important role in its development [185]. FCC comprise both cysts (macro and micro) and solid lesions, including adenosis, epithelial hyperplasia with or without atypia, apocrine metaplasia, radial scar, and papilloma (Figure 16). Because some of the more frequent types of adenosis, mild and florid usual ductal hyperplasia, papilloma and radial scar comprise lesions with proliferative activity, they are discussed later under the heading of proliferative lesions without atypia. The remaining components of FCC are discussed below.

Cysts

Cysts are fluid-filled, round or ovoid structures that are found in as many as one third of women between 35 and 50 years of age. Although the majority are subclinical "microcysts", in about 20–25% of cases, palpable (gross) cystic change is encountered, which generally presents as a simple cyst [15,186]. Cysts cannot reliably be distinguished from solid masses by clinical breast examination or mammography; in these cases, ultrasonography and fine-needle aspiration (FNA) cytology, which are highly accurate, are used. Cysts are derived from the terminal duct lobular unit. In the majority of cysts, the epithelial lining is either flattened or totally absent. An apocrine epithelial lining is observed in only a small number of cysts. Because gross cysts are not associated with an increased risk of carcinoma development, current consensus on the management of gross cysts is routine patient follow-up, without further therapy [186]. Complex (or complicated or atypical) cyst is a sonographic diagnosis that is characterized by internal echoes or thin septations, thickened and/or irregular wall, and absent posterior enhancement [187]. They are reported in approximately 5–5.5% of all breast Ultrasound (US) examinations. The malignancy rate of complex cysts, which is 0.3% as described by Venta et al., is lower than that for lesions classified as "probably benign." Patients with these cysts can be managed with follow-up imaging studies [187,188]. However, if the lesion also includes an intracystic mass (intracystic nodule), it should be regarded as "suspicious for neoplasm" and managed as a solid lesion. Either a CNB or a surgical biopsy is indicated for these lesions [187-189].

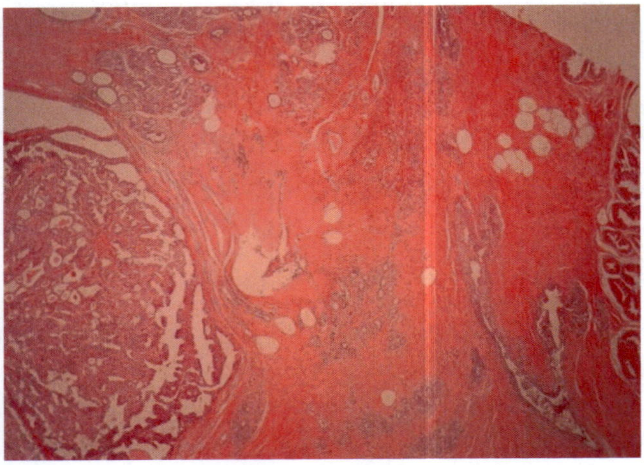

Figure 16. Fibrocystic changes: dilated ducts with apocrine metaplasia, periductal fibrosis, and an area of sclerosing adenosis are some of the features of this condition that were present in this specimen (40X HE).

Metaplasia

Apocrine metaplasia is characterized by the presence of columnar cells with abundant granular, eosinophilic cytoplasm and luminal cytoplasmic projections or apical snouts. These cells line dilated ducts or can be observed in papillary proliferations. They are more frequently found in younger women. All normal and metaplastic apocrine cells can be stained with gross cystic disease fluid protein 15. Atypical apocrine metaplasia should be diagnosed only when nuclei of the apocrine cells display significant cytologic atypia [190].

Clear cell metaplasia of the breast is a rare lesion. Its significance derives from its morphological similarity to clear-cell carcinoma. However, the similarity of its immunohistochemical staining profile with that of eccrine sweat glands suggests that clear-cell metaplasia may in fact represent "eccrine metaplasia" [191].

Benign Epithelial Proliferation

The main concern in patients with epithelial proliferative lesions is the risk of developing breast carcinoma. Early epidemiological studies to analyze this relationship resulted in clinical and histological parameters that allowed stratification of these lesions into different risk groups [10]. The presence of proliferative atypia emerged as an important histopathological marker of risk, as illustrated in Table 2.

Aside from the histological features, age at biopsy and degree of familial history of breast cancer are reported as the major determinants of the risk for breast cancer after the diagnosis of benign breast disease [192]. According to Hartmann et al. [192], after a diagnosis of atypical epithelial proliferation, the risk for breast cancer in young women is twice that of the observed among women >55 years of age. It was also reported, in the same study, that familial history of breast cancer is an independent risk factor and that a strong familial history may increase the risk for breast cancer even in patients with nonproliferative lesions [192]. Absolute risk, however, for both atypical and atypical epithelial proliferations is quite low. More than 80% of patients with a diagnosis of atypical hyperplasia do not develop invasive cancer during their lifetimes.

Table 2. Histologic category of benign epithelial breast lesions Associated with Relative risk (RR) for breast cancer

Histological category		RR
Nonproliferative lesions	Nonproliferative components of fibrocystic change (cysts, papillary apocrine change, epithelial-related calcifications, ductal dilatation/ectasia, periductal fibrosis)	1–1.27
Proliferative lesions without atypia	*Moderate or florid ductal hyperplasia of the usual type *Sclerosing adenosis *Radial scar, *intraductal papilloma, and papillomatosis	1.3–1.9
Atypical proliferative lesions	*Atypical lobular hyperplasia *Atypical ductal hyperplasia *Columnar cell lesions with atypia/Flat epithelial atypia	3.9–13.0

*Data from [10, 15,40].

Given such a scenario, we focus our discussion of benign proliferative disease on the main entities that may cause confusion with breast cancer due to the morphological features of the entities, and on those that point toward an increase in the risk of subsequent breast cancer.

Proliferative Lesions without Atypia

Adenosis

Adenosis of the breast is a proliferative lesion that is characterized by an increased number and/or size of glandular components, mainly involving lobular units, which maintain the luminal, epithelial, and myoepithelial components, as well as the basement membrane [15, 193,194].

Adenosis is usually grossly inapparent and most often is an incidental microscopic finding. At the histological level, various types of adenosis have been described, among which sclerosing, microglandular, and tubular adenosis merit detailed description [193–195].

Sclerosing adenosis. In sclerosing adenosis, there is preferential preservation of myoepithelial cells with variable, although sometimes profound atrophy, of epithelial cells, accompanied by lobular fibrosis. These features impart a disordered appearance of acinar, myoepithelial, and connective tissue elements in which abnormally dense, intralobular connective tissue compresses and distorts acinar structures, mimicking infiltrating carcinoma [15,194] (Figure 17).

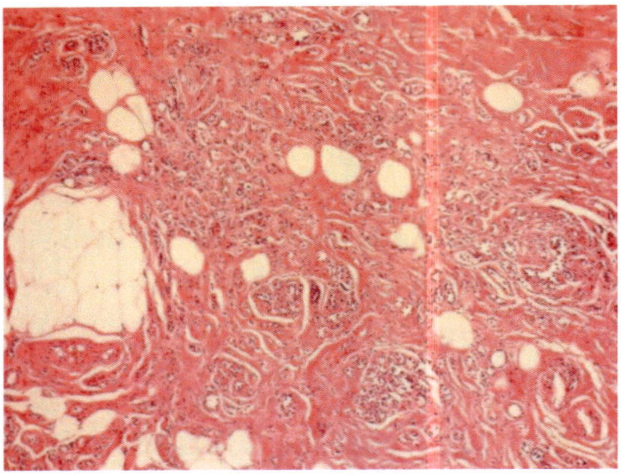

Figure 17. Sclerosing adenosis. Abnormally dense, intralobular connective tissue compresses and distorts acinar structures, the loss of the characteristic lobulocentric pattern makes more difficult to distinguish it from invasive carcinoma (100X HE).

Despite expansion and alteration of normal lobular configuration, a lobulocentric arrangement, recognizable on low-power examination, is usually retained [194]. Caution is recommended in cases where sclerosing adenosis is not limited to a lobulocentric pattern, which renders this lobulocentric arrangement more difficult to identify, affording it, at the same time, an infiltrative pattern in stroma and fat [193]. A similar situation presents with cases with confluence of lobules altered by sclerosing adenosis. In both situations, immunohistochemistry for myoepithelial cell markers such as p63, calponin, or other smooth-muscle differentiation antigens, which are not lost in sclerosing adenosis in contrast with carcinoma, allows the distinction of sclerosing adenosis [193] (Figure 18).

Sclerosing adenosis is strongly associated with various other proliferative lesions, including epithelial hyperplasias, intraductal or sclerosing papilloma, complex sclerosing lesion, calcifications, and apocrine changes. It can coexist with both invasive and *in situ* cancers [15, 193]. Additionally, some studies have found sclerosing adenosis to be a risk factor for invasive breast cancer, aside from its association with other proliferative lesions of the breast [196, 197].

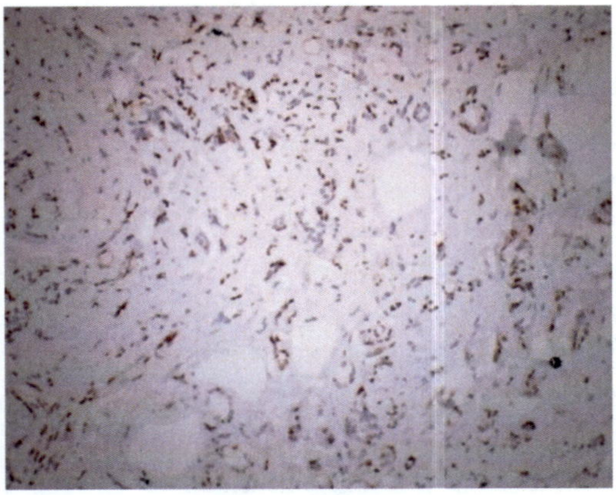

Figure 18. Myoepithelial markers in sclerosing adenosis. Inmmunohistochemistry for p63 shows the preservation of myoepithelial cells and partial atrophy (scarcity) of luminal cells. In this example the lobulocentric pattern is retained (200X).

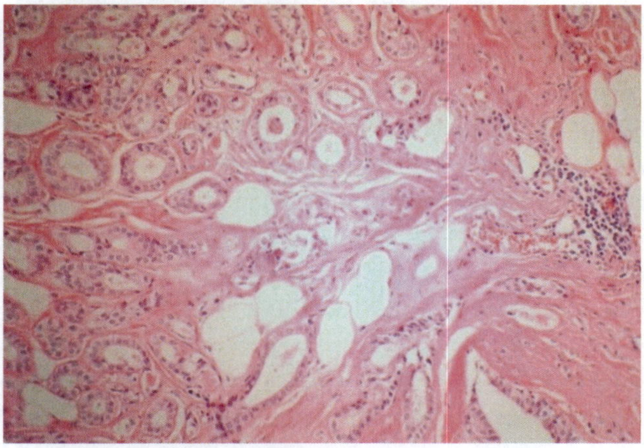

Figure 19. Microglandular adenosis. The proliferation of round, small glands, arranged in a rather infiltrative pattern, with a single layer of flat-to-cuboidal epithelial cells and lacking myoepithelial cells is evident (200X HE).

Microglandular adenosis. Microglandular adenosis of the breast is characterized by nonlobulocentric proliferation of round, small glands, with open lumina, arranged in a rather infiltrative pattern within a fibro-fatty stroma and composed of a single layer of flat-to-cuboidal epithelial cells, invested by basement membrane, and that most frequently lack myoepithelial cells [15,194,198](Figure 19).

Oncocytic differentiation and chondroid metaplasia may be observed in rare cases [194]. An atypical variant has been described that retains the glandular pattern but exhibits architectural atypia, mitoses, and higher expression of Ki 67 [199,200]. Lack of the myoepithelial layer renders it difficult to differentiate microglandular adenosis from tubular carcinoma. However, the presence of basal lamina encircling glandular structures, which can also be shown by laminin or type IV collagen immunohistochemical stains, and the absence of epithelial membrane antigen staining in the luminal epithelial cells, distinguish microglandular adenosis from tubular carcinoma [201]. Another feature of microglandular adenosis is its positivity for S-100 protein [202] (Figure 20).

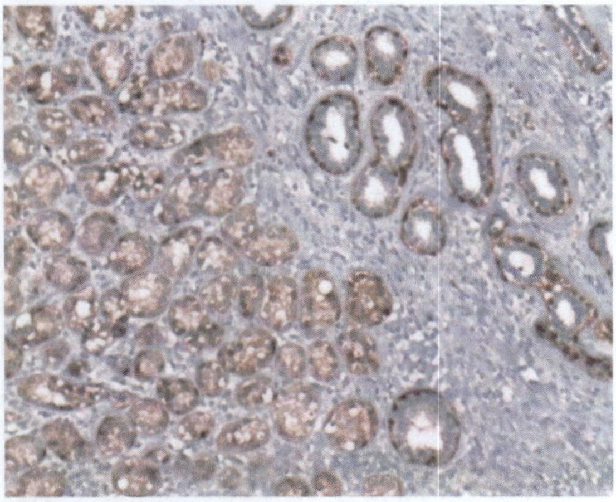

Figure 20. Microglandular adenosis, S-100 protein positivity in the epithelial cells by immunohistochemistry (200X).

Microglandular adenosis has a tendency to recur if not completely excised [15], perhaps with predilection for atypical cases [200].

Association of microglandular adenosis with carcinoma has been recognized for some time [199], and although microglandular adenosis continues to be classified as adenosis, there is evidence of similar copy-number alterations in microglandular adenosis and coexisting glandular carcinoma with some degree of accumulation of alterations from microglandular adenosis to carcinoma [198, 203]. Carcinomas associated with microglandular adenosis are mainly triple-negative and may possess the complete morphological spectrum of such carcinomas, including adenoid cystic carcinoma [200, 204,205].

Tubular adenosis. Tubular adenosis of the breast is another rare variant of adenosis that should be distinguished from tubular carcinoma [15]. It is characterized by a proliferation of elongated, noncrowded narrow tubules, sometimes branching, with no lobular arrangement or, at most, vague lobular grouping. Some of its tubules often extend into the fat, mimicking invasion. The tubules contain basophilic or granular eosinophilic secretion and are lined with bland-appearing ductal cells surrounded by an intact myoepithelial layer. The stroma around them is sclerotic-to-edematous. The presence of an intact myoepithelial layer around the tubules is the most helpful feature for separating it from invasive carcinoma [195].

Nodular adenosis/adenosis tumor. In a few cases, adenosis may assume grossly the appearance of a firm mass [193,194] (Figure 21A), which correlates with mammography or US findings and which may occasionally mimic carcinoma. Histological examination is often required, because even when benign-appearing, nodular adenosis can be indistinguishable from other ellipsoid, circumscribed, or hypodense masses identified by imaging [206,207].

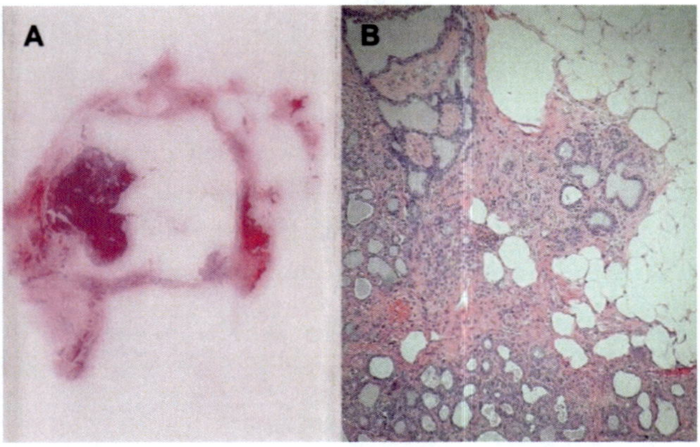

Figure 21. Nodular adenosis. The well delimited, clinically palpable mass is evident at gross level. Microscopically adenosis in a mixture of different patterns is observed (A, 1X HE, B, 100X HE).

Excised adenosis tumors may vary in gross appearance depending upon their microscopic composition. Lesions consisting of florid adenosis with a prominent glandular component are typically well-circumscribed nodules composed of gray or pale-tan, firm homogeneous tissue [193], while those with increasing sclerosis are likely to be grossly less well-defined at the borders, multinodular, and more fibrous in appearance [193]. Lesions with abundant calcifications may appear gritty when cut [194]. Gross cyst formation is infrequent [193].

Histologically, adenosis tumours characteristically show adenosis arranged in a mixture of different patterns, the most frequent and extensive being sclerosing adenosis [208] (Figure

21B). Other fibrocystic changes, such as apocrine metaplasia, microcysts, luminal histiocytes, and pseudopapillomas, may also be present within an adenosis tumor, as well as other proliferative lesions such as radial scar or rarely, even carcinoma *in situ*[208]. A conspicuous feature in adenosis tumors is their patchy growth, in contrast to the stellate configuration of tubular carcinoma, which aids in the differential diagnosis [208].

Microscopically, the most frequent growth pattern was classical sclerosing adenosis.

Radial Scar and Complex Sclerosing Lesion

Radial scar lesions (RSL) are benign pseudoinfiltrative lesions of uncertain significance that on imaging, gross examination, and low-power microscopy, may resemble invasive carcinoma [15, 194].

Over the years, many authors have studied the biological significance of radial scars. To date, there is no evidence that these lesions are premalignant. They have been related with benign breast disease with varying frequencies (4–26%), as well as with invasive carcinoma of the breast (1.7–28%) [209]. In studies with long-term follow-up, the association with an increased risk of breast cancer is rather modest (1.75 and 1.45), although present even after adjustment for the histological category of benign breast disease [210]. It appears that radial scars may serve as a milieu for the development of atypical epithelial proliferations, including atypical intraductal hyperplasia, atypical lobular hyperplasia, lobular carcinoma *in situ*, and DCIS [15].

Previously, radial scars comprised an incidental finding in breast specimens excised for other diagnostic reasons, but their incidence has increased dramatically as a result of population-based screening programs [211]. In current practice, these lesions are most frequently identified by mammography, while they are very rarely of sufficient size to produce a palpable mass [212].

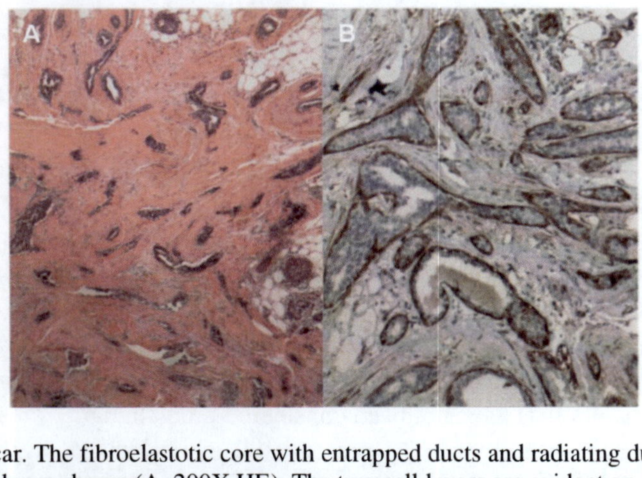

Figure 22. Radial Scar. The fibroelastotic core with entrapped ducts and radiating ducts on the periphery of the fields are shown (A, 200X HE). The two cell layers are evident on an smooth muscle actin immunohistochemistry stain (B, 200X).

Radial scars, when apparent on gross examination, produce an irregular area of firm breast tissue that exhibits a solid, retracted center with white or yellow streaks and pale, slender bands of stroma that extend into the surrounding tissue [194, 209]. The lesions can be multiple or bilateral [194, 209]. Some authors have suggested using the term "radial scar" for lesions measuring <1 cm, while reserving the term "complex sclerosing lesion" for lesions measuring 1 cm or larger [211,213].

The role of Fine-needle aspiration (FNA) cytology in diagnosis is limited. Recent publications have shown the importance of CNB of these lesions for diagnosis, but because malignancy cannot be reliably excluded with limited sampling, a spiculated lesion suggestive of radial scar or complex sclerosing lesion on mammography may be excised on the basis of its size and the amount of sampling performed by core biopsy [211,213,214].

Histologically, radial scar is a lobulocentric lesion characterized by a fibroelastotic core with entrapped ducts that is surrounded by radiating ducts and lobules displaying variable epithelial hyperplasia, adenosis, duct ectasia, and papillomatosis [15, 194].

The central fibrous tissue shows small, entrapped benign tubules that retain a two-cell layer, although this may not always visible on Hematoxylin & eosin (H&E) stains(Figure 22A). Immunohistochemical stains for myoepithelial markers should be used to make this distinction when there is substantial doubt concerning the benign nature of the lesion, and particularly in CNB [209] (Figure 22B). However caution is recommended because, in some cases, myoepithelial cells may be attenuated in such tubules [209]. Abundant elastin in the walls of ducts and throughout the stroma appears as a dense, sometimes granular eosinophilic or weakly basophilic, deposit that can be enhanced by an elastic tissue stain such as Verhoeff's or van Gieson's stain [209].

At the periphery of the lesion and especially in the larger and more complex sclerosing lesions, several of the proliferating epithelial lesions, or even normal epithelial structures, appear to intermingle in an asymmetrical manner [194, 209]. Sclerosing adenosis, sclerosing papillomas, and cysts are frequent components. A light, scattered infiltrate of lymphocytes and plasma cells is found in the stroma. Conspicuous lymphocytic aggregates are uncommon in typical Radial scar lesions (RSL) and their presence may indicate a low-grade carcinoma [209].

Intraductal Papilloma and Papillomatosis

Intraductal papilloma is a discrete benign tumor of the epithelium of mammary ducts. Any point in the ductal system can be affected, though the most frequent locations are the lactiferous sinuses and the terminal ductules [215] (Figure 23A). Central papillomas tend to be solitary, whereas the peripheral ones are usually multiple. The usual presenting symptom is serous or serosanguinous nipple discharge. Histologically, papillomas are composed of epithelial fronds supported by fibrovascular stroma and lined with two layers of epithelial cells: luminal and myoepithelial (Figure 23B-C). The epithelial component can be subject to a spectrum of morphologic changes ranging from metaplasia to hyperplasia, atypical intraductal hyperplasia, and *in situ* carcinoma (Figure 23C).

Central single papillomas have not been considered premalignant or markers of risk when they are not associated with atypia. The presence of atypical ductal hyperplasia within the papilloma is associated to the presence of invasive or preinvasive carcinoma of the breast in excisional biopsies [216,217]. However, epithelial atypia, even to the extent of low-grade DCIS, has no known prognostic significance or impact on outcome when it is confined to the central papilloma. Therefore, if atypia is encountered in a papilloma on an excisional biopsy, the surrounding breast tissue should be carefully examined for further follow-up of the patient [218].

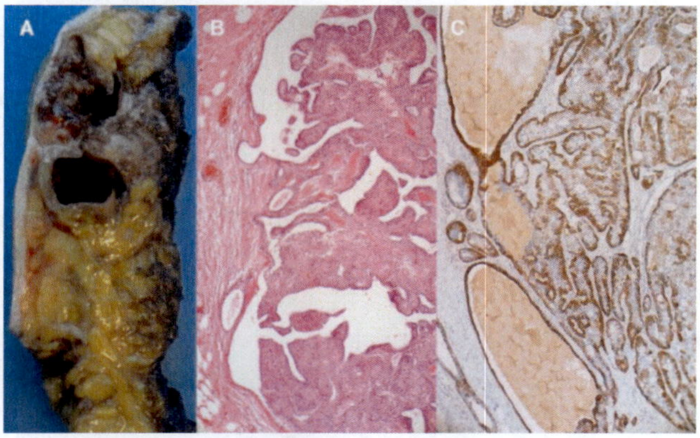

Figure 23. Intraductal papilloma. On gross examination the papillary lesion grows within a cavity formed by the cystically dilated duct (A). Microscopically the lesion is composed of epithelial fronds supported by fibrovascular stroma and lined with two layers of cells (B, 100X HE). With immunohistochemistry for cytokeratin 14, some areas of expansion of luminal negative cells (hyperplasia) is seen (C, 100X).

Papillomatosis (multiple papillomas) is defined as a minimum of five clearly separate papillomas within a localized segment of breast tissue, usually in a peripheral or subareolar location [15]. Multiple papillomas are more likely to occur bilaterally, and their probability of having an *in situ* or invasive carcinoma is higher than with the central papilloma. Therefore, in patients with multiple papillomas on excisional biopsy, thorough sampling of the specimen, as well as diagnostic radiographic imaging of contralateral breast tissue, is suggested to rule out malignancy [219]. All available data suggest that multiple papillomas may indicate a slightly elevated risk for subsequent breast cancer [220,221].

Juvenile papillomatosis of the breast is defined as severe ductal papillomatosis occurring in young women of <30 years of age. This disease is associated with a heightened risk for breast cancer. Because both a familial history of breast cancer and an increased risk for breast cancer are associated with the diagnosis of juvenile papillomatosis, long-term follow-up is recommended both for the patient and the family [222].

Nonatypical Epithelial Hyperplasia of the Ductal Type

Epithelial hyperplasia is the most common form of proliferative breast disease. Normally, breast ducts are lined by two layers of low cuboidal cells; these are luminal and basal myoepithelial cells. Any increase in cell number within the ductal space that leads to its dilatation is regarded as epithelial hyperplasia [15]. Some studies suggest that many of the proliferative changes commonly described as ductal hyperplasia arise from ductal structures of the lobules, and that the specific histological features of hyperplasia arising in a major duct or in the components of an unfolded lobule are not readily distinguishable in conventional histological sections [224]. If intraductal hyperplasia is traced in serial sections, it is often possible to observe the discontinuous, multifocal nature of the condition along the course of a single duct. Enlargement of the entire affected glandular structure is also frequently observed and results in a sinuous structure [225].

Usual ductal hyperplasia or simple hyperplasia denotes an increase in the number of epithelial cells, but is devoid of atypical cytologic features of the proliferating cells. Usual ductal hyperplasia does not increase the risk for breast cancer. It can be classified into three categories: mild; moderate, or florid. The most important cytologic features of mild, moderate, or florid epithelial hyperplasia are an admixture of cell types (epithelial cells, myoepithelial cells, and metaplastic apocrine cells) and variation in the appearances of epithelial cells and their nuclei, which impart an heterogeneous aspect to the lesion [226,227]. In mild hyperplasia of the usual type, proliferating epithelial cells are a 3–4-cell layer mainly only thickening the epithelium in the duct, whereas moderate hyperplasia describes epithelial proliferation >4 cells thick, often with accompanying bridging of the luminal space [15, 225]. Micropapillary structures may be, when present, usually have a broad base and a narrow tip with hyperchromatic, nearly, pyknotic, nuclei[223]. In florid hyperplasia, the lumen is severely distended and most frequently filled with the epithelial proliferation [15, 225]. Foci of florid hyperplasia may fill the duct lumen in solid or fenestrated (cribriform) fashion. The cells are often distributed in a streaming pattern in solid or in fenestrated areas [228]. A part of the original duct lumen may remain as a crescentic space or spaces at the edge of the duct. The predominantly peripheral distribution of microlumens that characterizes moderate and florid hyperplasia is an important feature to separate it from cribriform intraductal carcinoma, in which microlumens tend to be distributed more evenly across the entire duct cross section [225]. The spaces in a given hyperplastic duct usually have varied shapes. In contrast, in cribriform carcinoma, they tend to be rounded. The nuclei of cells surrounding spaces tend to run parallel to them [225, 223] (Figure 24). Foamy histiocytes and calcifications may be observed and more rarely, foci of necrosis. Occasional mitotic figures do not preclude the diagnosis of usual ductal hyperplasia [223].

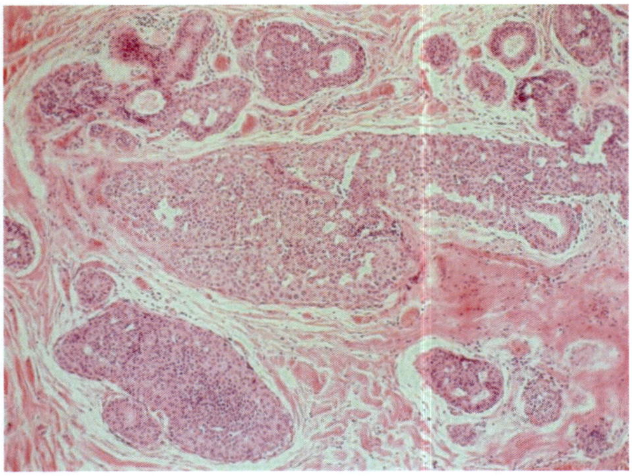

Figure 24. Usual ductal hyperplasia. Duct distended by the epithelial proliferation with a fenestrated pattern, with irregular micro lumens mainly at the periphery, with nuclei oriented in parallel to this spaces solid foci with a streaming pattern of the cells, and heterogeneity in the appaerance of the epithelial cells (100X HE).

Atypical Proliferative Lesions

It can be difficult to distinguish between usual ductal or lobular hyperplasias and their atypical counterparts—atypical ductal hyperplasia and atypical lobular hyperplasia/lobular neoplasia. The distinction, however, is guaranteed given the increases in risk of invasive breast cancer in the latter two.

Lobular Neoplasia

Lobular-type epithelial proliferations, in contrast with ductal lesions that possess subtle but distinctive morphological features, are very similar among themselves, and the sole difference between atypical lobular hyperplasia and lobular carcinoma *in situ* is the extent and degree of epithelial proliferation. Consequently, both atypical lobular hyperplasia and lobular carcinoma *in situ* are collectively termed lobular neoplasia. Because both lesions are regarded and managed as a risk factor rather than as well-established precursor lesions, lobular neoplasia terminology has gained general acceptance [15]. Subsequent increase in the risk for the development of invasive carcinoma is of about 4-fold for atypical lobular hyperplasia and 10-fold for lobular carcinoma *in situ*[15].

Lobular neoplasia is a relatively rare breast lesion. It is most often identified as an incidental finding in biopsies excised for other abnormalities, because it rarely manifests itself as a palpable mass and not frequently gives rise to calcifications [15]. Proliferative fibrocystic changes are usually the site of mammographic abnormalities that lead to a biopsy in which Lobular carcinoma *in situ* (LCIS) is detected [229]. In retrospective reviews, each involving several thousand "benign" breast specimens, the frequency of LCIS ranged from 0.5–1.5% [229]. Incidence rates have been reported to be steadily rising, most probably as a consequence of mammographic screening [230]. Lobular neoplasia is most prevalent in peri- and menopausal women [15, 229].

Lobular neoplasia is multifocal [229, 15], with many patients having lesions involving multiple quadrants of the breast [15]. Women with LCIS also have a significant risk of having bilateral involvement, often at the same time [229]. Although subsequent carcinomas can occur in either breast without a direct relationship with the previous site-of-biopsy, a recent retrospective study reports ipsilateral association as three times more likely [231]. Invasive carcinomas may arise as late as 20 years after diagnosis [15].

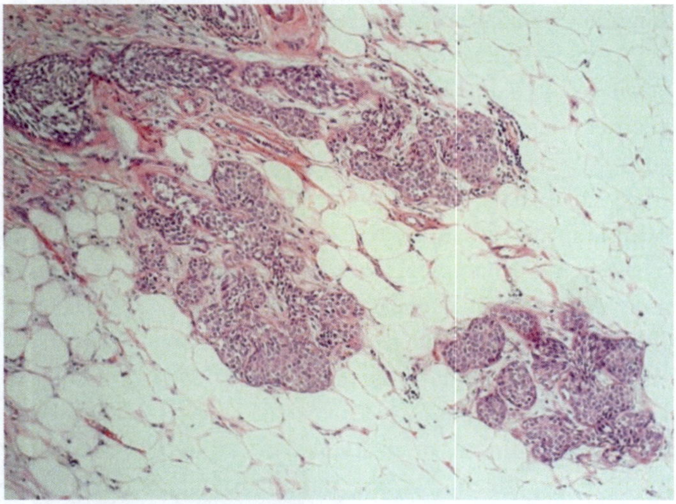

Figure 25. Lobular neoplasia. Terminal ductolobular unit involved by an epithelial proliferation of small sized, homogeneous, discohesive cells with scant cytoplasm (100X HE).

Histopathologically, lobular neoplasia is a proliferation within the terminal ductolobular unit. It may have pagetoid involvement of terminal ducts. Involved lobules are expanded by monomorphic proliferation of discohesive epithelial cells with uniform round nuclei, indistinct nucleoli, uniform chromatin, and scant cytoplasm (Figure 25). Intracytoplasmic lumina and or signet ring cells are often present [232].

Classic lobular *in situ* carcinoma is diagnosed if more than one half of the acini of a lobular unit are distended and distorted by the lesion. Below this threshold, the diagnosis should be atypical lobular hyperplasia [232].

Pleomorphic lobular *in situ* carcinoma is a variant of lobular neoplasia in which there is marked pleomorphism (equivalent to that observed in high-grade ductal *in situ* carcinoma). It may be associated with apocrine features or comedo-type necrosis [232].

The majority of lobular *in situ* carcinomas, even of the pleomorphic subtype, are typically negative for E-cadherin. However, 10–16% of cases may show aberrant positivity, which should not be used to diagnose ductal *in situ* carcinoma [232].

Systemic follow-up and appropriate risk assessment is recommended for patients with lobular neoplasia. Management of lobular neoplasia diagnosed in a core biopsy is controversial. Excision should be performed if there is another lesion that in itself warrants excision, or if comedo necrosis, pleomorphic LCIS, or a bulky lesion are present [232]. In general, lobular carcinoma *in situ* does not warrant surgical therapy, in that it is considered a risk marker rather than an obligate precursor lesion of invasive breast cancer. However, in patients with other risk factors, such as a high-risk familial history, prophylactic bilateral mastectomy would be a consideration, given the fact that the risk for developing invasive cancer appears to be similar in both the ipsilateral and contralateral breasts. Chemoprevention may be the preferred approach for patients with moderate risk associated with the diagnosis of lobular carcinoma *in situ* [15].

Atypical Ductal Hyperplasia

Ductal hyperplasia is defined as atypical when it morphologically mimics low-grade ductal carcinoma *insitu*. With the increasing use of mammography, atypical ductal hyperplasias are being diagnosed more frequently, mainly associated with the identification of microcalcifications. Atypical ductal hyperplasia is observed in only 4% of symptomatic benign biopsies taken for a palpable mass, in contrast with 31% of biopsies performed because of microcalcifications that show this same condition [233].

The significance of atypical ductal hyperplasia derives from the fact that the patient has a 4–5-times greater risk for invasive breast cancer than that of the general population. Further, this risk is nearly 10-fold if the patient has a first-degree relative with breast cancer [233,234], and premenopausal women with atypical ductal hyperplasia have a substantially higher risk than postmenopausal women with that same diagnosis [15]. The risk for breast cancer is higher in the ipsilateral breast, but the contralateral breast is also at risk [192,235–237]. Women with atypical ductal hyperplasia develop cancer usually within 10–15 years of the diagnosis. The risk for cancer declines after 15 years [235,238].

From the morphological point of view, atypical ductal hyperplasia characteristically has a uniform population of cells, given that the mixture of epithelial and myoepithelial cells observed in usual ductal hyperplasia is replaced by a monotonous clonal proliferation of luminal cells. The involved duct is distended, and its lumen is partially or totally obliterated by the proliferating cells in a solid or cribriform pattern. Microlumens in the case of cribriform proliferations are evenly distributed and have rigid contours [225, 223] (Figure 26).

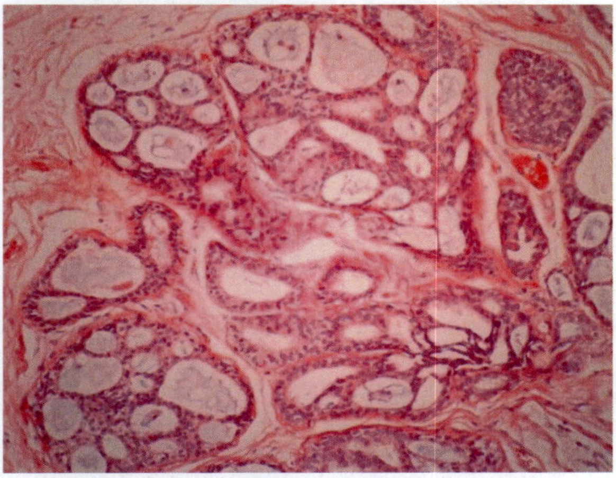

Figure 26. Atypical ductal hyperplasia. Duct distended by the epithelial proliferation with a cribriform pattern, with rigid evenly distributed lumens and homogeneity in the appaerance of the epithelial cells (200X HE).

In short, the microscopic features of atypical ductal hyperplasia are those of low-grade *in situ* ductal carcinoma. The distinction between these two entities relies only on the extent of the lesion. According to some authors, the proliferation is termed atypical ductal hyperplasia when the affected duct is not entirely involved by the proliferation, while for other authors, atypical ductal hyperplasia is limited to only a few small ducts measuring <2 mm. In any instance, the majority of lesions of atypical ductal hyperplasia are small and focal [223,226].

Molecular data also support the concept that atypical ductal hyperplasia and low-grade ductal *in situ* carcinoma are two stages of the same pathological process only differing in the size of the lesion. Ma et al. profiled atypical ductal hyperplasias and low-grade ductal *in situ* carcinomas and found that transcriptional alterations are maintained from atypical ductal hyperplasia throughout purported later stages of progression as ductal *in situ* carcinoma [239]. However, the main differences between these two lesions may be observed in the expression profiles of the surrounding stroma [239,240].

Perhaps more important than the distinction from *in situ* carcinoma, is the identification of atypical ductal hyperplasia as opposed to usual ductal hyperplasia. This is relevant given the associated risk of invasive breast cancer of atypical ductal hyperplasia. Immunohistochemistry is a useful adjunct of histopathology for this aim. As already stated, in atypical ductal hyperplasia the mixture of epithelial and myoepithelial cells observed in usual ductal hyperplasia is replaced by a monotonous clonal proliferation of luminal cells. In this way, a combination of markers for luminal and myoepithelial cells, such as CK7, CK8, or CK18 (luminal), and CK17, CK14, CK34bE12, CK5/6, p63, smooth muscle actin, or calponin (myoepithelial), helps to separate both entities and increases interobserver reproducibility of these diagnoses [241]. With these stains, a mosaic pattern is observed in usual ductal hyperplasia (Figure 27A). In contrast, atypical ductal hyperplasia shows a homogeneous stain with luminal markers and with attenuated peripheral positivity for myoepithelial markers (Figure 27B).

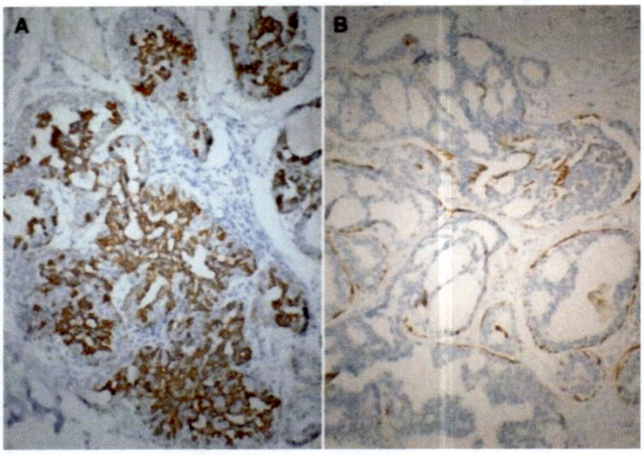

Figure 27. Diferential diagnosis between usual ductal hyperplasia and atypical ductal hyperplasia by immunohistochemistry. Usual ductal hyperplasia shows a mosaic pattern with high-molecular weight cytokeratin (A, 200X) in contrast with the negativity on atypical ductal hyperplasia with only peripherally located positive cells (B, 200X).

Routine follow-up for both breasts is recommended on identification of atypical ductal hyperplasia. Therapy options, such as chemoprevention, should be determined on the basis of other risk factors for breast cancer and the expression of hormonal receptors in the lesion [15].

Columnar Cell Lesions

Another spectrum of lesions that have been encountered with increasing frequency in core needle breast biopsies because of their association with microcalcifications detected by mammographic screening are columnar cell lesions. Schnitt and Vincent-Salomon proposed a working classification of these lesions as "columnar cell change" and "columnar cell hyperplasia", each of which may have atypia or not [242].

Atypical columnar cell lesions merit further mention given their association with invasive carcinoma. A variety of names have been given to these lesions, including ''columnar cell change or hyperplasia with atypia'',''columnar alteration with prominent apical snouts and secretions with atypia'',''ductal intraepithelial neoplasia 1-flat type'',''atypical cystic lobule'',''atypical cystic duct'',''small ectatic ducts lined with atypical ductal cells with apocrine snouts'', and ''clinging *in situ* duct carcinoma flat type'', among others [243]. Although the World Health Organization Working Group on Breast Tumors has recently adopted the term "flat epithelial atypia" for these lesions, their designation as columnar cell lesions with atypia has achieved notable popularity [243].

Studies on the clinical significance of atypical columnar cell lesions have shown that the likelihood of local recurrence or progression to invasive breast cancer is exceedingly low [15]. So although there is good evidence pointing toward a precursor role of FEA in the development of tubular (or other low-grade) carcinomas [244, 245], looking at the follow-up data on patients with FEA, this risk is only 4.7% of DCIS in locally excised lesions in all published series. Consequently, experts consider FEA as a risk lesion in the great majority of cases [246].

There are four main histologic features of flat epithelial atypia: 1) the involved terminal duct-lobular units are enlarged and dilated (Figure 28); 2) the ductal cells display low-grade cytologic atypia characterized by evenly distributed monomorphic, hyperchromatic, and mildly enlarged nuclei (Figure 29A); 3) a flat layer of ductal cells lines the distended glands, and 4) the myoepithelial cells are often attenuated (Figure 29B). The second and third histological features listed strike at the morphologic definition of flat epithelial atypia, namely, a proliferation of ductal cells demonstrating the presence of low-grade cytologic atypia in the absence of important architectural atypia [243]. Applying these criteria, fairly good interobserver agreement may be achieved for the distinction of atypical columnar cell lesions vs. nonatypical counterparts [247].

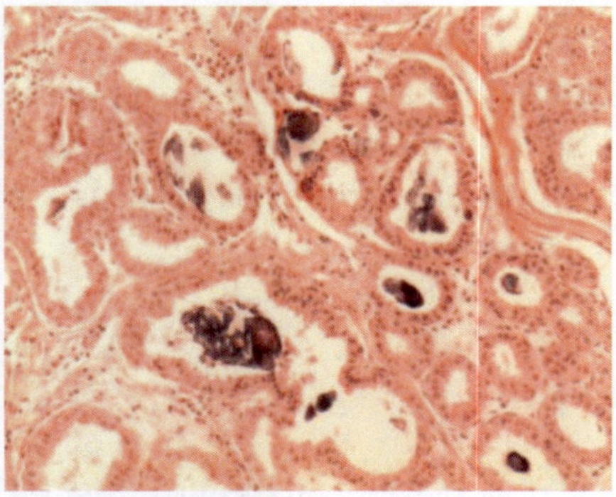

Figure 28. Flat epithelial atypia. Terminal-ductlobular units are enlarged and dilated. Associated calcifications are common (100X HE).

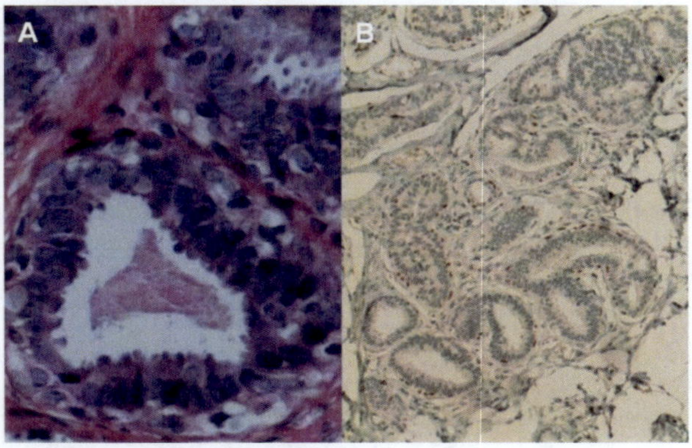

Figure 29. Low-grade cytologic atypia with mildly enlarged nuclei with fine granular chromatin (A, 400X HE), and attenuated myoepithelial cells on immunohistochemstry for p63 (B, 200X).

When an atypical columnar lesion is encountered in a core needle biopsy, excision is suggested to exclude more advanced lesions such as *in situ* or invasive cancer. On obtaining an excisional biopsy specimen, a careful histological search for areas with diagnostic features of *in situ* or invasive cancer should be performed. Because this lesion has been referred to by several different names in the literature, it is difficult to assess its significance as a risk marker for development of invasive cancer. Without having firm data, close follow-up of the patient with columnar cell changes is recommended at this point [245, 248].

Benign Epithelial Neoplasms

Tubular Adenoma (TA)

This is a nodule formed by compact proliferation of tubular structures lined by epithelial and myoepithelial cells.

Macroscopy

TA are firm, well-circumscribed, and homogeneous, with a uniform, yellowish or tan-brown cut surface.

Microscopy

The tumors are well-circumscribed and entirely composed of small, round tubules, lined by uniform epithelial cells with surrounding myoepithelial cells. Tubular lumina rarely contain proteinaceous material or mucin. Stroma may contain a few lymphocytes. Carcinoma only rarely involves a tubular adenoma.

Lactanting Adenoma (LA)

During pregnancy and lactation, the epithelial cells of the FA of TA may show extensive secretory changes. The majority of lesions classified as "lactating adenoma" represent nodular areas of hyperplastic lobules with secretory or lactational changes.

Macroscopy

LA vary in size, and in some cases reach large dimensions.

Microscopy

Localization of lobules comprising the lesion show lactational changes, and infarction and hemorrhage may be present.

Apocrine Adenoma (AA)

AA is a nodular collection of cysts or glands lined with apocrine metaplasia or papillary apocrine changes.

Macroscopy

The lesion has well-defined margins. Size ranges from 3 mm to 1.7 cm.

Microscopy

AA is characterized by a nodular collection of glands lined with apocrine epithelium and no atypia. One case has been reported associated with breast cancer.

Ductal Adenoma (DA)

Proliferation within a duct lumen, which is well- circumscribed.

Macroscopy

Lesions can be unilateral, single or multiple nodules. Dimensions range from 0.5–4.0 cm. Bilateral lesions has been observed in Carney syndrome.

Microscopy

These are glandular structures with a typical, dual cell layer of epithelial and myoepithelial cells within a central area of dense, scar-like fibrosis and surrounded by a thick fibrous wall. In some cases, myoepithelial cell proliferation is prominent, and DA can resemble adenomyoepithelioma. DA do not predispose to carcinoma.

Tumors of the Nipple

Nipple Adenoma

Nipple adenoma was first recognized as a distinctive entity in 1955 by Jones, who referred to it as "florid papillomatosis" of the nipple duct [249]. This lesion is also known as duct adenoma, papillary adenoma, erosive adenomatosis, florid papillomatosis, or superficial papillomatosis of the nipple [250,251]. Papillary adenomatosis occurs most frequently in women aged 40–50 years [250]. The most frequent clinical symptoms are swelling, erythema, crusting, and erosion or ulceration of the nipple, usually accompanied by a discrete palpable tumor. Bloody nipple discharge may also present. Because of this presentation, nipple adenoma clinically mimics Paget's disease [15,252]. Histologically, nipple adenoma is characterized by proliferating ductal structures that spread with an infiltrative pattern into the surrounding stroma. A double layer of epithelium lines these ductal structures. Papillary proliferation is another important feature in nipple adenoma, and is reported by some authors to be even the most frequent pattern [252] (Figure 30). The presence of keratin cysts and tiny apical snouts are other distinguishing features of the disease [253]. Nipple adenoma may be misinterpreted as a tubular adenocarcinoma. Differential diagnosis also includes nipple syringomatous adenoma [254].

Generally, a biopsy is necessary for diagnosis. Nipple adenoma can be successfully treated by complete excision of the tumor with normal surgical margins. Recurrences of incompletely excised lesions have been documented. Nipple adenoma is considered a benign lesion but malignant changes within nipple adenoma have been rarely defined [252,253]. Coexistent invasive carcinoma is generally considered an incidental finding, although some authors have described invasive carcinomas arising from nipple adenomas [252,255].

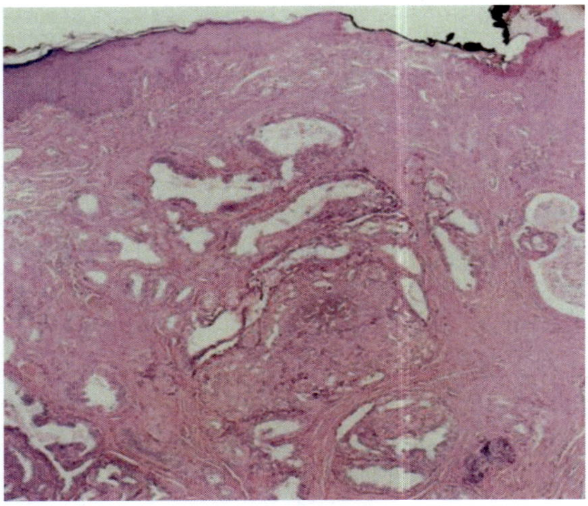

Figure 30. Nipple adenoma. Proliferating ductal structures that with an infiltrative pattern in the stroma of the nipple. These ductal structures are lined with a double layer of epithelium, papillary proliferation was also observed in this case (right side) (40X HE).

References

[1] Cole P, Mark Elwood J, Kaplan SD. Incidence rates and risk factors of benign breast neoplasms. *Am. J. Epidemiol.* 1978;108:112-120.

[2] Bartow SA, Pathak DR, Black WC, et al. Prevalence of benign, atypical, and malignant breast lesions in populations at different risk for breast cancer. A forensic autopsy study. *Cancer 1*987;60:2751-2760.

[3] Sangma MM, Panda K, Dasiah S. *A* clinico-pathological study on benign breast diseases. J. Clin. Diagn. Res. *2013 Mar; 7(3):503-506.*

[4] Sainsbury RC. Breast. In: Norman WS, Bulstrode CJK, P. Ronan O'Connel, Editors. Bailey and Love's Short Practice of Surgery. 25th ed. London: Edward Arnold Ltd.; 2008. pp. 827-835.

[5] Courtillot C, Plu-Bureau G, Binart N, et al. Benign breast diseases. *J. Mammary Gland Biol. Neoplasia* 2005;10:325-335.

[6] Harris JR, Osborne CK, Morrow M, et al. Breast anatomy and development, In: Diseases of the Breast. Philadelphia, PA, USA: Lippincott, Williams & Wilkins; 2000. pp. 1-13.

[7] Santen RJ and Mansel R. Benign breast disorders. *NEJM* 2005;353:275-285.

[8] Goehring C and Morabia A. Epidemiology of benign breast disease, with special attention to histologic types. *Epidemiol. Rev.* 1997;19:310-327.

[9] Sitruk-Ware R and Plu-Bureau G. Epidemiology and treatment of benign breast disease: effect of progestins on breast disease. In: Progestins and Antiprogestins in Clinical Practice. New York: Marcel Dekker; 2000. pp. 327-340.

[10] Dupont WD and Page DL. Risk factors for breast cancer in women with proliferative breast disease. *NEJM* 1985;312:146-151.

[11] Lopez-Garcia MA, Geyer FC, Lacroix-Triki M, et al. Breast cancer precursors revisited: molecular features and progression pathways. *Histopathology* 2010;57(2):171-192.
[12] Spencer JP. Management of mastitis in breastfeeding women. *Am. Fam. Physician* 2008;78(6):727-731.
[13] Stafford I1, Hernandez J, Laibl V, et al. Community-acquired methicillin-resistant *Staphylococcus aureus* among patients with puerperal mastitis requiring hospitalization. *Obstet Gynecol* 2008;112(3):533-537.
[14] Wambach KA. Lactation mastitis: a descriptive study of the experience. *J. Hum. Lact.* 2003;19(1):24-34.
[15] Guray M and Sahin AA. Benign breast diseases: classification, diagnosis, and management. *Oncologist* 2006;11:435-449.
[16] Department of Child and Adolescent Health and Development. Mastitis: causes and management. Geneva, Switzerland: World Health Organization; 2000. http://whqlibdoc.who.int/hq/2000/WHO_FCH_CAH_00.13. pdf
[17] Walker M. Mastitis and the Lactating Woman. Schaumburg, IL, USA: La Leche League International; 2004. Unit 2. Lactation Consultant, Series Two, No. 1603-19.
[18] Osterman KL and Rahm VA. Lactation mastitis: bacterial cultivation of breast milk, symptoms, treatment, and outcome. *J. Hum. Lact.* 2000;16(4):297-302.
[19] Kvist LJ, Larsson BW, Hall-Lord ML, et al. The role of bacteria in lactational mastitis and some considerations of the use of antibiotic treatment. *Int. Breastfeed J.* 2008;3:6.
[20] Delgado S, Arroyo R, Martín R, et al. PCR-DGGE assessment of the bacterial diversity of breast milk in women with lactational infectious mastitis. *BMC Infect Dis.* 2008;8:51.
[21] Fahrni M, Schwarz EI, Stadlmann S, et al. Breast abscesses: diagnosis, treatment and outcome. *Breast Care* 2012;7:32-38.
[22] Rosen PP. Inflammatory and reactive tumors, In: Rosen's Breast Pathology. Philadelphia, PA, USA: Lippincott Williams & Wilkins; 2009. pp. 33-65.
[23] Dener C and Inan A. Breast abscesses in lactating women. *World J. Surg*. 2003;27:130-133.
[24] Barbosa-Cesnik C, Schwartz K, Foxman B. Lactation mastitis. *JAMA* 2003;289:1609-1612.
[25] Cornejo-Juárez P, Vilar-Compte D, Pérez-Jiménez C, et al. Granulomatous mastitis. Experience at a cancer center. (In press 2014).
[26] Petersen L, Graversen HP, Andersen JA. The duct ectasia syndrome- an overlooked disease entity. *Ugeskr Laeger* 1993;155(20):1540-1545.
[27] Dixon JM, Ravisekar O, Chetty U, et al. Periductal mastitis and duct ectasia: different conditions with different aetiologies. *Br. J. Surg*. 1996;83(6):820-822.
[28] Petersen L, Graversen HP, Andersen JA. The duct ectasia syndrome- an overlooked disease entity. *Ugeskr Laeger* 1993;155(20):1545-1549.
[29] Furlong AJ1, al-Nakib L, Knox WF, et al. Periductal inflammation and cigarette smoke. *J. Am. Coll. Surg*. 1994;179(4):417-420.
[30] Dixon JM. Periductal mastitis/duct ectasia. World J Surg 1989 Nov-Dec;13(6):715-720.
[31] Paredes López A, Moreno G. Mastitis no puerperales: investigación clínica de 30 pacientes/Non puerperal mastitis: clinical research in 30 patients. *Ginecol. Obstet. Mex* 1995;63:226-230.

[32] Dixon JM, Anderson TJ, Lumsden AB, et al. Mammary duct ectasia. *Br. J. Surg.* 1983;70(10):601-603.

[33] Wilhelmus JL, Schrodt GR, Mahaffey LM. Cholesterol granulomas of the breast. A lesion which clinically mimics carcinoma. *Am. J. Clin. Pathol* 1982;77:592-597.

[34] Payne RI, Strauss AF, Glasser RD. Mastitis obliterans. Surgery 1943;14:719-727.

[35] Hartley MN, Stewart J, Benson EA. Subareolar dissection for duct ectasia and periareolar sepsis. *Br. J. Surg* 1991;78(10):1187-1188.

[36] Sakorafas GH. Nipple discharge: current diagnostic and therapeutic approaches. *Cancer Treat Rev*. 2001;27:275-282.

[37] Taylor GB, Paviour SD, Musaad S, et al. A clinicopathological review of 34 cases of inflammatory breast disease showing an association between corynebacteria infection and granulomatous mastitis. *Pathology* 2003;35(2):109-119.

[38] Ang LM and Brown H. *Corynebacterium accolens* isolated from breast abscess: possible association with granulomatous mastitis. *J. Clin. Microbiol*. 2007;45(5):1666-1668.

[39] Tewari M, Shukla HS. Breast tuberculosis: diagnosis, clinical features & management. *Indian J. Med. Res* 2005;122:103-110.

[40] Kok KY and Telisinghe PU. Granulomatous mastitis: presentation, treatment and outcome in 43 patients. *Surgeon* 2010;8:197-201.

[41] Azlina AF, Ariza Z, Arni T, et al. Chronic granulomatous mastitis: diagnostic and therapeutic considerations. *World J. Surg*. 2003;27:515-518.

[42] Patel RA, Strickland P, Sankara IR, et al. Idiopathic granulomatous mastitis: case reports and review of literature. *J. Gen. Intern. Med*. 2009;25:270-273.

[43] Diesing D, Axt-Fliedner R, Hornung D, et al. Granulomatous mastitis. *Arch. Gynecol. Obstet.* 2004;269:233-236.

[44] Dupont WD, Page DL, Parl FF, et al. Long-term risk of breast cancer in women with fibroadenoma. *NEJM* 1994;331(1):10-15.

[45] Ozzello L and Gump FE. The management of patients with carcinomas in fibroadenomatous tumors of the breast. *Surg. Gynecol. Obstet*. 1985;160(2):99-104.

[46] Kuijper A, Preisler-Adams SS, Rahusen FD, Gille JJ, van der Wall E, vanDiest PJ. Multiple fibroadenomas harbouring carcinoma *in situ* in a woman with a family history of breast/ovarian cancer. *J. Clin. Pathol*. 2002;55(10):795-797.

[47] Kuijper A, Mommers EC, van der Wall E, et al. Histopathology of fibroadenoma of the breast. *Am. J. Clin. Pathol.* 2001;115:736-742.

[48] Yang X,, Kandil D, Cosar EF, Khan AF. Fibroepithelial tumors of the breast. Pathologic and immunohistochemical features and molecular mechanisms. *Arch. Pathol. Lab. Med.* 2014;138:25-36.

[49] Baxi M, Agarwal A, Mishra A, et al. Multiple bilateral giant juvenile fibroadenomas of breast. *Eur. J. Surg*. 2000;166:828-830.

[50] Greydanus DE, Parks DS, Farrel EG. Breast disorders in children and adolescents. *Pediatr. Clin. North Am*. 1989;36:601-639.

[51] Davis C and Patel V. Surgical problems in the management of giant fibroadenoma of the breast. *Am. J. Obstet. Gynecol*. 1985;152:1010-1005.

[52] Raganoonan C, Fairbain JK, Williams S, et al. Giant breast tumours of adolescence. *Aust. NZ J. Surg*. 1987;57:243-247.

[53] Greydanus DE, Matytsina L, Gains M. Breast disorder in children and adolescent. *Primary Care* 2006;33(2):455-502.

[54] Courcoutsakis NA, Chow CK, Shawker TH, et al. Syndrome of spotty skin pigmentation, myxomas, endocrine overactivity, and schwannomas (Carney complex): breast imaging findings. *Radiology* 1997;205(1):221-227.

[55] Carney JA and Toorkey BC. Myxoid fibroadenoma and allied conditions (myxomatosis) of the breast: a heritable disorder with special associations including cardiac and cutaneous myxomas. *Am. J. Surg. Pathol.* 1991;15:713-721.

[56] Koerner FC. Fibroepithelial lesions, In: Diagnostic Problems in Breast Pathology. 1st ed. USA: Saunders Elsevier; 2009. pp. 321-328.

[57] Heneghan HM, Martin ST, Casey M, et al. Case report**.** A diagnostic dilemma in breast pathology - benign fibroadenomawith multinucleated stromal giant cells. *Diagn. Pathol.* 2008:3:33.

[58] Rao BR, Meyer JS, Fry CG. Most cystosarcoma phyllodes and fibroadenomas have progesterone receptor but lack estrogen receptor: stromal localization of progesterone receptor. *Cancer* 1981;47:2016-2021.

[59] Rosen PP and Urban JA. Coexistent mammary carcinoma and cystosarcoma phyllodes. *Breast* 1975;1:9-15.

[60] Umekita Y and Yoshida H. Immunohistochemical study of hormone receptor and hormone-regulated protein expression in phyllodes tumour: comparison with fibroadenoma. *Virchows Arch.* 1998;433:311-314.

[61] Mechtersheimer G, Kruger KH, Born IA, et al. Antigenic profile of mammary fibroadenoma and cystosarcoma phyllodes. A study using antibodies to estrogen and progesterone receptors and to a panel of cell surface molecules. *Pathol. Res. Pract.* 1990;186:427-438.

[62] Giani C, D'Amore E, Delarue JC, et al. Estrogen and progesterone receptors in benign breast tumors and lesions: relationship with histological and cytological features. *Int. J. Cancer* 1986;37:7-10.

[63] Moore T and Lee AH. Expression of CD34 and bcl-2 in phyllodes tumours, fibroadenomas and spindle cell lesions of the breast. Histopathology 2001;38:62-67.

[64] Umekita Y and Yoshida H. Immunohistochemical study of MIB1 expression in phyllodes tumor and fibroadenoma. *Pathol. Int.* 1999;49:807-810.

[65] Ozisik YY, Meloni AM, Stephenson CF, et al. Chromosome abnormalities in breast fibroadenomas. *Cancer Genet. Cytogenet* 1994;77:125-128.

[66] Petersson C, Pandis N, Risou H, et al. Karyotypic abnormalities in fibroadenomas of the breast. *Int. J. Cancer* 1997;70:282-286.

[67] Calabrese G, Di Virgilio C, Cianchetti E, et al. Chromosome abnormalities in breast fibroadenomas. *Gene Chromosome Cancer* 1991;3:202-204.

[68] Tibiletti MG, Sessa F, Bernasconi B, et al. A large 6q deletion is a common cytogenetic alteration in fibroadenomas, pre-malignant lesions, and carcinomas of the breast. *Clin. Cancer Res.* 2000;6:1422-1431.

[69] Lakhani SR, Ellis IO, Schnitt SJ, et al. Fibroepithelial Tumors. In: World Health Organization Classification of Tumours of the Breast. Lyon, France: *IARC Press*; 2011. pp. 143-147.

[70] Tan PH, Thike AA, Tan WJ, et al. Predicting clinical behaviour of breast phyllodes tumours: a nomogram based on histological criteria and surgical margins. *J. Clin. Pathol.* 2012;65(1):69-76.

[71] Barrio AV, Clark BD, Goldberg JI, et al. Clinicopathologic features and long-term outcomes of 293 phyllodes tumors of the breast. *Ann. Surg. Oncol.* 2007;14(10):2961-2970.

[72] Lenhard MS, Kahlert S, Himsl I, Ditsch N, Untch M, Bauerfeind I. Phyllodes tumour of the breast: clinical follow-up of 33 cases of this rare disease. *Eur. J. Obstet. Gynecol. Reprod. Biol.* 2008;138(2):217-221.

[73] Geisler DP, Boyle MJ, Malnar KF, et al. Phyllodes tumors of the breast: a review of 32 cases. *Am. Surg.* 2000;66(4):360-366.

[74] Kapiris I, Nasiri N, A'Hern R, Healy V, Gui GP. Outcome and predictive factors of local recurrence and distant metastases following primary surgical treatment of high-grade malignant phyllodes tumours of the breast. *Eur. J. Surg. Oncol.* 2001;27(8):723-730.

[75] Alberti O, Brentani MM, Goes JCS, et al. Carcinoembryonic antigen. A possible predictor of recurrence on cystosarcoma phyllodes. *Cancer* 1986;57:1042-1045.

[76] Tse GMK, Lee CS, Kung FYL, et al. Hormonal receptors expression in epithelial cells of mammary phyllodes tumors correlates with pathologic grade of the tumor. *Am. J. Clin. Pathol.* 2002;118:522-526.

[77] Aranda FI, Laforga JB, Lopez JL. Phyllodes tumor of the breast. An immunohistochemical study of 28 cases with special attention to the role of myofibroblasts. *Pathol. Res. Pract.* 1994;190:474-481.

[78] Auger M, Hanna W, Kahn HJ. Cystosarcoma phyllodes of the breast and its mimics. An immunohistochemical and ultrastructural study. *Arch. Pathol. Lab. Med.* 1989;113:1231-1235.

[79] Kuroda N, Sugimoto T, Ueda S, et al. Malignant phyllodes tumor of the breast with expression of osteonectin and vinculin. *Pathol. Int.* 2001;51:277-282.

[80] Shpitz B, Bomstein Y, Sternberg A, et al. Immunoreactivity of p53, Ki-67, and c-erbB-2 in phyllodes tumors of the breast in correlation with clinical and morphologic features. *J. Surg. Oncol.* 2000;79:86-92.

[81] Chen CM, Chen CJ, Chang CL, et al. CD34, CD117, and actin expression in phyllodes tumor of the breast. *J. Surg. Res.* 2000;94:84-91.

[82] Sawyer EJ, Poulsom R, Hunt FT, et al. Malignant phyllodes tumours show stromal overexpression of c-myc and c-kit. *J. Pathol.* 2003;200:59-64.

[83] Kleer CG, Giordano TJ, Braun T, et al. Pathologic, immunohistochemical, and molecular features of benign and malignant phyllodes tumors of the breast. *Mod. Pathol.* 2001;14:185-190.

[84] Birdsall SH, MacLennan KA, Gusterson BA. t(6;12)(q23;q13) and t(10;16)(q22;p11) in a phyllodes tumor of breast. *Cancer Genet. Cytogenet.* 1992;60:74-77.

[85] Ladesich J, Damjanov I, Persons D, et al. Complex karyotype in a low grade phyllodes tumor of the breast. *Cancer Genet. Cytogenet.* 2002;132:149-151.

[86] Polito P, Cin PD, Pauwels P, et al. An important subgroup of phyllodes tumors of the breast is characterized by rearrangements of chromosomes 1q and 10q. *Oncol. Rep.* 1998;5:1099-1102.

[87] Kuenen-Boumeester V, Henzen-Logmans SC, Timmermans MM, et al. Altered expression of p53 and its regulated proteins in phyllodes tumours of the breast. *J. Pathol.* 1999;189:169-175.

[88] Lu YJ, Birdsall S, Osin P, et al. Phyllodes tumors of the breast analyzed by comparative genomic hybridization and association of increased 1q copy number with stromal overgrowth and recurrence. *Genes. Chromosomes Cancer* 1997;20:275-281.

[89] Jee KJ, Gong G, Hyun Ahn S, et al. Gain in 1q is a common abnormality in phyllodes tumours of the breast. *Anal. Cell. Pathol.* 2003;25:89-93.

[90] Arrigoni MG, Dockerty MB, Judd ES. The identification and treatment of mammary hamartoma. *Surg. Gynecol. Obstet.* 1971;133:577-582.

[91] Lee EH, Wylie EJ, Barke AG, Bastiaan De Boer W. Invasive ductal carcinoma arising in a breast hamartoma: two case reports and a review of the literature. *Clin. Radiol.* 2003;58:80-83.

[92] Moinfar F. Mesenchymal lesions/tumors. In: Essentials of Diagnostic Breast Pathology. Heidelberg, Germany: Springer-Verlag; 2007. p. 383.

[93] Rosen PP. Benign mesenchymal neoplasms. In: Rosen's Breast Pathology. Philadelphia, PA, USA: Lippincott Williams & Wilkins; 2009. p. 864.

[94] Jones MW, Norris HJ, Wargotz ES. Hamartomas of the breast. *Surg. Gynecol. Obstet.* 1991;173:54-56.

[95] Tavassoli FA and Devilee P. Fibroepithelial tumors, In: World Health Organization: Pathology & Genetics: Tumours of the Breast and Female Genital. Organs. Lyon, France: IARC Press; 2003. p. 103.

[96] Mester J, Simmons RM, Vazquez MF, Rosenblatt R: *In situ* and infiltrating ductal carcinoma arising in a breast hamartoma. AJR Am. J. Roentgenol. 2000;175:64-66.

[97] Barbaros U, Deveci U, Erbil Y, Budak D. Breast hamartoma: a case report. *Acta. Chir. Belg.* 2005;105:658-659.

[98] Davies JD and Riddell RH. Muscular hamartomas of the breast. *J. Pathol.* 1973;111:209-211.

[99] Daroca PJ, Reed RJ, Love GL, Kraus SD. Myoid hamartomas of the breast. *Hum. Pathol.* 1985;16:212-219.

[100] Vuitch MF, Rosen PP, Erlandson RA. Pseudoangiomatous hyperplasia of mammary stroma. *Hum. Pathol.* 1986;17:185-191.

[101] Bowman E, Oprea G, Okoli J, et al. Pseudoangiomatous stromal hyperplasia (PASH) of the breast: a series of 24 patients. *Breast J.* 2012; 8(3):242-247.

[102] Castro CY, Whitman GJ, Sahin AA. Pseudoangiomatous stromal hyperplasia of the breast. *Am. J. Clin. Oncol.* 2002;25:213-216.

[103] Ibrahim RE, Sciotto CG, Weidner N. Pseudoangiomatous hyperplasia of mammary stroma: some observations regarding its clinicopathologic spectrum. *Cancer* 1989;63(6):1154-1160.

[104] Milanezi MF, Saggioro FP, Zanati SG, Bazan R, Schmitt FC. Pseudoangiomatous hyperplasia of mammary stroma associated with gynaecomastia. *J. Clin. Pathol.* 1998;51(3):204-206.

[105] Powell CM, Cranor ML, Rosen PP. Pseudoangiomatous stromal hyperplasia (PASH): a mammary stromal tumor with myofibroblastic differentiation. *Am. J. Surg. Pathol.* 1995;19(3):270-277.

[106] Ferreira M, Albarracin CT, Resetkova E. Pseudoangiomatous stromal hyperplasia tumor: a clinical, radiologic and pathologic study of 26 cases. *Mod. Pathol.* 2008;21(2):201-207.

[107] Vuitch MF, Rosen PP, Erlandson RA. Pseudoangiomatous hyperplasia of mammary stroma. *Hum. Pathol.* 1986;17(2):185-191.

[108] Virk RK and Khan A. Pseudoangiomatous stromal Hyperplasia. An overview. *Arch. Pathol. Lab. Med.* 2010;134:1070-1074.

[109] Magro G, Michal M, Bisceglia M. Benign spindle cell tumors of the mammary stroma: diagnostic criteria, classification, and histogenesis. *Pathol. Res. Pract.* 2001;197:453-466.

[110] Magro G, Bisceglia M, Michal M, Eusebi V. Spindle cell lipoma-like tumor, solitary fibrous tumor and myofibroblastoma of the breast: a clinicopathological analysis of 13 cases in favor of a unifying histologic concept. *Virchows Arch.* 2002;440:249-260.

[111] Gocht A, Bosmuller HC, Bassler R, et al. Breast tumors with myofibroblastic differentiation: clinico-pathological observations in myofibroblastoma and myofibrosarcoma. *Pathol. Res. Pract.* 1999;195:1-10.

[112] Nucci MR and Fletcher CDM. Myofibroblastoma of the breast: a distinctive benign stromal tumor. *Pathol. Case Rev.* 1999;4:214-219.

[113] Julien M, Trojani M, Coindre JM. Myofibroblastoma of the breast: report of 8 cases. *Ann. Pathol.* 1994;14:143-147.

[114] Hamele-Bena D, Cranor M, Sciotto C, Erlandson R, Rosen PP. Uncommon presentation of mammary myofibroblastoma. *Mod. Pathol.* 1996;9:786-790.

[115] Salomao DR, Crotty TB, Nascimento AG. Myofibroblastoma and solitary fibrous tumors of the breast: histopathological and immunohistochemical studies. *Breast*2001;10:49-54.

[116] Drijkoningen M, Tavassoli FA, Magro G, et al. Mesenchymal tumours. In: Tavassoli FA, Devilee P, Editors. Pathology and Genetics of Tumors of the Breast and Female Genital Organs. World Health Organization Classification of Tumors. Lyon, France: IARC Press; 2003. pp. 89-98.

[117] Ali S, Teichberg S, DeRisi DC, Urmacher C. Giant myofibroblastoma of the male breast. *Am. J. Surg. Pathol.* 1994;18:1170-1176.

[118] McMenamin ME, Fletcher CDM. Mammary-type myofibroblastoma of soft tissue: a tumor closely related to spindle cell lipoma. *Am. J. Surg. Pathol.* 2001;25:1022-1029.

[119] Magro G. Stromal tumors of the lower female genital tract: histogenetic, morphological and immunohistochemical similarities with the "benign spindle cell tumors of the mammary stroma." *Pathol. Res. Pract.* 2007;203:827-829.

[120] Lopez-Rios F, Burgos F, Madero S, Ballestín C, Martınez-Gonzalez MA, de Agustın P. Fine needle aspiration of breast myofibroblastoma: a case report. *Acta. Cytol.* 2001;45:381-384.

[121] Magro G, Gangemi P, Villari L, Greco P. Deciduoid-like stromal cells in a diabetic patient with bilateral gynecomastia: a potential diagnostic pitfall. *Virchows Arch.* 2004;445:659-660.

[122] Magro G, Gangemi P, Greco P. Deciduoid-like myofibroblastoma of the breast: a potential pitfall of malignancy. *Histopathology* 2008;52:652.654.

[123] Rosen PP. Myofibroblastoma. In: Rosen PP, Editor. Rosen's Breast Pathology, 2nd ed. Philadelphia, PA, USA: Lippincott Williams & Wilkins; 2001. pp. 766-774.

[124] Magro G, Gurrera A, Bisceglia M. H-caldesmon expression in myofibroblastoma of the breast: evidence supporting the distinction from leiomyoma. *Histopathology* 2003;42:233-238.

[125] Lee AH, Sworn MJ, Theaker JM, Fletcher CD. Myofibroblastoma of breast: an immunohistochemical study. *Histopathology* 1993;22:75-78.

[126] Fukunaga M and Ushigome S. Myofibroblastoma of the breast with diverse differentiation. *Arch. Pathol. Lab. Med.* 1997;121:599-603.

[127] Wargotz ES, Weiss SW, Norris HJ. Myofibroblastoma of the breast: sixteen cases of a distinctive benign mesenchymal tumor. *Am. J. Surg. Pathol.* 1987;11: 493-502.

[128] Morgan MB and Pitha JV. Myofibroblastoma of the breast revisited: an aetiologic association with androgens? *Hum. Pathol.* 1998;29:347-351.

[129] Magro G, Bisceglia M, Michal M. Expression of steroid hormone receptors and their regulated proteins and bcl-2 protein in myofibroblastoma of the breast. *Histopathology* 2000;36:515-521.

[130] Pauwels P, Sciot R, Croiset F, Rutten H, van den Berghe H, Dal Cin P. Myofibroblastoma of the breast: genetic link with spindle cell lipoma. *J. Pathol.* 2000;191:282-285.

[131] Maggiani F, Debiec-Rychter M, Verbeeck G, Sciot R. Extramammary myofibroblastoma is genetically related to spindle cell lipoma. *Virchows Arch.* 2006;449:244-247.

[132] Abrikossoff AI. ÜberMyome, Ausgehend von der quergestreiftenwillkurlichenmuskulatur. *Virchow Arch. Pathol. Anat. Physiol.* 1926; 260:215-233.

[133] Lack EE, Worsham GF, Callihan MD, et al. Granular cell tumor: a clinicopathologic study of 110 patients. *J. Surg. Oncol.* 1980;13:301-316.

[134] Kanabe S, Watanabe I, Lotuaco L. Multiple granular-cell tumors of the ascending colon: microscopic study. *Dis. Colon. Rectum.* 1978;21:322-328.

[135] Becelli R, Perugini M, Gasparini G, et al. Abrikossoff's tumor. *J. Craniofac. Surg.* 2001;12:78-81.

[136] Vance SF III and Hudson RP Jr. Granular cell myoblastoma. Clinicopathologic study of forty-two patients. *Am. J. Clin. Pathol.* 1969;52:208-211.

[137] Ordóñez NG. Granular cell tumor: review and update. *Adv. Anat. Pathol.* 1999;6:186-203.

[138] Lauwers K, Bestman TJ, Bergmans G, et al. Granular cell tumor of the male breast. *Acta. Chir. Belg.* 2008;108:112-114.

[139] Sonobe H, Iwata J, Furihata M, et al. Malignant granular cell tumor: report of a case and review and the literature. *Pathol. Res. Pract.* 1998;194:507-513.

[140] Khansur T, Balducci L, Tavassoli M. Granular cell tumor. Clinical spectrum of the benign and malignant entity. *Cancer* 1987;60:220-222.

[141] Fanburg-Smith JC, Meis-Kindblom JM, Fante R, et al. Malignant granular cell tumor of soft tissue: diagnostic criteria and clinicopathologic correlation. *Am. J. Surg. Pathol.* 1998;22:779-794.

[142] Kataoka A, Koike M, Kuranuki K, et al. A case of malignant granular cell tumor arisen in the chest wall. *J. Jpn. Surg. Assoc.* 2005;66:2403-2406.

[143] Lanng C, Eriksen BO, Hoffmann J. Lipoma of the breast: a diagnostic dilemma. *Breast* 2004;13:408-411.

[144] Salvatore C, Antonio B, Del Vecchio W, et al. Giant infiltrating lipoma of the face: CT and MR imaging findings. *AJNR Am. J. Neuroradiol*. 2003;24:283-286.
[145] Hakim E, Kolander Y, Meller Y, et al. Gigantic lipomas. *Plast. Reconstr. Surg*. 1994;94:369-371.
[146] Ramírez-Montaño L, Vargas-Tellez E, Dajer-Fadel W, Espinosa Maceda S. Giant lipoma of the breast. *Arch. Plast. Surg*. 2013;40:244-246.
[147] Kryvenko ON, Chitale DA, VanEgmond EM, et al. Angiolipoma of the female breast. Clinicomorphological correlation of 52 cases. *Int. J. Surg. Pathol*. 2011;19:35-43.
[148] Damiani S, Chiodera P, Guaragni M, et al. Mammary angiomyolipoma. Virchows Arch 2002;440:551-552.
[149] Jozefczyk MA, Rosen PP. Vascular tumors of the breast II. Perilobular hemangiomas and hemangiomas. *Am. J. Surg. Pathol*. 1985;9:491-503.
[150] Rosen PP. Benign mesenchymal neoplasms. In: Rosen's Breast Pathology. Philadelphia, PA, USA: Lippincott Williams & Wilkins; 2009. pp. 872-888.
[151] Lesueur GC, Brown RW, Bhathal PS. Incidence of perilobular hemangioma in the female breast. *Arch. Pathol. Lab. Med*. 1983;107:308-310.
[152] Rosen PP and Ridolfi RL. The perilobular hemangioma. A benign vascular lesion of the breast. *Am. J. Clin. Pathol*. 1977;68:21-23.
[153] Lakhani SR, Ellis IO, Schnitt SJ et al. Mesenchymal tumors, In: World Health Organization Classification of Tumours of the Breast. Lyon, France: IARC Press, 2011. pp. 127-129.
[154] Nagar H, Marmor S, Hammar B. Haemangiomas of the breast in children. *Eur. J. Surg*. 1992;158(9):503-505.
[155] Webb LA and Young JR. Case report: Haemangioma of the breast—appearances on mammography and ultrasound. *Clin. Radiol*. 1996;51:523-524.
[156] Glazenbrook KN, Morton MJ, Reynolds C. Vascular tumors of the breast: mammographic, sonographic, and MRI appearances. *AJR Am. J. Roentgenol*. 2005;184:331-338.
[157] Rosen PP. Vascular tumors of the breast. III. Angiomatosis. *Am. J. Surg. Pathol*. 1985;9(9):652-658.
[158] Rao VK and Weiss SW. Angiomatosis of soft tissue. An analysis of the histologic features and clinical outcome in 51 cases. *Am. J. Surg. Pathol*. 1992;16:764-771.
[159] Mandrell J, Mehta S, McClure S. Atypical vascular lesion of the breast. *J. Am. Acad. Dermatol*. 2010;63(2):337-340.
[160] Lucas DR. Angiosarcoma, radiation-associated angiosarcoma and atypical vascular lesion. *Arch. Pathol. Lab. Med*. 2009;133(11):1804-1809.
[161] Tan PH and Ellis IO. Myoepithelial and epithelial-myoepithelial, mesenchymal and fibroepithelial breast lesions: updates from the WHO Classification of Tumours of the Breast 2012. *J. Clin. Pathol*. 2013; 66:465-470.
[162] Tavassoli FA and Devilee P. Myoepithelial lesions, In: World Health Organization: Pathology & Genetics: Tumours of the Breast and Female Genital Organs. Lyon, France: IARC Press; 2003. pp. 86-88.
[163] Tavassoli FA. Myoepithelial lesions of the breast. Myoepitheliosis, adenomyoepithelioma, and myoepithelial carcinoma. *Am. J. Surg. Pathol*. 1991;15:554-568.

[164] Hayes MM, Adenomyoepithelioma of the breast: a review stressing its propensity for malignant transformation. *J. Clin. Pathol.* 2011;64:477-484.

[165] Resetkova E, Albarracin C, Sneige N. Collagenous spherulosis of the breast: morphologic study of 59 cases and review of the literature. *Am. J. Surg. Pathol.* 2006;30:20-27.

[166] Reiss-Filho JS, Fulford LG, Crebassa B, et al. Collagenous spherulosis in an adenomyoepithelioma of the breast. *J. Clin. Pathol.* 2004;57:83-86.

[167] Clement PB, Young RH, Azzopardi JG. Collagenous spherulosis of the breast. *Am. J. Surg. Pathol.* 1987;11:411-417.

[168] Pia-Foschini M, Reiss-Filho JS, Eusebi V, et al. Salivary gland-like tumours of the breast: surgical and molecular pathology. *J. Clin. Pathol.* 2003;6:497-506.

[169] Thakur B, Misra V, Dhingra V, et al. Myoepithelioma breast: clinically masquerading as breast carcinoma. *Rare Tumors* 2012;4:e50.

[170] Díaz NM, McDivitt RW, Wick MR. Pleomorphic adenoma of the breast: a clinicopathologic and immunohistochemical study of 10 cases. *Hum. Pathol.* 1991;22:1206-1214.

[171] Ballance WA, Ro JY, el-Naggar AK, et al. Pleomorphic adenoma (benign mixed tumor) of the breast. An immunohistochemical, flow cytometric, and ultrastructural study and review of the literature. *Am. J. Clin. Pathol.* 1990;93:795-801.

[172] Reid-Nicholson M, Bleiweiss I, Pace B, et al. Pleomorphic adenoma of the breast. A case report and distinction from mucinous carcinoma. *Arch. Pathol. Lab. Med.* 2003; 127:474-477.

[173] Lecene AL. Observation d'un cas de tumeur "mixte" du sein. *Rev. Chir.* (Paris) 1906;33:434-468.

[174] Mizukami Y, Takayama T, Takemura A, et al. Pleomorphic adenoma of the breast. *Radiat. Med.* 2008;26:442-445.

[175] Tavassoli FA. Benign lesions, In: Pathology of the Breast. Stamford, CT, USA: *Appleton & Lange;* 1999. pp. 115-204.

[176] Padilla-Rosciano A, Castillero-Pinilla C, Chanon-Vilchis JG, et al. Adenoma pleomórfico de mama. *Rev. Inst. Nal. Cancerol. Mex.* 1998;44:148-151.

[177] Chen KT. Pleomorphic adenoma of the breast. *Am. J. Clin. Pathol.* 1990;93:792-794.

[178] Hamperl H. The myothelia (myoepithelial cells): normal state; regressive changes; hyperplasia; tumors. *Curr. Top Pathol.* 1970;53:161-220.

[179] Yoon JY and Chitale D. Adenomyoepithelioma of the breast. A brief diagnostic review. *Arch. Pathol. Lab. Med.* 2013;137:725-729.

[180] Rosen PP. Adenomyoepithelioma of the breast. *Hum. Pathol.* 1987;18(12):1232-1237.

[181] Fitzgibbons PL, Henson DE, Hutter RV. Benign breast changes and the risk for subsequent breast cancer: an update of the 1985 Consensus Statement. Cancer Committee of the College of American Pathologists. *Arch. Pathol. Lab. Med.* 1998;122:1053-1055.

[182] Bartow SA, Pathak DR, Black WC, et al. Prevalence of benign, atypical, and malignant breast lesions in populations at different risk for breast cancer. A forensic autopsy study. *Cancer* 1987;60:2751-2760.

[183] Love SM, Gelman RS, Silen W. Fibrocystic "disease" of the breast- a nondisease? NEJM 1982;307:1010-1014.

[184] Rosai J. Breast. In: Rosai and Ackerman's Surgical Pathology. Philadelphia, PA, USA: Mosby; 2004. pp. 1763-1876.

[185] Vorherr H. Fibrocystic breast disease: pathophysiology, pathomorphology, clinical picture, and management. *Am. J. Obstet. Gynecol.* 1986;154:161-179.

[186] O'Malley FP and Bane AL. The spectrum of apocrine lesions of the breast. *Adv. Anat. Pathol.* 2004;11:1-9.

[187] Houssami N, Irwig L, Ung O. Review of complex breast cysts: implications for cancer detection and clinical practice. *ANZ J. Surg.* 2005;75:1080-1085.

[188] Venta LA, Kim JP, Pelloski CE, et al. Management of complex breast cysts. *AJR Am. J. Roentgenol.* 1999;173:1331-1336.

[189] Vargas HI, Vargas MP, Gonzalez KD, et al. Outcomes of sonography-based management of breast cysts. *Am. J. Surg.* 2004;188:443-447.

[190] Tavassoli FA. Benign lesions. In: Pathology of the Breast. Stamford, CT, USA: Appleton & Lange; 1999. pp. 115-204.

[191] Vina M and Wells CA. Clear cell metaplasia of the breast: a lesion showing eccrine differentiation. *Histopatholog*y 1989;15:85-92.

[192] Hartmann LC, Sellers TA, Frost MH, et al. Benign breast disease and the risk of breast cancer. *NEJM* 2005;353:229-237.

[193] Rosen PP. Adenosis and microglandular adenosis, In: Rosen's Breast Pathology. Philadelphia, PA., USA: Lippincott Williams & Wilkins; 2009. pp. 161-186.

[194] Lakhani SR, Ellis IO, Schnitt SJ, et al. Benign epithelial proliferations, In: World Health Organization Classification of Tumours of the Breast. Lyon, France: IARC Press; 2011. pp. 112-118.

[195] Lee K, Chan JKC, Gwi E. Tubular adenosis of the breast: a distinctive benign lesion mimicking invasive carcinoma. *Am. J. Surg. Pathol.* 1996;20:46-54.

[196] Jensen RA, Page DL, Dupont WD, et al. Invasive breast cancer risk in women with sclerosing adenosis. *Cancer* 1989;64:1977-1983.

[197] Bodian CA, Perzin KH, Lattes R, et al. Prognostic significance of benign proliferative breast disease. *Cancer* 1993;71:3896-3907.

[198] Geyer FC, Lacroix-Triki M, Colombo P, et al. Molecular evidence in support of the neoplastic and precursor nature of microglandular adenosis. *Histopathology* 2012;60:E115-E130.

[199] Rosenblum MK, Purrazzella R, Rosen PP. Is microglandular adenosis a precancerous disease? A study of carcinoma arising therein. *Am. J. Surg. Pathol.* 1986;10(4):237-245.

[200] Khalifeh IM, Albarracin C, Diaz LK, et al. Clinical, histopathologic, and immunohistochemical features of microglandular adenosis and transition into *in situ* and invasive carcinoma. *Am. J. Surg. Pathol.* 2008;32(4):544-552.

[201] Eusebi V, Foschini MP, Betts CM, et al. Microglandular adenosis, apocrine adenosis, and tubular carcinoma of the breast. An immunohistochemical comparison. *Am. J. Surg. Pathol.* 1993;17(2):99-109.

[202] Salarieh A and Sneige N. Breast carcinoma arising in microglandular adenosis. A review of the literature. *Arch. Pathol. Lab. Med. 2007*;131:1397-1399.

[203] Shin SJ, Simpson PT, Da Silva L, et al. Molecular evidence for progression of microglandular adenosis (MGA) to invasive carcinoma. *Am. J. Surg. Pathol.* 2009;33(4):496-504.

[204] Shui R and Yang W. Invasive breast carcinoma arising in microglandular adenosis: a case report and review of the literature. *Breast J.* 2009;15(6):653-656.

[205] Acs G, Simpson JF, Bleiweiss IJ, et al. Microglandular adenosis with transition into adenoid cystic carcinoma of the breast. *Am. J. Surg. Pathol.* 2003;27(8):1052-1060.

[206] DiPiro PJ, Gulizia JA, Lester SC, et al. Mammographic and sonographic appearances of nodular adenosis. *AJR Am. J. Roentgenol.* 2000;175(1):31-34.

[207] Nielsen NS and Nielsen BB. Mammographic features of sclerosing adenosis presenting as a tumour. *Clin. Radiol.* 1986;37(4):371-373.

[208] Nielsen BB. Adenosis tumour of the breast- a clinicopathological investigation of 27 cases. *Histopathology* 1987;11(12):1259-1275.

[209] Rosen PP. Papilloma and benign related tumors. In: Rosen's Breast Pathology. Philadelphia, PA, USA: Lippincott Williams & Wilkins; 2009. pp. 100-107.

[210] Jacobs TW, Byrne C, Colditz G, et al. Radial scars in benign breast-biopsy specimens and the risk of breast cancer. *NEJM* 1999;340:430-436.

[211] Kennedy M, Masterson AV, Kerin M, et al. Pathology and clinical relevance of radial scars: a review. *J. Clin. Pathol.* 2003;56:721-724.

[212] Sloane JP and Mayers MM. Carcinoma and atypical hyperplasia in radial scars and complex sclerosing lesions: importance of lesion size and patient age. *Histopathology* 1993;23(3):225-231.

[213] Patterson JA, Scott M, Anderson N, et al. Radial scar, complex sclerosing lesion and risk of breast cancer. Analysis of 175 cases in Northern Ireland. *Eur. J. Surg. Oncol.* 2004;30:1065-1068.

[214] Fasih T, Jain M, Shrimankar J, et al. All radial scars/complex sclerosing lesions seen on breast screening mammograms should be excised. *Eur. J. Surg. Oncol.* 2005;31:1125-1128.

[215] Oyama T and Koerner FC. Noninvasive papillary proliferations. *Semin. Diagn. Pathol.* 2004;21:32-41.

[216] Agoff SN and Lawton TJ. Papillary lesions of the breast with and without atypical ductal hyperplasia: can we accurately predict benign behavior from core needle biopsy? *Am. J. Clin. Pathol.* 2004;122:440-443.

[217] Ivan D, Selinko V, Sahin AA, et al. Accuracy of core needle biopsy diagnosis in assessing papillary breast lesions: histologic predictors of malignancy. *Mod. Pathol.* 2004;17:165-171.

[218] MacGrogan G, Tavassoli FA. Central atypical papillomas of the breast: a clinicopathological study of 119 cases. *Virchows Arch.* 2003;443:609-617.

[219] Ali-Fehmi R, Carolin K, Wallis T, et al. Clinicopathologic analysis of breast lesions associated with multiple papillomas. *Hum. Pathol.* 2003;34:234-239.

[220] Krieger N, Hiatt RA. Risk of breast cancer after benign breast diseases. Variation by histologic type, degree of atypia, age at biopsy, and length of follow-up. *Am. J. Epidemiol.* 1992;135:619-631.

[221] Page DL, Salhany KE, Jensen RA, et al. Subsequent breast carcinoma risk after biopsy with atypia in breast papilloma. *Cancer* 1996;78:258-266.

[222] Bazzocchi F, Santini D, Martinelli G, et al. Juvenile papillomatosis (epitheliosis) of the breast: a clinical and pathologic study of 13 cases. *Am. J. Clin. Pathol.* 1986;86:745-748.

[223] Lakhani SR, Ellis IO, Schnitt SJ, et al. Intraductal proliferative lesions, In: World Health Organization Classification of Tumours of the Breast. Lyon, France: IARC Press; 2011. pp. 82-89.

[224] Wellings SR, Jensen HM and Marcum RG. An atlas of subgross pathology of the human breast with special reference to possible precancerous lesions. *J. Natl. Cancer Inst.* 1975;55:231-273.

[225] Rosen PP. Ductal hyperplasia: usual and atypical. In: Rosen's Breast Pathology. Philadelphia, PA, USA: Lippincott Williams & Wilkins; 2009. pp. 231-262.

[226] Tavassoli FA. Ductal intraepithelial neoplasia. In: Pathology of the Breast. Stamford, CT, USA: Appleton & Lange; 1999. pp. 205-323.

[227] Koerner FC. Epithelial proliferations of ductal type. *Semin. Diagn. Pathol.* 2004;21:10-17.

[228] Ozaki D and Kondo Y. Comparative morphometric studies of benign and malignant intraductal proliferative lesions of the breast by computerized image analysis. *Hum. Pathol.* 1995;26:1109-1113.

[229] Rosen PP. Lobular carcinoma *in situ* and atypical lobular hyperplasia, In: Rosen's Breast Pathology. Philadelphia. PA, USA: Lippincott Williams & Wilkins; 2009. pp. 637-689.

[230] Li CI, Anderson BO, Daling JR, et al. Changing incidence of lobular carcinoma *in situ* of the breast. *Breast Cancer Res. Treat.* 2002;75:259-268.

[231] Page DL, Schuyler PA, Dupont WD, et al. Atypical lobular hyperplasia as a unilateral predictor of breast cancer risk: a retrospective cohort study. *Lancet* 2003;361:125-129.

[232] Lakhani SR, Ellis IO, Schnitt SJ, et al. Lobular neoplasia. In: World Health Organization Classification of Tumours of the Breast. Lyon, France: IARC Press; 2011. pp. 78-80.

[233] Pinder SE and Ellis IO. The diagnosis and management of pre-invasive breast disease: ductal carcinoma *in situ* (DCIS) and atypical ductal hyperplasia (ADH)- current definitions and classification. *Breast Cancer Res.* 2003;5:254-257.

[234] Webb PM, Byrne C, Schnitt SJ, et al. Family history of breast cancer, age, and benign breast disease. *Int. J. Cancer* 2002;100:375-378.

[235] Page DL, Dupont WD, Rogers LW, et al. Atypical hyperplastic lesions of the female breast. A long-term follow-up study. *Cancer* 1985;55:2698-2708.

[236] Tavassoli FA and Norris HJ. A comparison of the results of long-term followup for atypical intraductal hyperplasia and intraductal hyperplasia of the breast. *Cancer* 1990;65:518-529.

[237] Collins L, Baer H, Tamimi R, et al. Magnitude and laterality of breast cancer risk in women with atypical hyperplasia of ductal and lobular types. *Lab. Invest.* 2006;86(Suppl 1):24A.

[238] Dupont WD and Page DL. Relative risk of breast cancer varies with time since diagnosis of atypical hyperplasia. *Hum. Pathol.* 1989;20:723-725.

[239] Ma XJ, Salunga R, Tuggle JT, et al. Gene expression profiles of human breast cancer progression. *Proc. Natl. Acad. Sci. U S A* 2003;100:5974-5979.

[240] Sgroi DC. Preinvasive breast. *Annu. Rev. Pathol. Mech. Dis.* 2010;5:193-221.

[241] Jain RK, Mehta R, Dimitrov R, et al. Atypical ductal hyperplasia: interobserver and intraobserver variability. *Mod. Pathol.* 2011;24:917-923.

[242] Schnitt SJ and Vincent-Salomon A. Columnar cell lesions of the breast. *Adv. Anat. Pathol.* 2003;10:113-124.
[243] Moinfar F. Flat ductal intraepithelial neoplasia of the breast. A review of diagnostic criteria, differential diagnoses, molecular-genetic findings, and clinical relevance—It is time to appreciate the Azzopardi concept! *Arch. Pathol. Lab. Med.* 2009;133:879-892.
[244] Sinn H, Elsawaf Z, Helmchen B, et al. Early breast cancer precursor lesions: lessons learned from molecular and clinical studies. *Breast Care* 2010;5:218-226.
[245] Schnitt SJ. The diagnosis and management of pre-invasive breast disease: flat epithelial atypia- classification, pathologic features and clinical significance. *Breast Cancer Res.* 2003;5:263-268.
[246] Pinder SE and Reis-Filho JS. Non-operative breast pathology: columnar cell lesions. *J. Clin. Pathol.* 2007;60:1307-1312.
[247] O'Malley FP, Mohsin SK, Badve S, et al. Interobserver reproducibility in the diagnosis of flat epithelial atypia of the breast. *Mod. Pathol.* 2006;19:172-179.
[248] Nasser SM. Columnar cell lesions: current classification and controversies. *Semin. Diagn. Pathol.* 2004;21:18-24.
[249] Jones DB. Florid papillomatosis of the nipple ducts. *Cancer* 1955;8:315-319-322.
[250] Wagner N, Schmidt S, Yerlikaya G, et al. Superficial papillary adenomatosis of the nipple: a rare disease diagnosed by sonography and histopathologically confirmed by nipple-preserving total excision. *J. Ultrasound. Med.* 2013;32(2):373-374.
[251] Shioi Y, Nakamura S, Kawamura S, et al. Nipple adenoma arising from axillary accessory breast: a case report. *Diagn. Pathol.* 2012;7:162.
[252] Rosen PP and Caicco JA. Florid papillomatosis of the nipple. A study of 51 patients, including nine with mammary carcinoma. *Am. J. Surg. Pathol.* 1986;10:87-101.
[253] Montemarano AD, Sau P, James WD. Superficial papillary adenomatosis of the nipple: a case report and review of the literature. *J. Am. Acad. Dermatol.* 1995;33:871-875.
[254] Oo KZ and Xiao PQ. Infiltrating syringomatous adenoma of the nipple. Clinical presentation and literature review. *Arch. Pathol. Lab. Med.* 2009;133:1487-1489.
[255] Jones MW and Tavassoli FA. Coexistence of nipple duct adenoma and breast carcinoma: a clinicopathologic study of five cases and review of the literature. *Mod. Pathol.* 1995;8(6):633-636.

Index

B

C

D

E

F

G

H

I

J

K

L

M

N

R

S

T

U

V

W

X

Y